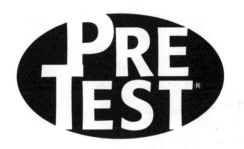

Neuroscience
PreTest® Self-Assessment and Review

Notice

Medicine is an ever-changing science. As new research and clinical experience broaden our knowledge, changes in treatment and drug therapy are required. The authors and the publisher of this work have checked with sources believed to be reliable in their efforts to provide information that is complete and generally in accord with the standards accepted at the time of publication. However, in view of the possibility of human error or changes in medical sciences, neither the authors nor the publisher nor any other party who has been involved in the preparation or publication of this work warrants that the information contained herein is in every respect accurate or complete, and they disclaim all responsibility for any errors or omissions or for the results obtained from use of the information contained in this work. Readers are encouraged to confirm the information contained herein with other sources. For example and in particular, readers are advised to check the product information sheet included in the package of each drug they plan to administer to be certain that the information contained in this work is accurate and that changes have not been made in the recommended dose or in the contraindications for administration. This recommendation is of particular importance in connection with new or infrequently used drugs.

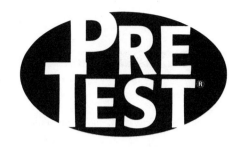

Neuroscience
PreTest® Self-Assessment and Review
Fifth Edition

Allan Siegel, Ph.D.
Departments of Neuroscience and Psychiatry
New Jersey Medical School
Newark, New Jersey

Heidi Siegel, M.D.
Formerly of the Epilepsy Research Branch
National Institute of Neurological Disorders and Stroke
National Institutes of Health
Bethesda, Maryland
Department of Neurology
Mt. Sinai School of Medicine
New York, New York

McGraw-Hill
Medical Publishing Division
New York   Chicago   San Francisco   Lisbon   London   Madrid   Mexico City
Milan   New Delhi   San Juan   Seoul   Singapore   Sydney   Toronto

Neuroscience: PreTest® Self-Assessment and Review, Fifth Edition

Copyright © 2005 by **The McGraw-Hill Companies**, Inc. All rights reserved. Printed in the United States of America. Except as permitted under the United States Copyright Act of 1976, no part of this publication may be reproduced or distributed in any form or by any means, or stored in a data base or retrieval system, without the prior written permission of the publisher.

Previous editions copyright © 2002, 1999, 1996, and 1993 by The McGraw-Hill Companies, Inc.

2 3 4 5 6 7 8 9 0   DOC/DOC   0 9 8 7 6 5

ISBN 0-07-143651-0

This book was set in Berkeley by North Market Street Graphics.
The editor was Catherine A. Johnson.
The production supervisor was Phil Galea.
Project management was provided by North Market Street Graphics.
The cover designer was Li Chen Chang/Pinpoint.
RR Donnelley was printer and binder.

This book is printed on acid-free paper.

Library of Congress Cataloging-in-Publication Data
Siegel, Allan.
  Neuroscience: PreTest self-assessment and review / Allan Siegel, Heidi Siegel.—5th ed.
    p. cm.
  Includes bibliographical references and index.
  ISBN 0-07-143651-0
    1. Neurophysiology—Examinations, questions, etc. 2. Neurosciences—Examinations, questions, etc. I. Siegel, Heidi. II. Title.

QP356 .S49 2004
612.8'076—dc22

                                                                    2004040264

Student Reviewers

J. Brandon Hill
Saint Louis University School of Medicine
St. Louis, Missouri
Class of 2003

Alisa A. Meny
UMDNJ—Robert Wood Johnson Medical School
Piscataway, New Jersey
Class of 2004

Michael Wolf
UMDNJ—Robert Wood Johnson Medical School
Piscataway, New Jersey
Class of 2004

To Carla, wife and mother, whose patience, support, and understanding made this book possible, and to David Eliahu, Tzipporah Hannah, Matan Dov, Nadav David, and Adi Hila.

Contents

Preface xi
Introduction xiii

High-Yield Facts

High-Yield Facts in Neuroscience 1

Gross Anatomy of the Brain

Questions 45
Answers, Explanations, and References 55

Development

Questions 61
Answers, Explanations, and References 65

The Neuron

Questions 67
Answers, Explanations, and References 75

The Synapse

Questions 86
Answers, Explanations, and References 89

Neurochemistry/Neurotransmitters

Questions 95
Answers, Explanations, and References 109

The Spinal Cord

Questions 119
Answers, Explanations, and References 133

The Autonomic Nervous System

Questions 145
Answers, Explanations, and References 148

The Brainstem and Cranial Nerves

Questions. 151
Answers, Explanations, and References. 186

Sensory Systems

Questions. 209
Answers, Explanations, and References. 220

Anatomy of the Forebrain

Questions. 231
Answers, Explanations, and References. 240

Motor Systems

Questions. 245
Answers, Explanations, and References. 257

Higher Functions

Questions. 269
Answers, Explanations, and References. 293

Bibliography 311

Index. 313

Preface

The study of the neurosciences has undergone remarkable growth over the past two decades. To a large extent, such advancements have been made possible through the development of new methodologies, especially in the fields of neuropharmacology, molecular biology, and neuroanatomy. Neuroscience courses presented in medical schools and related schools of health professions generally are unable to cover all the material that has evolved in recent years. For this reason, *Neuroscience: PreTest® Self-Assessment and Review* was written for medical students preparing for licensing examinations as well as for undergraduate students in the health professions.

The subject matter of this book is mainly the anatomy and physiology of the nervous system. Also, an attempt was made to encompass the subjects of molecular and biophysical properties of membranes, neuropharmacology, and higher functions of the nervous system. Moreover, clinical correlations for each part of the central nervous system, often using MRI and CT scans, are presented. Although it is virtually impossible to cover all aspects of neuroscience, the objective of this book is to include its most significant components as we currently understand them.

The authors wish to express their gratitude to Leo Wolansky, M.D., and Alan Zimmer, M.D., of blessed memory, for providing the MRI and CT scans.

Introduction

Each *PreTest® Self-Assessment and Review* allows medical students to comprehensively and conveniently assess and review their knowledge of a particular basic science, in this instance, neuroscience. The 500 questions parallel the format and degree of difficulty of the questions found in the United States Medical Licensing Examination (USMLE) Step 1. Practicing physicians who want to hone their skills before USMLE Step 3 or recertification may find this to be a good beginning in their review process.

Each question is accompanied by an answer, a paragraph explanation, and a specific page reference to an appropriate textbook or journal article. A bibliography listing the sources can be found following the last chapter of this text.

An effective way to use this PreTest® is to allow yourself one minute to answer each question in a given chapter. As you proceed, indicate your answer beside each question. By following this suggestion, you approximate the time limits imposed by the step. After you finish going through the questions in the section, spend as much time as you need verifying your answers and carefully reading the explanations provided. Pay special attention to the explanations for the questions you answered incorrectly, but read every explanation. The authors of this material have designed the explanations to reinforce and supplement the information tested by the questions. If you feel you need further information about the material covered, consult and study the references indicated.

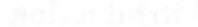

High-Yield Facts

GROSS ANATOMY OF THE BRAIN

Lateral view of the brain (Fig. 1). The loci of key motor and sensory structures of the cerebral cortex are indicated in this figure. Anatomical definitions: anterior—toward the front (rostral end) of the forebrain; posterior—toward the back (caudal end) of the forebrain; dorsal—toward the superior surface of the forebrain; ventral—toward the inferior surface of the forebrain. Note that with respect to the brainstem and spinal cord, the terms *anterior* and *ventral* are synonymous; likewise, *posterior* and *dorsal* are also synonymous. Here, the term *rostral* means toward the midbrain, and the term *caudal* means toward the sacral aspect of the spinal cord.

Midsagittal view of the brain (Fig. 2). Magnetic resonance image: T2-weighted, high-resolution, fast spin echo image.

Horizontal (transaxial) view of the brain (Fig. 3). Magnetic resonance image: Fast inversion recovery for myelin suppression image.

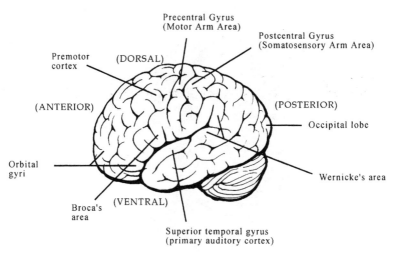

Figure 1

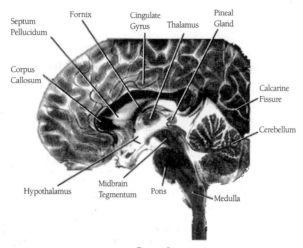

Figure 2
(Courtesy of Leo J. Wolansky, M.D.)

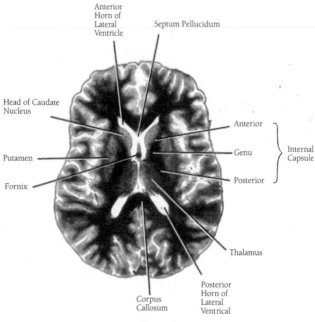

Figure 3
(Courtesy of Leo J. Wolansky, M.D.)

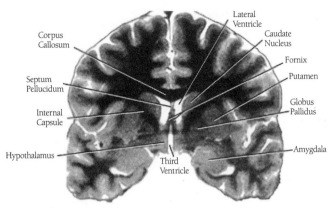

Figure 4
(Courtesy of Leo J. Wolansky, M.D.)

Frontal view of the brain (Fig. 4). Magnetic resonance image: Fast inversion recovery for myelin suppression image.

I. Cerebral cortex and adjoining structures
   A. Lateral surface of the brain
      1. Frontal lobe
         a. Motor functions
            (1) Precentral gyrus: primary motor cortex for head region and upper limbs
            (2) Premotor cortex: assists in integrating complex motor responses
            (3) Broca's area: motor speech area
         b. Areas regulating cognitive and emotional behavior
            (1) orbital (prefrontal) cortex
      2. Parietal lobe
         a. Postcentral gyrus: primary somatosensory cortex
         b. Inferior and superior parietal lobules: areas mediating complex perceptual discriminations
         c. Inferior parietal lobule and adjoining aspect of the superior temporal gyrus: area mediating speech perception
      3. Temporal lobe
         a. Primary and secondary auditory receiving areas
      4. Occipital cortex
         a. Secondary visual receiving areas and region for the integration of visual signals

B. Medial surface of the brain
1. Subcortical structures
   a. Corpus callosum: commissure connecting the hemispheres of the cerebral cortex
2. Areas of the cerebral cortex
   a. Frontal lobe
      (1) Medial prefrontal cortex and anterior cingulate gyrus: regions regulating intellectual, emotional, and autonomic processes
      (2) Medial aspect of the precentral gyrus: region mediating motor functions of the lower limbs
   b. Parietal lobe
      (1) Primary and secondary somatosensory receiving areas for the lower limb
   c. Occipital lobe
      (1) Primary visual cortex
C. Inferior surface of the brain
1. Frontal lobe: the part of the prefrontal cortex that relates to control of emotional and autonomic processes
2. Olfactory bulb and cortex: receiving areas for olfactory signals
3. Temporal lobe
   a. Superior temporal gyrus: primary auditory receiving area
   b. Limbic cortex: pyriform and entorhinal areas, receiving areas for olfactory signals; also serves as afferent sources of signals to the amygdala and hippocampal formation
II. Other forebrain structures
A. Ventricular system of the brain: lateral and third ventricles; the most important function includes cerebrospinal fluid formation
B. Septum pellucidum: membranous structure separating the lateral ventricles on each side of the hemisphere
C. Fornix: fiber pathway that passes in a dorsomedial direction from the hippocampal formation to the diencephalon
D. Diencephalon
1. Thalamus: large group of nuclei that serve as relays for signals from different regions of the nervous system to the cerebral cortex
2. Hypothalamus: structure situated below the thalamus; mediates a number of important visceral functions, such as endocrine and autonomic regulation, control of sexual behavior, aggression, and feeding and drinking behavior

E. Anterior commissure: connects the olfactory bulbs of each side of the brain; aids in the integration of olfactory signals

F. Basal ganglia: group of structures, seen best from horizontal and frontal sections, that serve primarily to regulate motor regions of the cortex
  1. Caudate nucleus
  2. Putamen
  3. Globus pallidus

G. Limbic structures: important group of structures, situated mainly within the temporal lobe, that regulate emotional behavior and autonomic and visceral functions associated with the hypothalamus
  1. Amygdala
  2. Hippocampal formation
  3. Cingulate gyrus

III. Cerebellum and brainstem

A. Cerebellum
  1. Attached to the brainstem by three pairs of peduncles (superior, inferior, and middle cerebellar peduncles) that serve primarily as communicating links between the cerebellum and the brainstem
  2. Anterior, posterior, and flocculonodular lobes: the three lobes of the cerebellum
  3. Vermis: midline structure of the cerebellum, to which the cerebellar hemispheres are attached

B. Midbrain
  1. Superior and inferior colliculus, situated dorsally in the roof of the midbrain (tectum); mediate visual and auditory functions, respectively
  2. Cerebral aqueduct: tubular portion of the ventricular system connecting the third and fourth ventricles; the aqueduct is surrounded by the periaqueductal gray, a group of compact cells that are continuous with similar cell populations surrounding the other ventricles
  3. Tegmentum: part of the core of the brainstem and a continuation of the tegmentum of lower regions of the brainstem
  4. Peduncular region: includes the cerebral peduncle, axons of cortical origin terminating in the brainstem and spinal cord, and the substantia nigra, a structure functionally associated with the basal ganglia

C. Pons
   1. Tegmentum: core of the brainstem, functionally linked with corresponding regions of the medulla and midbrain
   2. Basilar region: contains descending fiber bundles from the cerebral cortex, in addition to numerous cells and transversely oriented fibers that communicate with the cerebellum
   3. Fourth ventricle: lies on the dorsal surface of the pons and upper medulla
D. Medulla
   1. Open part of the medulla: rostral half of the medulla; contains many different cell groups, including some cranial nerve nuclei and ascending and descending fiber bundles
   2. Closed part of the medulla: caudal half of the medulla; contains many different cell and fiber groups, including those of cranial nerves
IV. Cranial nerves
   A. Forebrain: cranial nerves I and II
   B. Midbrain: cranial nerves III and IV
   C. Pons: cranial nerves V–VII
   D. Medulla: cranial nerves VIII–X and XII (note that cranial nerve XI is mainly a spinal nerve but does have a cranial root that functions as a component of cranial nerve X)

DEVELOPMENT

The sulcus limitans divides the alar plate, from which sensory regions of the spinal cord and brainstem are formed, from a basal plate, from which motor regions of the spinal cord and brainstem are formed.

THE NEURON

The neuron consists of a cell body, dendrites (which extend from the cell body), and an axon. Activation of sodium channels is associated with membrane depolarization, while activation of potassium and chloride channels is associated with membrane hyperpolarization. After information is received from a presynaptic neuron, depolarization occurs in the postsynaptic neuron; then the action potential is initiated and propagated down the axon from the initial segment.

Myelin formation is produced in the peripheral nervous system by numerous Schwann cells, while a similar function in the central nervous system (CNS) is carried out by an oligodendrocyte, which can wrap itself around numbers of neurons. Myelination in the nervous system allows for rapid conduction of ac-

DIFFERENTIATION OF THE NEURAL TUBE

Embryonic Derivative	Spinal Cord	Rhombencephalon (Hindbrain) Myelencephalon (Medulla) and Metencephalon (Pons and Cerebellum)	Mesencephalon (Midbrain)	Prosencephalon (Diencephalon and Telencephalon)
Roof plate	Region of posterior median septum.	Superior medullary velum.	Commissures of the superior and inferior colliculi.	Choroid tela and choroid plexus of the lateral and third ventricles.
Alar plate	Dorsal gray columns.	Sensory nuclei of cranial nerves: V, VII, VIII, IX, X; cerebellum, deep pontine nuclei, inferior olivary nucleus, mesencephalic nucleus (cranial Nerve [CN] V; but displaced to midbrain).	Superior and inferior colliculi, red nucleus, substantia nigra, main sensory nucleus (CN V). Some nuclei of reticular formation?	It has been suggested that diencephalon (thalamus and hypothalamus) telencephalic structures are derived from alar plate, but derivation is still unclear at this time.
Basal plate	Ventral gray columns; nucleus of cranial nerve XI.	Motor nuclei of cranial nerves: V, VI, VII, IX, X, XII; nuclei of reticular formation.	Motor nuclei of cranial nerves: III, IV; nuclei of reticular formation.	—
Floor plate	Region of ventral median fissure.	?	—	—

tion potentials by a process of saltatory conduction, in which the signals skip along openings in the myelin called *nodes of Ranvier.* Neurons that are myelinated (e.g., the pyramidal tracts and dorsal column–medial lemniscal system) are rapidly conducting, whereas those that are poorly or nonmyelinated (e.g., certain pain-afferent fibers to the spinal cord) are slowly conducting. Damage to such myelinated neurons typically disrupts the transmission of neural signals and is frequently seen in autoimmune diseases such as multiple sclerosis (MS), in which sensory and motor functions are severely compromised.

I. Different components of the neuron

   A. The plasma membrane forms the external boundary of the neuronal cell body and its processes. It consists of a double layer of lipids in which proteins, including ion channels, are embedded. Inorganic ions enter and leave the neuron through the ion channels.

   B. The nerve cell body (soma) consists of a mass of cytoplasm, which contains the nucleus and various organelles. The synthesis of most proteins, phospholipids, and other macromolecules occurs in the soma. The genetic material of the nucleus, consisting of deoxyribonucleic acid (DNA), is called *chromatin.* The nucleus contains a prominent (relatively large) nucleolus, which is concerned with the synthesis of ribonucleic acid (RNA). In the female, the Barr body represents one of the two X chromosomes and is located at the inner surface of the nuclear membrane. The cytoplasm contains the following organelles: Nissl substance or bodies, consisting of RNA granules called *ribosomes*—many ribosomes are attached to the membrane of the endoplasmic reticulum (rough endoplasmic reticulum); mitochondria, which are involved in the generation of energy; and Golgi apparatus, where proteins are modified, packaged into vesicles, and transported to other intracellular locations. Lysosomes, membrane-bound vesicles, are formed from the Golgi apparatus and contain hydrolytic enzymes. They serve as scavengers in the neurons. The cytoskeleton determines the shape of the neuron; it consists of the following filamentous elements: microtubules, neurofilaments, and microfilaments.

   C. Dendrites: short processes arising from the cell body. Their primary function is to increase the surface area for receiving signals from axonal projections of other neurons.

   D. Axon: a single long, cylindrical, and slender process arising usually from the soma. The axon usually arises from a small, conical elevation on the soma of a neuron that does not contain Nissl substance and is called an *axon hillock.* The first 50 to 100μm of the axon, after it emerges from the axon hillock, is known as the *initial segment*. This segment is the site where the action potential originates. Axons are either myelinated or unmyelinated. At their distal ends, the axons branch extensively, and their terminal ends, which are mostly enlarged, are called *synaptic terminals*.

II. Axonal transport

A. Fast anterograde transport: Precursors of peptide neurotransmitters, lipids, and glycoproteins, which are necessary to reconstitute the plasma membrane, are carried from the cell body to the terminals by this mechanism.

B. Slow anterograde axonal transport: Neurofilaments and microtubules are synthesized in the cell body and are transported by this mechanism to the terminals.

C. Fast retrograde axonal transport: Rapid retrograde transport carries materials from the nerve terminals to the cell body. Fast retrograde transport is involved in some pathological conditions. For example, herpes simplex, polio, and rabies viruses and tetanus toxin are taken up by the axon terminals in peripheral nerves and carried to their cell bodies in the CNS by rapid retrograde transport.

D. Neuroanatomical applications: In anterograde tracing techniques, amino acids are taken up by the perikarya of the neurons (receiving the microinjection of the given label) for protein synthesis and are then transported anterogradely to their axon terminals. The labeled axons and their terminals are then visualized by autoradiography. Anterograde transport of carbohydrate-binding proteins, called *lectins,* has been used for investigating neuronal connections.

1. Retrograde tracing technique: This procedure involves the microinjection of an enzyme (e.g., horseradish peroxidase [HRP]), fluorescent dyes (e.g., Fluoro-Gold), cholera toxin, or viruses at the desired site. The injected substance is taken up by axon terminals and transported retrogradely into the neuronal cell bodies. The labeled neurons are then visualized by a chemical reaction. Likewise, fluorescent substances such as Fluoro-Gold, microinjected at the desired site, are taken up by axon terminals and transported to the cell bodies, where they are visualized under a fluorescent microscope.

III. Types of neurons: multipolar neurons, bipolar neurons, pseudo-unipolar neurons, and unipolar neurons. Neurons can also be grouped as principal or projecting neurons (also known as type I or Golgi type I) and intrinsic neurons (also known as type II or Golgi type II neurons). Principal neurons (type I neurons, e.g., motor neurons in the ventral horn of the spinal cord) possess very long axons. Intrinsic neurons (type II neurons) have very short axons.

IV. Neuroglia (glial cells): These are supporting cells located in the CNS. They are nonexcitable and more numerous than neurons. They have been classified into the following groups: astrocytes (fibrous and protoplasmic), oligodendrocytes, and microglia and ependymal cells (ependymocytes, choroidal epithelial cells, and tanycytes).

V. Myelination: Myelinated axons are present in the peripheral nervous system as well as the CNS. In the peripheral nervous system, Schwann cells provide myelin sheaths around axons. The myelin sheaths are interrupted along the length of the axons at regular intervals at the nodes of Ranvier. The action potential becomes regenerated at uninsulated nodes of Ranvier. Therefore, the action potential traveling along the length of the axon jumps from one node of Ranvier to another (saltatory conduction). In the CNS, oligodendrocytes form the myelin sheaths around neurons. The intervals between adjacent oligodendrocytes are devoid of myelin sheaths and are called the nodes of Ranvier.

VI. Composition of peripheral nerves: Each peripheral nerve consists of epineurium, perineurium, endoneurium, and nerve fibers.

VII. Neuronal injury: *Wallerian degeneration* refers to the changes that occur distal to the site of damage on an axon. Initially, the axon swells up and becomes irregular. Later, it is broken down into fragments (which are phagocytosed by adjacent macrophages and Schwann cells). When an axon is damaged, alterations may be restricted to the proximal segment of the axon up to the first node of Ranvier. Retrograde degeneration occurs when sectioning of an axon produces changes in the cell body, and if the injury is close to the cell body, the neuron may degenerate. The cell body swells up due to edema and becomes round in appearance, and the Nissl substance gets distributed throughout the cytoplasm (chromatolysis). The nucleus moves from its central position to the periphery due to edema. Transneuronal degeneration occurs in the CNS when damage to one group of neurons results in the degeneration of another set of neurons closely associated with the same function.

VIII. Recovery of neuronal injury (regeneration): If the damage to the neurons is not severe, regeneration is possible, but complete recovery may take as long as three to six months. Although sprouting occurs in axons in the CNS, this process ceases within a short time (about two weeks). Function of the neurons in the CNS is not restored. However, in peripheral nerves, an axon can regenerate satisfactorily if the endoneurial sheaths are intact. In this situation, the regenerating axons reach the correct destination and the chances of recovery of function are reasonable.

IX. Neuronal membrane
  A. The neuronal membrane, like other cell membranes, consists of a lipid bilayer in which proteins, including ion channels, are embedded.
  B. The lipid bilayer determines the basic structure of the neuronal membrane, while the proteins embedded in it are responsible for most of the membrane functions, such as serving as specific receptors, enzymes, and transport proteins.
X. Permeability of the neuronal membrane
  A. The neuronal membrane is permeable to all lipid soluble substances and some polar (lipid-insoluble, water-soluble) molecules, provided they are uncharged and small in volume.
  B. The neuronal membrane is impermeable to most polar and charged molecules (even if they are very small).
  C. Cations and anions contain electrostatically bound water (waters of hydration). The attractive forces between the ions and the water molecules make it difficult for the ions to move from a watery environment into the hydrophobic lipid bilayer of the neuronal membrane.
XI. Carrier proteins (carriers or transporters)
  A. When a specific solute binds to a carrier protein, a reversible conformational change occurs in the protein, which, in turn, results in the transfer of the solute across the lipid bilayer of the membrane.
  B. When a carrier protein transports a solute from one side of the membrane to the other, it is called a *uniport.*
  C. A carrier protein that moves one solute in a particular direction and another solute in the opposite direction is called an *antiport.*
  D. A carrier protein that carries one solute in a particular direction and another solute in the same direction is called a *symport.*
XII. The channel proteins: The channel proteins span the neuronal membrane and contain water-filled pores. The inorganic ions of suitable size and charge (e.g., Na^+, K^+) can pass through the pore when it is in open state and, thus, pass through the membrane.
XIII. Simple diffusion: The substances that pass through the neuronal membrane by simple diffusion include all lipid-soluble substances and some polar (lipid-insoluble or water-soluble) molecules, provided they are uncharged and small in volume.
XIV. Passive transport (facilitated diffusion): In this type of transport, solutes are transported across the neuronal membrane passively.
XV. Active transport: Some carrier proteins transport certain solutes by active transport (i.e., the solute is moved across the neuronal membrane

against its electrochemical gradient). This type of transport requires coupling of the carrier protein to a source of metabolic energy.

XVI. Intracellular and extracellular ionic concentrations: The concentration of sodium ions is much greater outside the neuron as compared to that inside the neuron. On the other hand, the concentration of potassium ions is greater inside the cell than outside.

XVII. Na^+,K^+-ATPase

A. The differences in intracellular and extracellular concentrations of different ions are maintained by Na^+,K^+-ATPase (also known as Na^+,K^+ pump), which is located in the neuronal membrane.

B. It transfers three Na^+ ions out of the neuron for every two K^+ ions that are taken in. A net outward ionic current is generated because of this unequal flow of Na^+ and K^+ ions across the neuronal membrane. Because of the generation of this current, the Na^+,K^+ pump is said to be *electrogenic*.

XVIII. Ion channels

A. Ion channels are made up of proteins and are embedded in the lipid bilayer of the neuronal membrane across which they span.

B. Nongated channels: These are always open and control the flow of ions during the resting membrane potential. Examples include non-gated Na^+ and K^+ channels that contribute to the resting membrane potential.

C. Gated channels: All gated channels are allosteric proteins. At rest, these channels are mostly closed, and they open in response to different stimuli (e.g., change in membrane potential, ligand binding, or mechanical forces).

D. Voltage-gated channels: They are opened or closed by a change in the membrane potential. Examples: Voltage-gated Na^+ channels, voltage-gated Ca^{2+} channels, and voltage-gated K^+ channels.

E. Ligand-gated channels: Noncovalent binding of chemical substances (transmitters or second messengers) with their receptors on the neuronal membrane opens these channels.

F. Mechanically gated channels: These channels open by a mechanical stimulus and include the channels involved in producing generator potentials of stretch and touch receptors.

XIX. Nernst equation: The equilibrium potential of any ion, which is present both inside and outside the cell where the cell membrane is permeable to that ion, is calculated by this equation.

XX. Goldman equation: This equation is used to determine the membrane potential when the membrane is permeable to more than one ion species.

XXI. The ionic basis of the resting membrane potential

A. When the neuron is at rest, the potential difference across its membrane is called the *resting membrane potential.*

B. In the resting state, the neuron has a more negative charge inside relative to outside.

C. If the neuronal membrane contained only K^+ channels, the resting membrane potential would be determined by the K^+ concentration gradient and would be equal to the equilibrium potential for K^+ ions (approximately −90 mV).

D. However, neurons at rest are selectively permeable to Na^+ ions also. The Na^+ ions tend to flow into the neuron. Due to influx of Na^+ ions, the resting membrane potential deviates somewhat from that of the K^+ equilibrium potential, but it does not reach the equilibrium potential for Na^+. The reason for the inability of the neuron to attain a resting membrane potential closer to the Na^+ equilibrium potential is that the number of open nongated Na^+ channels is much smaller than the number of open nongated K^+ channels in the resting state of a neuron.

XXII. The ionic basis of the action potential

A. When a neuron receives an excitatory input, the neuronal membrane is depolarized, resulting in an opening of some voltage-gated Na^+ channels and influx of Na^+.

B. The accumulation of positive charges due to influx of Na^+ promotes further depolarization of the neuronal membrane.

C. When the membrane potential reaches a threshold level, a large number of voltage-gated Na^+ channels open and the permeability of Na^+ increases during the rising phase of the action potential. The depolarization continues so that the membrane potential approaches the Na^+ equilibrium potential.

D. The neuron is then repolarized by slow inactivation of voltage-gated Na^+ channels, which stops influx of Na^+ through these channels, and delayed opening of voltage-gated K^+ channels, which allows increased efflux of K^+ through voltage-gated K^+ channels (delayed rectifiers). It should be noted that influx of Na^+ and efflux of K^+ through the nongated channels continues throughout these events.

XXIII. Propagation of action potentials

A. When a region of the axonal membrane is depolarized sufficiently to reach a threshold, voltage-gated Na^+ channels open, Na^+ flows into the axoplasm, and an action potential is generated in that region.

B. The local depolarization spreads electronically (passively) to an adjacent region, where an action potential is generated by the opening of voltage-gated Na^+ channels and the influx of Na^+ into the axoplasm. The passive spread of voltage along the length of an axon results in an active regeneration process.

C. In vertebrates, nodes of Ranvier (bare segments of the axonal membrane) are present in between the segments of the myelin sheath.

D. The passive spread of current can generate an intense current at the nodes of Ranvier due to the presence of a high density of voltage-gated Na^+ channels.

E. The action potential propagates along an axon by saltatory conduction without decrement (i.e., the jumping of an action potential from one node to another).

THE SYNAPSE AND NEUROTRANSMITTERS

The binding of the neurotransmitter to the receptor molecule is determined by the postsynaptic receptor, which serves a gating function for particular ions. The receptor is responsible for opening or closing ligand-gated channels, which are regulated by noncovalent binding of compounds such as neurotransmitters. The neurotransmitter, which is contained in presynaptic vesicles and released onto the postsynaptic terminal, causes activation of the receptor, which in turn produces postsynaptic potentials.

	NEURONAL INTRACELLULAR AND EXTRACELLULAR CONCENTRATIONS OF SOME IMPORTANT IONS	
Ion	Extracellular Concentration, Millimolar (mM)	Intracellular Concentration (mM)
Cations (positively charged):		
Na^+	140–145	5–15
K^+	4–5	140
Ca^{2+}	1–2	10^4
Cl^-	110	4–30
Anions: A^- (fixed anions; organic acids and proteins)	—	385

The sequence of events in synaptic transmission is as follows: transmitter synthesis → release of transmitter into synaptic cleft → binding of transmitter to postsynaptic receptor → removal of transmitter.

Major excitatory transmitters include substance P, acetylcholine, and excitatory amino acids; major inhibitory transmitters include GABA, enkephalin, and glycine. Disruption of neurotransmitter function can lead to different diseases of the nervous system. One such example involves the role of acetylcholine at the neuromuscular junction. When antibodies are formed against the acetylcholine receptor at the neuromuscular junction, transmission is disrupted and the autoimmune disease called *myasthenia gravis* occurs. This disorder includes symptoms such as weakness and fatigue of the muscles.

I. Synaptic transmission

   A. Characteristics of electrical transmission

      1. Current generated by an impulse in one neuron spreads to another neuron through a pathway of low resistance. Such a pathway has been identified at gap junctions.

      2. Current generated by voltage-gated channels at the presynaptic neuron flows directly into the postsynaptic neuron. Therefore, transmission at such a synapse is very rapid (<0.1 ms).

      3. Electrical transmission is not very common in the CNS.

   B. Characteristics of chemical transmission

      1. At chemical synapses, the pre- and postsynaptic cells are separated by synaptic clefts, which are fluid-filled gaps (about 20 to 40 nm). The presynaptic terminal contains synaptic vesicles, which are filled with several thousand molecules of a specific chemical substance, the neurotransmitter.

      2. An action potential depolarizes the presynaptic nerve terminal, the permeability to Ca^{2+} increases, and Ca^{2+} enters the terminal. These events cause the vesicles to fuse with the cytoplasmic membrane and then release the neurotransmitter into the synaptic cleft (exocytosis).

II. Characteristics of receptors: They consist of membrane-spanning proteins. The recognition sites for the binding of the chemical transmitter are located on the extracellular components of the receptor. The binding of the neurotransmitter to its receptor results in opening or closing of ion channels on the postsynaptic membrane.

III. Characteristics of ion channels

   A. Indirectly gated ion channels: In this type of channel, the ion channel and the recognition site for the transmitter (receptor) are separate.

This type of receptor is called a *metabotropic receptor.* When a transmitter binds to the receptor, a guanosine-5'-triphosphate (GTP)-binding protein (G-protein) is activated, which in turn activates a second messenger system. The second messenger can either act directly on the ion channel to open it or activate an enzyme, which in turn opens the channel by phosphorylating the channel protein. Activation of this type of channel elicits slow synaptic actions, which are long lasting (seconds or even minutes).

B. Directly gated ion channels: In this type of ion channel, several protein subunits (four or five) are arranged in such a way that the recognition site for the neurotransmitter is part of the ion channel. This type of receptor is called an *ionotropic receptor.* A transmitter binds to its receptor and brings about a conformational change, which results in the opening of the ion channel. Receptors of this type usually bring about fast synaptic responses lasting for only a few milliseconds.

C. Directly gated synaptic transmission at a peripheral synapse (nerve-muscle synapse): At the neuromuscular junction, the axons of motor neurons whose cell bodies are located in the CNS innervate skeletal muscle fibers. As the motor axon reaches a specialized region on the muscle membrane, called the *end plate,* it loses its myelin sheath and gives off several fine branches. Many varicosities (swellings), called *synaptic boutons,* are present at the terminals of these branches. The presynaptic boutons contain the synaptic vesicles containing acetylcholine. When the motor axon is stimulated, an action potential reaches the axon terminal and depolarizes the membrane of the presynaptic bouton, which results in the opening of the voltage-gated Ca^{2+} channels. Influx of Ca^{2+} into the terminal promotes fusion of the vesicle with the terminal membrane and subsequent release of acetylcholine by exocytosis. Acetylcholine acts on the nicotinic cholinergic receptors located at the crest of the junctional folds to produce an end plate potential (EPP). The amplitude of the EPP is large enough (about 70 mV) to activate the voltage-gated Na^+ channels in the junctional folds and generate an action potential, which then propagates along the muscle fiber and brings about muscle contraction.

D. Directly gated transmission at a central synapse: A synaptic potential that excites a postsynaptic cell in the CNS is called an *excitatory postsynaptic potential* (EPSP). This EPSP is generated by opening of directly gated ion channels, which permit influx of Na^+ and efflux of K^+. If the depolarization produced by the EPSP is large enough, the membrane potential of the axon hillock of the spinal motor neuron is raised to a threshold and an action potential results. A synaptic potential that inhibits a postsynaptic cell in the CNS system is called an *inhibitory postsynaptic potential* (IPSP). An IPSP usually hyperpolarizes the neuronal membrane.

IV. Diseases affecting the chemical transmission at the nerve-muscle synapse
   A. Myasthenia gravis: This is an autoimmune disease in which the number of functional nicotinic acetylcholine receptors is reduced by an antibody. This results in muscular weakness. The symptoms include weakness of eyelids, eye muscles, oropharyngeal muscles, and limb muscles. Antibodies, probably produced by T and B lymphocytes, against the acetylcholine receptors are present in the serum of such patients. Acetylcholinesterase-inhibiting drugs (e.g., neostigmine) can reverse the muscle weakness.
   B. Lambert-Eaton syndrome: In this disorder, antibodies are developed to voltage-gated Ca^{2+} channels on presynaptic terminals. The loss of voltage-gated Ca^{2+} channels is expected to impair the release of acetylcholine from the nerve terminals. Standard treatment consists of administration of guanidine and calcium gluconate, which elicit or facilitate acetylcholine release from the presynaptic nerve terminals.

V. Major classes of neurotransmitters
   A. Small molecule neurotransmitters: acetylcholine, excitatory amino acids (glutamate, aspartate), inhibitory amino acids (GABA, glycine), catecholamines (dopamine, norepinephrine, epinephrine), indoleamines (serotonin), imidazoleamines (histamine), and purines (adenosine).
   B. Large molecule neurotransmitters: opioid peptides (e.g., endomorphins, enkephalins, nociceptin), substance P.

VI. Steps in neurotransmitter release
   A. Depolarization of presynaptic terminal
   B. Ca^{2+} entry into the terminal
   C. Fusion of vesicles containing the neurotransmitters with the presynaptic terminal membrane
   D. Release of the neurotransmitter into the synaptic cleft

VII. Individual neurotransmitters
   A. Acetylcholine
      1. Synthesis
         a. Choline present in the plasma enters the nerve terminal by active transport.
         b. Acetylcholine is synthesized in the cytoplasm from choline and acetylcoenzyme-A by choline acetyltransferase.
         c. Acetylcholine is transported into vesicles and stored there.

2. Release and removal
   a. Acetylcholine is released into the synaptic cleft.
   b. It is hydrolyzed by acetylcholinesterase.
3. Distribution
   a. The basal forebrain constellation including the basal nucleus of Meynert
   b. Cholinergic neurons in the dorsolateral tegmentum of the pons
4. Physiological and clinical considerations
   a. Cholinergic neurons have been implicated in the regulation of forebrain activity and sleep-wakefulness cycles.
   b. In Alzheimer's disease, there is a dramatic loss of cholinergic neurons in the basal nucleus of Meynert.

B. Glutamate
1. Synthesis
   a. Glucose enters the neuron, undergoes glycolysis in the cytoplasm to generate pyruvic acid, which enters into the mitochondria. In the mitochondria, pyruvic acid generates an acetyl group that combines with coenzyme-A present in the mitochondria to form acetylcoenzyme-A.
   b. The acetyl group is regenerated from acetylcoenzyme-A; it enters the Krebs cycle in the mitochondria.
   c. Alpha-ketoglutaric acid, generated in the Krebs cycle, is transaminated to form glutamate. .
   d. Glutamate released into the synaptic cleft is recaptured by neuronal-type and glial-type Na^+-coupled glutamate transporters.
   e. In the nerve terminal, glutamate is repackaged into vesicles.
   f. In the glial cell, glutamate is converted to glutamine by an enzyme, glutamine synthetase. Glutamine in the glial cells is then transported into the neighboring nerve terminals and converted to glutamate, which is then packaged into vesicles.
2. Release and removal: Glutamate is taken up by a high-affinity sodium-dependent reuptake mechanism into the nerve terminals and glial cells.
3. Physiological and clinical considerations
   a. Glutamate has been implicated as a transmitter in several circuits in the brain.
   b. Alteration in glutamate levels has been implicated in Huntington's chorea and amyotrophic lateral sclerosis (ALS).
   c. Prolonged stimulation of neurons by excitatory amino acids results in neuronal death or injury. This effect is known as *excitotoxicity*.

C. GABA

1. Synthesis: It is formed by alpha-decarboxylation of L-glutamate. This reaction is catalyzed by L-glutamic acid-1-decarboxylase (GAD), which is present almost exclusively in GABAergic neurons.

2. Release and removal

   a. In the brain, after its release, GABA is taken up into presynaptic terminals as well as glia.

   b. Most of GABA is metabolized to yield glutamate and succinic semialdehyde by an enzyme, GABA-oxoglutarate transaminase (GABA-T).

3. Physiological and clinical considerations

   a. GABA is found in high concentrations in the brain and spinal cord; it is an inhibitory transmitter in many brain circuits.

   b. Alteration of GABAergic circuits has been implicated in neurological disorders like epilepsy, Huntington's chorea, Parkinson's disease, senile dementia, Alzheimer's disease, and schizophrenia.

   c. Barbiturates act as agonists or modulators on postsynaptic GABA receptors; they are used to treat epilepsy.

   d. Valproic acid (dipropylacetic acid) is an anticonvulsant. It inhibits GABA-transaminase, an enzyme that metabolizes GABA, and increases GABA levels in the brain. Since epileptic seizures can be facilitated by lack of neuronal inhibition, increase in the inhibitory transmitter, GABA, is helpful in terminating them.

D. Glycine

1. Synthesis

   a. In the nerve tissue, serine is formed from glucose via the intermediates, 3-phosphoglycerate and 3-phosphoserine.

   b. Glycine is formed from serine by an enzyme, serine transhydroxy-methylase.

2. Release and removal: After its release, glycine is taken up by neurons by means of an active sodium-dependent mechanism involving specific membrane transporters.

3. Distribution: Glycine is found in all body fluids and tissue proteins in substantial amounts. It is not an essential amino acid, but it is an intermediate in the metabolism of proteins, peptides, and bile salts. It is also a neurotransmitter in the CNS.

4. Physiological and clinical considerations

   a. Glycine has been implicated as a neurotransmitter in the spinal cord, the lower brainstem, and perhaps the retina.

   b. Mutations of genes coding for some of the membrane transporters needed for removal of glycine result in hyperglycinemia, which is a devastating neonatal disease characterized by lethargy, seizures, and mental retardation.

E. Catecholamines

1. Dopamine

   a. Synthesis

      (1) Tyrosine enters the neuron by active transport.

      (2) Tyrosine is converted into dihydroxyphenylalanine (DOPA) by tyrosine hydroxylase enzyme. DOPA is converted to dopamine by an enzyme, aromatic L-amino acid decarboxylase (DOPA-decarboxylase). These steps occur in the cytoplasm.

      (3) Dopamine is then actively transported into the storage vesicles.

   b. Release and removal

      (1) Dopamine released into the synaptic cleft is removed by reuptake into the presynaptic terminal.

      (2) It diffuses into the circulation and is destroyed in the liver by two enzymes, catechol-O-methyltransferase (COMT) and monoamine oxidase (MAO).

   c. Distribution

      (1) Substantia nigra: The axons of these neurons ascend rostrally in the nigrostriatal projection and provide dopaminergic innervation of·neurons located in the corpus striatum (caudate nucleus and putamen).

      (2) Ventral tegmental area: This paired area lies adjacent to the substantia nigra, and the dopaminergic neurons located in this area project to different brain areas via the following pathways: (a) the mesolimbic pathway and (b) the mesocortical pathway. In the mesolimbic pathway, the axons of the dopaminergic neurons supply limbic structures (i.e., amygdala, septal area, hippocampal formation) and the nucleus accumbens (ventral striatum). In the mesocortical pathway, the axons of the dopaminergic neurons provide innervation to the frontal and cingulate cortex.

      (3) Arcuate nucleus of hypothalamus: Dopaminergic neurons in this area project to the median eminence. They release dopamine directly into the hypophyseal portal circulation, which is then carried to the anterior lobe of the pituitary to inhibit the release of prolactin.

d. Physiological and clinical considerations
   (1) Parkinson's disease: This disease is characterized by tremor at rest, slowness of movement (bradykinesia), rigidity of extremities and neck, and an expressionless face. Dopaminergic neurons located in the substantia nigra are degenerated in this disease, and the release of dopamine in the caudate putamen is decreased. Treatment: oral administration of a combination of L-dopa and carbidopa (Sinemet).
   (2) Psychotic disorders: Many adult psychotic disorders, including schizophrenia, are believed to involve increased activity at dopaminergic synapses. Many drugs that are effective in the treatment of these disorders are believed to mediate their action through the D_2-dopamine receptors.

2. Norepinephrine
   a. Synthesis
      (1) In the noradrenergic neurons, dopamine stored in the vesicles is converted into norepinephrine by the enzyme dopamine-β-hydroxylase (DBH).
   b. Release and removal: Norepinephrine released into the synaptic cleft is removed by the following mechanisms:
      (1) Reuptake-1: Norepinephrine is transported back into the terminal of the noradrenergic neuron.
      (2) Reuptake-2: Norepinephrine is actively transported into the effector cells (about 10%), where it is inactivated primarily by COMT.
      (3) Norepinephrine diffuses into the circulation from the synaptic cleft and is destroyed in the liver by two enzymes, COMT and MAO.
   c. Distribution: Noradrenergic neurons are located in the locus coeruleus. These neurons project to the thalamus, hypothalamus, limbic forebrain structures (cingulate and parahippocampal gyri, hippocampal formation, amygdaloid complex), and the cerebral cortex, where norepinephrine modulates a wide variety of functions associated with these regions.
   d. Physiological and clinical considerations
      (1) Norepinephrine is released as a transmitter from postganglionic sympathetic nerve terminals.
      (2) It is believed to play a role in psychiatric disorders such as depression.

3. Epinephrine
   a. Synthesis
      (1) About 10% of norepinephrine stored in the vesicles leaks out into the cytoplasm.
      (2) In the adrenergic neuron, it is converted into epinephrine by the enzyme phenyl-ethanolamine-N-methyltransferase (PNMT).
      (3) Epinephrine thus formed is actively transported into storage vesicles in the nerve terminal (or chromaffin granules in the adrenal medulla) and stored for subsequent release.
   b. Release and removal: The mechanisms for removal of epinephrine are the same as those for norepinephrine.
   c. Distribution:
      (1) C1 neurons located in the rostral ventrolateral medulla
      (2) C2 neurons located in the nucleus tractus solitarius
   d. Physiological and clinical considerations: The function of adrenergic neurons in the CNS has not been clearly established.

F. Indoleamines
   1. Serotonin (5-hydroxytryptamine)
      a. Synthesis
         (1) Plasma tryptophan enters the brain by an active uptake process and is hydroxylated at the 5 position, by tryptophan hydroxylase, to form 5-hydroxytryptophan.
         (2) 5-hydroxytryptophan is immediately decarboxylated to form serotonin. Serotonin is then actively taken up and stored in vesicles, where it is ready for release.
      b. Release and removal
         (1) Serotonin is removed from the synaptic cleft by reuptake mechanisms.
         (2) It is also metabolized by monoamine oxidase (MAO).
      c. Distribution
         (1) Serotonin-containing neurons are located in the midline or raphe regions of the medulla, pons, and upper brainstem.
         (2) The rostral serotonin-containing cell groups of the dorsal, median, and central superior raphe project to the diencephalon and telencephalon.
         (3) 5-HT neurons in the caudal raphe nuclei project to the spinal cord.
      d. Physiological and clinical considerations
         (1) Serotonin-containing cells in the raphe regions of the

brainstem are believed to play a role in descending-pain-control systems.

(2) Serotonin-containing neurons may play a role in mediating affective processes such as aggressive behavior and arousal.

(3) Serotonin synthesized in the pineal gland serves as a precursor for the synthesis of melatonin, which in turn serves as a neurohormone regulating sleep patterns.

(4) Serotonin is also believed to play an important role in depression. Fluoxetine (Prozac) selectively blocks reuptake of serotonin and enhances 5-HT levels in the brain. It may produce beneficial effects in mental depression via enhancement of transmission through 5-HT_{1A} receptors. Sumatriptan (Imitrex), a 5-HT_{1D} receptor agonist, is a vasoconstrictor and has proved useful in treating migraine headaches.

(5) Some drugs of abuse mediate their effects through serotonin-containing neurons. For example, ecstasy (3,4,methylene-dioxy-methamphetamine, or MDMA) is believed to release 5-HT.

G. Imidazoleamines
  1. Histamine
    a. Synthesis
      (1) Histidine enters the brain by active transport.
      (2) It is then decarboxylated, by histidine decarboxylase, to form histamine.
    b. Release and removal
      (1) Histamine utilizes catecholamine uptake processes in certain tissues.
      (2) It is metabolized to 1-methylhistamine and imidazole acetic acid.
    c. Distribution
      (1) The highest density of histamine-containing neurons has been found in the median eminence and premammillary regions of the hypothalamus.
      (2) These neurons project to many areas of the brain and spinal cord.
    d. Physiological and clinical considerations: Histamine has been implicated as a transmitter in the regulation of food and water intake, thermoregulation, autonomic function, and hormone release.

H. Purines
   1. Recently, ATP (adenosine triphosphate) has been implicated as a neurotransmitter.
   2. ATP has been implicated in pain mechanisms in the spinal cord.
   3. Purinergic transmission has been demonstrated in autonomic neurons innervating the bladder, vas deferens, and muscle fibers of the heart.
I. Opioid peptides
   1. Synthesis
      a. β-endorphin: The pre-propeptide (pre-proopiomelanocortin) is present in the rough endoplasmic reticulum (RER) of neurons in the anterior pituitary, the intermediate lobe of the pituitary, and the arcuate nucleus of the hypothalamus. It is converted into the propeptide proopiomelanocortin, which is transported to the axon terminal by fast axonal transport. β-endorphin is derived from proopiomelanocortin.
      b. Enkephalins: The pre-propeptide (pre-proenkephalin A) is present in the RER of neurons predominantly in the hindbrain. It is converted to the propeptide, proenkephalin A, which is transported to the axon terminal by fast axonal transport. Further proteolytic processing in the terminal results in the generation of active peptides, methionine, and leucine enkephalin. Both of them are pentapeptides.
      c. Dynorphins (1–13): These peptides can be isolated from the pituitary and consist of C-terminally extended forms of Leu^5-enkephalin.
   2. Release and removal: In the CNS, the action of most of the peptides is terminated by their degradation due to the presence of peptidases.
   3. Physiological and clinical considerations: Opioid peptides have been implicated in regulating blood pressure, temperature, feeding, and sexual behavior.
J. Tachykinins
   1. Substance P is an undecapeptide (11 amino acids) and is present in the substantia nigra, caudate putamen, amygdala, hypothalamus, and cerebral cortex. Substance P neurons in the striatum project to the dopamine-containing neurons in the substantia nigra.
   2. Physiological and clinical considerations
      a. Substance P has been implicated as one of the transmitters in mediating pain sensation.

    b. Substance P levels are reduced in the substantia nigra in patients suffering from Huntington's chorea, which is characterized by movement and psychological disorders.

K. Gaseous neurotransmitters

  1. Nitric oxide (NO)

    a. Synthesis

      (1) Glutamate, released from a presynaptic neuron, acts on NMDA receptors located on the postsynaptic neuron; calcium ions enter the postsynaptic neuron and bind with calmodulin (calcium-binding protein), which results in the activation of nitric oxide synthase (NOS).

      (2) NOS then generates NO and citrulline from L-arginine.

      (3) NO stimulates soluble guanylate cyclase, which results in the formation of cGMP from GTP. Increased levels of cGMP in the postsynaptic neuron elicit a physiological response.

    b. Physiological and clinical considerations

      (1) In the CNS, the role of nitric oxide as a transmitter is still under investigation.

      (2) The relaxation of blood vessels caused by cholinergic agonists may be mediated by NO.

VIII. Receptors

A. Ligand-gated or ionotropic receptors, which consist of multimeric proteins directly linked to ion channels

  1. Nicotinic acetylcholine receptors (nAChR) are located at the neuromuscular junction (NMJ) as well as at central neurons. ACh binds to the alpha subunits and opens the channel to allow influx of Na^+ and efflux of K^+.

  2. N-methyl-D-aspartic acid (NMDA) receptor: The activity of this receptor can be altered through the following binding sites:

    a. Transmitter binding site: L-glutamate and related agonists bind at the transmitter binding site and promote opening of a high conductance channel through which sodium and calcium ions enter the target cells.

    b. The strychnine-insensitive glycine modulatory site: This site is very important because unless it is occupied, L-glutamate is ineffective at this receptor.

    c. The phencyclidine binding site: This is located within the channel. Noncompetitive blockers of NMDA receptor-ionophore complex (e.g., ketamine) also bind at the same site.

    d. Voltage-dependent magnesium binding site: The channel associated with an NMDA receptor is blocked by Mg^{2+} at normal resting potentials or when the cell is hyperpolarized. When the cell is depolarized, Mg^{2+} is dislodged and Na^+ and Ca^{2+} enter while K^+ leaves the cell through the same channel.

3. Kainate receptor: Binding of kainic acid to this ionotropic glutamate receptor results in the opening of an ion channel permitting influx of Na^+ (but not Ca^{2+}) and efflux of K^+ through the same channel and efflux of K^+ ion; the neuron is depolarized.

4. AMPA/quisqualate receptor: AMPA and quisqualic acid are agonists for this ionotropic glutamate receptor. Binding of these agonists to their receptors results in the opening of an ion channel permitting influx of Na^+ (but not Ca^{2+}) and efflux of K^+; the neuron is depolarized.

5. $GABA_A$ receptors: The following major binding sites are present on these receptors:
    a. For agonists (e.g., GABA, muscimol).
    b. For antagonists (e.g., bicuculline).
    c. For benzodiazepines (e.g., diazepam or Valium).
    d. For barbiturates.
    e. GABA agonists open the chloride channels and thus hyperpolarize the neurons. Drugs that bind to the benzodiazepine site enhance the electrophysiological effects of GABA (e.g., diazepam or Valium, an anxiolytic drug). Barbiturates bind to another site and prolong the opening of the chloride channel.

6. Glycine receptor: Activation of glycine receptors results in an influx of chloride ions into the neuron, which is then hyperpolarized. Strychnine blocks the glycine receptors.

7. Serotonin receptors: At least seven subtypes of serotonin receptors have been identified. Only $5\text{-}HT_3$ receptors are ionotropic receptors. All other subtypes are metabotropic receptors.

B. Metabotropic receptors
1. They consist of a single protein (monomeric) molecule that usually has seven membrane-spanning domains.
2. G-proteins bind to an intracellular loop of these domains.
3. Binding of the neurotransmitter to the receptor results in the replacement of GDP by GTP on the α-subunit of the G-protein. The activated GTP-α-subunit complex can have the following results: (1) it can open the ion channels directly, or (2) they can bind to

effector molecules (e.g., adenylyl cyclase), generate second messengers (e.g., cAMP) and, later, effectors (e.g., protein kinase A), which then finally phosphorylate the ion channel to open it. Ions flow across the membrane and a postsynaptic response is elicited.

4. Some examples of metabotropic receptors are as follows:
   a. Cholinergic muscarinic receptors:
   b. Acetylcholine (ACh) binds with muscarinic receptors, a G-protein (G_o) is activated, phospholipase C is generated, and two second messengers—IP_3 and diacylglycerol (DAG)—are produced.
      (1) IP_3 releases Ca^{2+} from intracellular stores, which leads to opening of Ca^{2+}-activated K^+ and Cl^- channels.
      (2) DAG activates protein kinase C, which can directly open Ca^{2+}-activated K^+ channels.
      (3) These events result in hyperpolarization and then inhibition of the neuron.
   c. Metabotropic glutamate receptors (mGLURs): mGLURs have been assigned to three groups. Group I mGLURs stimulate phospholipase C and phosphoinositide hydrolysis. Group II and III mGLURs inhibit adenylyl cyclase and cAMP formation.
   d. Dopamine receptors: At least five subtypes of dopamine receptors (D_1–D_5) have been identified. All of them are metabotropic receptors.
   e. Adrenergic receptors
      (1) Norepinephrine and epinephrine mediate their actions via adrenergic receptors. These receptors are divided into two major classes: α and β. These classes have been further subdivided into many subtypes of adrenergic receptors.
      (2) Binding of norepinephrine with β-adrenergic receptors results in the activation of a stimulatory G-protein (G_s).
      (3) Adenylyl cyclase enzyme is activated, which generates the second messenger cAMP.
      (4) The latter activates protein kinase A, which phosphorylates appropriate channels and opens them.
      (5) The neurons are depolarized, the amplitude of neurotransmitter-induced EPSPs is increased, and the neuron is made more excitable.
   f. $GABA_B$ receptors
      (1) They are coupled to calcium or potassium channels via second messenger systems.

(2) Activation of presynaptic $GABA_B$ receptors by baclofen decreases calcium conductance and reduces transmitter release.

(3) Postsynaptic $GABA_B$ receptors are indirectly coupled to potassium channels via G-proteins, and they mediate delayed IPSPs.

g. Serotonin receptors

  (1) At least five subtypes of serotonin receptors have been identified. As stated earlier, all of them except $5\text{-}HT_3$ receptors are metabotropic.

  (2) $5\text{-}HT_1$ receptors are located primarily in the CNS.

  (3) $5\text{-}HT_2$ receptors are located in the CNS, gastrointestinal tract, and vascular smooth muscle.

  (4) $5\text{-}HT_4$ receptors are located in the CNS, gastrointestinal tract, heart, and urinary bladder.

  (5) Identification of the function of 5-HT receptors in the CNS remains an active area of research.

h. Histamine receptors

  (1) At least three subtypes of histamine receptors (H_1, H_2, and H_3) have been identified. All of them are metabotropic.

  (2) The stimulation of histamine receptors results in the formation of cyclic adenosine monophosphate.

i. Adenosine receptors

  (1) At least three adenosine receptors (A_1–A_3) have been identified.

  (2) All of them are metabotropic receptors.

  (3) Identification of their function in the CNS is an active area of research at present.

j. Opioid receptors

  (1) Three major classes of opioid receptors have been identified in the CNS: mu (μ), delta (δ), and kappa (κ) receptors.

  (2) Morphine and endogenous opioid peptides produce their supraspinal analgesic (pain-relieving) effect via μ-receptors.

  (3) Endomorphin-1 and endomorphin-2 are endogenous μ opiate receptor ligands. Naloxone blocks the effect of these peptides.

  (4) A new opiate receptor, called ORL_1 receptor, has been identified. Its endogenous ligand is nociceptin. Naloxone does not block this receptor.

MAJOR CLASSES OF NEUROTRANSMITTERS

Small molecule neurotransmitters:
  Acetylcholine
  Excitatory amino acids: glutamate, aspartate
  Inhibitory amino acids: γ-aminobutyric acid (GABA), glycine
  Biogenic amines:
    Catecholamines: dopamine, norepinephrine, epinephrine
    Indoleamine: serotonin (5-hydroxytryptamine)
    Imidazoleamine: histamine
  Purines (ATP, adenosine)
Neuropeptides
  Opioid peptides: β-endorphin, methionine enkephalin, leucine-enkephalin, endomorphins, nociceptin
  Substance P
Gaseous neurotransmitters: nitric oxide

ISOFORMS OF NITRIC OXIDE SYNTHASE (NOS)

Property	Isoform I	Isoform II	Isoform III
Name	cNOS or nNOS	iNOS	eNOS
Expression	Constitutive	Inducible by cytokines	Constitutive
Calcium dependence	Yes	No	Yes
Tissue	Neurons, epithelial cells	Macrophages smooth muscle cells	Endothelial cells

IONOTROPIC AND METABOTROPIC RECEPTORS FOR DIFFERENT NEUROTRANSMITTERS		
Neurotransmitter	**Ionotropic Receptor**	**Metabotropic Receptor**
Acetylcholine	Cholinergic nicotinic	Cholinergic muscarinic
Glutamate	NMDA, AMPA, Kainate	$mGlu_1$–$mGlu_8$
GABA	$GABA_A$	$GABA_B$
Glycine	Strychnine-sensitive glycine receptor	—
Dopamine	—	D_1–D_5
Norepinephrine	—	α and β adrenergic receptors
Epinephrine	—	α and β adrenergic receptors
Serotonin	$5\text{-}HT_3$	$5\text{-}HT_1$–$5\text{-}HT_2$, $5\text{-}HT_4$–$5\text{-}HT_7$
Histamine	—	H_1, H_2, H_3
Adenosine	—	A_1–A_3
Opioid peptides	—	μ, δ, κ ORL_1

SPINAL CORD

Major ascending tracts of the spinal cord and their functions include (see questions relating to pathways of spinal cord and related diagram in section entitled "The Spinal Cord"):

Dorsal columns. Mediates conscious proprioception, two-point discrimination, and some tactile sensation ipsilaterally to the dorsal column nuclei and then contralaterally from the dorsal column nuclei to the postcentral gyrus from the VPL of the thalamus.

Lateral spinothalamic tract. Mediates pain and temperature inputs contralaterally to the VPL and posterior complex of the thalamic nuclei and then to the postcentral gyrus.

Anterior spinothalamic tract. Mediates tactile impulses contralaterally to the VPL and then to the postcentral gyrus.

Posterior spinocerebellar tract. Mediates unconscious proprioception from muscle spindles and Golgi tendon organs of the lower limbs through the inferior cerebellar peduncle ipsilaterally to the anterior lobe of the cerebellar cortex.

Cuneocerebellar tract.   Mediates unconscious proprioception from muscle spindles and Golgi tendon organs of the upper limbs from the accessory cuneate nucleus through the inferior cerebellar peduncle to the anterior lobe of the cerebellar cortex.

Anterior spinocerebellar tract.   Mediates unconscious proprioception from the Golgi tendon organs of the lower limbs bilaterally to the anterior lobe of the cerebellar cortex. This tract initially crosses in the spinal cord and then crosses again through the superior cerebellar peduncle.

Major descending tracts of the spinal cord and their functions include:

Lateral corticospinal tract.   Mediates voluntary control of motor functions from the contralateral cerebral cortex to all levels of the spinal cord.

Rubrospinal tracts.   Mediates descending excitation of flexor motor neurons at both the cervical and the lumbar levels of the contralateral spinal cord.

Reticulospinal tracts.   The lateral reticulospinal tract arises from the medulla and descends bilaterally to the cervical and lumbar levels of the spinal cord, mediating inhibition upon the spinal reflexes, mainly of extensors; the medial reticulospinal tract arises from the pons and descends mainly ipsilaterally to the cervical and lumbar levels of the spinal cord and facilitates extensor reflexes.

Vestibulospinal tracts.   The lateral vestibulospinal tract arises from the lateral vestibular nucleus and descends ipsilaterally to the cervical and lumbar levels of the spinal cord, mediating powerful excitation of the extensor motor neurons; the medial vestibulospinal tract arises from the medial vestibular nucleus and descends mainly to the cervical levels of the spinal cord, mediating postural reflexes of the head and neck.

Major disorders of the spinal cord include:

Brown-Séquard's syndrome.   Hemisection of the spinal cord often due to a bullet or knife wound—contralateral loss of pain and temperature below the level of the lesion; bilateral segmental loss of pain and temperature at the level of the lesion; ipsilateral loss of conscious proprioception below the level of the lesion; ipsilateral upper motor neuron (UMN) paralysis below the level of the lesion; ipsilateral lower motor neuron (LMN) paralysis at the level of the lesion.

Tabes dorsalis.   Damage to the dorsal root ganglion and dorsal columns resulting from syphilis—ipsilateral loss of conscious proprioception and tendon reflexes.

Amyotrophic lateral sclerosis (ALS).   A disease whose etiology is not yet known that destroys both corticospinal fibers and ventral horn cells, causing abnormal reflexes, muscle weakness, atrophy, and ultimately death.

Syringomyelia.   Caused by abnormal closure of the central canal during development, by trauma, or by a tumor, the result of which is an enlargement of the central canal, causing a segmental bilateral loss of pain and temperature due to damage to the decussating spinothalamic fibers.

Combined systems disease.   Results from pernicious anemia associated with a deficiency in vitamin B_{12}; there is degeneration of both the dorsal columns and the corticospinal tracts, resulting in a loss of conscious proprioception, position sense, UMN symptoms, and muscle weakness.

AUTONOMIC NERVOUS SYSTEM

The sympathetic nervous system arises from the thoracic and lumbar cords (T1–L2), and the parasympathetic nervous system arises from S2–S4 and cranial nerves III, VII, IX, and X. All preganglionic neurons are cholinergic as well as parasympathetic postganglionic neurons. In addition, sympathetic postganglionic innervation of sweat glands and blood vessels in skeletal muscle is also cholinergic. Most other postganglionic sympathetic endings are adrenergic. Examples of functions of the sympathetic nervous system include pupillary dilation, acceleration of heart rate, constriction of blood vessels of the trunk and extremities, and inhibition of gastric motility. Examples of functions of the parasympathetic nervous system include pupillary constriction, decrease in heart rate, secretion of the salivary and lacrimal glands, and stimulation of gastric motility.

  I. Divisions of the autonomic nervous system
    A. Sympathetic division: The neurons from which the outflow of the sympathetic division originates (preganglionic neurons) are located in the intermediolateral cell column of the first thoracic to second lumbar (T1–L2) spinal cord. This division of the autonomic nervous system is activated in stressful situations, and the individual is prepared for fight or flight.
    B. Parasympathetic division: Parasympathetic preganglionic neurons are located in the brainstem (Edinger-Westphal nucleus, superior salivatory nucleus of the facial nerve, inferior salivatory nucleus, nucleus ambiguus, and dorsal motor nucleus of vagus) and the sacral region of the spinal cord (second, third, and fourth segments). Activation of this division of the autonomic nervous system results in conservation and restoration of body energy.
    C. Enteric nervous system: This consists of two layers of neurons that are present in the smooth muscle of the gut: the myenteric (Auerbach's) and submucosal (Meissner's) plexuses. The neurons of the myenteric (Auerbach's) plexus control gastrointestinal motility, while

the neurons of the submucosal (Meissner's) plexus control water and ion movement across the intestinal epithelium.

II. Autonomic innervation of different organs

   A. Eye

     1. Iris and ciliary body: The iris and the circumferential muscles of the ciliary body receive parasympathetic innervation from the preganglionic parasympathetic neurons located in the Edinger-Westphal nucleus via the oculomotor nerve (cranial nerve III) and the ciliary ganglion. Activation of the parasympathetic innervation to the eye results in contraction of circular muscles of the iris, causing constriction of the pupil (miosis) and contraction of circumferential muscles of the ciliary body, causing the relaxation of the suspensory ligaments of the lens and making it more suitable for near vision. The preganglionic neurons providing sympathetic innervation to the radial smooth muscle fibers of the iris are located in the intermediolateral column at the T1 level. Activation of the sympathetic nervous system results in contraction of the radial muscles of the iris, which brings about pupillary dilatation (mydriasis).

     2. Upper eyelid. The tarsal muscle (a small portion of the levator palpebrae superioris muscle) and the orbital muscle of Müller receive sympathetic innervation from the preganglionic sympathetic neurons from the intermediolateral cell column at the T1 level via the superior cervical ganglion. Interruption of the sympathetic innervation to the tarsal muscle results in pseudoptosis (partial drooping of the upper eyelid), and damage to the orbital muscle of Müller results in enophthalmos (sinking of eyeball). These symptoms are characteristic of Horner's syndrome.

   B. Salivary glands

     1. Sublingual and submandibular glands: These glands receive parasympathetic innervation from the superior salivatory nucleus via the chorda tympani branch of the facial nerve and the submandibular ganglion. Activation of these parasympathetic fibers (secretomotor fibers) results in the secretion of watery saliva. They receive sympathetic innervation from preganglionic sympathetic neurons located in the T1 level of the intermediolateral cell column via the superior cervical ganglion. Activation of the sympathetic innervation to these glands produces viscous salivary secretions.

     2. Parotid glands: These receive parasympathetic innervation from the inferior salivatory nucleus via the lesser petrosal branch of the

glossopharyngeal nerve and the otic ganglion. Activation of these fibers results in secretion of watery saliva from the parotid gland into the oral cavity. Sympathetic innervation to these glands is similar to that for the sublingual and submandibular glands. Activation of the sympathetic nervous system produces viscous saliva.

3. Lacrimal glands: These receive parasympathetic innervation from the superior salivatory nucleus (lacrimal nucleus) via the greater petrosal branch of the facial nerve and the pterygopalatine ganglion. Activation of these postganglionic parasympathetic fibers results in secretion of tears. Sympathetic innervation to these glands is the same as that described for the sublingual and submandibular glands.

C. Heart: The heart receives parasympathetic innervation from the preganglionic neurons located in the dorsal motor nucleus of the vagus and a region surrounding the compact zone of the nucleus ambiguus via the vagus nerve. The preganglionic sympathetic neurons innervating the heart are located in the intermediolateral cell column (IML) at T1–T3 spinal segments.

D. Blood vessels: Arterioles in most of the organs do not receive parasympathetic innervation. The preganglionic sympathetic neurons innervating the blood vessels are located in the thoracolumbar cord.

E. Lungs: The preganglionic parasympathetic neurons innervating the lungs are located in the dorsal motor nucleus of the vagus, and their axons travel to the thoracic cavity in the vagus nerves. The preganglionic sympathetic neurons innervating the lungs are located in the intermediolateral cell column at T2–T4 level.

F. Kidney: The preganglionic parasympathetic fibers descending in the vagus nerves enter the kidney along the renal artery. The preganglionic sympathetic neurons innervating the kidneys are located in the IML at the T7–T11 level.

G. Adrenal medulla: The adrenal medulla is functionally analogous to a sympathetic ganglion; the adrenal medullary cells are directly innervated by the sympathetic preganglionic neurons, which are located in the intermediolateral column at the T7–T11 level.

H. Gastrointestinal tract (GIT)

1. Stomach, small intestine, and proximal part of large intestine: The preganglionic neurons providing parasympathetic innervation to these organs are located in the dorsal motor nucleus of the vagus. These preganglionic fibers descend in the vagus nerves and synapse on postganglionic neurons located in the myenteric (Auer-

bach's) and submucosal (Meissner's) plexuses. The sympathetic preganglionic neurons innervating these regions of the GIT are located in the intermediolateral cell column at the T5–T11 level.

2. Descending colon and rectum, parasympathetic innervation: The preganglionic parasympathetic neurons innervating these regions of the GIT are located in the intermediolateral column of the sacral spinal cord at the S2–S4 level. The sympathetic preganglionic neurons innervating this region of the GIT are located in the intermediolateral cell column at the L1–L2 level.

I. Urinary bladder: The preganglionic parasympathetic neurons innervating the bladder are located in the intermediolateral column of the sacral spinal cord at the S2–S4 level. Their axons travel via the pelvic nerves, and synapse on postganglionic neurons located in the pelvic plexus and in the wall of the urinary bladder. The sympathetic preganglionic neurons innervating the urinary bladder are located in the intermediolateral column at the T11–L2 level. The preganglionic sympathetic fibers reach the urinary bladder through the hypogastric plexuses.

1. Role of the sphincter vesicae in ejaculation: The sympathetic nerves innervating the sphincter located at the bladder neck (sphincter vesicae) play an important role during ejaculation in the male. Sympathetic activation contracts the sphincter located at the bladder neck during ejaculation and prevents seminal fluid from entering the bladder.

2. Somatic innervation: The external urethral sphincter is innervated by alpha motor neurons located in the ventral horn in the sacral segments S2–S4 (Onuf's nucleus).

3. Micturition: Urination results from activation of sacral parasympathetic neurons innervating the bladder and temporary inhibition of alpha motor neurons innervating the external urethral sphincter.

J. Male reproductive system: The preganglionic parasympathetic neurons innervating the erectile tissue in the penis are located in the IML at the S2–S4 level. Activation of the parasympathetic nervous system results in the dilation of the arteries in the erectile tissue, causing erection of the penis. The preganglionic sympathetic neurons innervating the vas deferens, seminal vesicles, and prostate glands are located in the IML at the L1–L2 level. Activation of the sympathetic nervous system causes ejaculation of the spermatozoa along with the secretions of the prostate and the seminal vesicles.

K. Female reproductive system: The innervation and the mechanism of vasodilation in the erectile tissue of the clitoris are similar to those described for the penis. The location of the preganglionic parasympathetic neurons and the pathways they follow to innervate the uterus are similar to those described for the penis. Parasympathetic stimulation causes relaxation of the uterine smooth muscle. The preganglionic sympathetic neurons innervating the smooth muscle of the uterine wall are located in the IML at the T12–L1 level. Activation of the sympathetic nervous system results in contraction of the uterus.

III. Neurotransmitters in the autonomic nervous system

A. Preganglionic terminals: Within the autonomic ganglia, acetylcholine is the transmitter released at the terminals of the sympathetic as well as the parasympathetic preganglionic fibers.

B. Postganglionic terminals: At the terminals of most sympathetic postganglionic neurons, norepinephrine is the transmitter liberated, with the exception of those innervating sweat glands and blood vessels of the skeletal muscles, where acetylcholine is the neurotransmitter. At the terminals of all the parasympathetic postganglionic neurons, acetylcholine is the neurotransmitter liberated.

IV. Receptors

A. Cholinergic receptors

1. Muscarinic receptors: Cholinergic receptors located in the visceral effector organ cells (smooth and cardiac muscle and exocrine glands) are called *muscarinic cholinergic receptors.*

2. Nicotinic receptors: Cholinergic receptors located in the adrenal medulla and autonomic ganglia are called *nicotinic receptors.*

B. Adrenergic receptors: At the present time, adrenergic receptors are divided into two major classes: α and β. These classes have been further subdivided into α_1 and α_2 and β_1 and β_2.

V. Other autonomic functions

A. Cardiovascular regulatory mechanisms in the CNS

1. Solitary nucleus (nTS): Baroreceptor afferent fibers (sensing blood pressure changes) and chemoreceptor fibers (sensing changes in blood gases and pH) arising from the carotid sinus make their first synapse in the middle and caudal regions of the nTS.

2. Caudal ventrolateral medullary depressor area (CVLM): These neurons are located in the ventrolateral medulla and send GABAergic projections to a pressor region (RVLM) located rostral to it.

3. Rostral ventrolateral medullary pressor area (RVLM): The RVLM is located caudal to the facial nucleus. It is believed to be one of the most important sources of vasomotor tone. RVLM neurons send monosynaptic projections to the IML.

4. Intermediolateral cell column of the spinal cord (IML): Sympathetic preganglionic neurons are located in the IML.

5. Baroreceptor reflex: The responses to stimulation of baroreceptors are hypotension and bradycardia. Activation of baroreceptors results in excitation of neurons located in the nTS and CVLM via excitatory amino acid receptors. Activation of CVLM neurons results in the release of GABA in the RVLM. Inhibition of RVLM neurons results in a decrease in the excitatory input to the sympathetic preganglionic neurons in the IML. Consequently, blood pressure and heart rate are decreased.

B. Respiratory regulatory mechanisms in the CNS

1. The ventral respiratory group (VRG)
   a. The caudal part (called the cVRG) contains mostly expiratory neurons.
   b. The part immediately rostral to the cVRG (called the rVRG) contains mostly inspiratory neurons. The neurons located rostral to the rVRG (called the Botzinger complex) are mostly expiratory.
   c. An area just caudal to the Botzinger complex, termed the pre-Botzinger complex, has been implicated as the site of respiratory rhythm generation.
   d. The phrenic motor nucleus (PMN), located in the ventral horn of the cervical spinal cord (C3–C5 level), innervates the diaphragm.

2. The dorsal respiratory group (DRG): These respiratory neurons are located in the ventrolateral nucleus of the solitary tract. The pneumotaxic center, located in the dorsolateral pontine tegmentum, is considered to be essential for maintaining a normal breathing pattern.

VI. Selected disorders of the autonomic nervous system

A. Horner's syndrome: This is characterized by drooping of the upper eyelid (ptosis), constriction of the pupil (miosis), enophthalmos (sinking of the eyeball in the orbit), dilation of arterioles of the skin, and anhydrosis (loss of sweating) at the face. It is caused by lesions of the brainstem and upper cervical cord, which interrupt the sympathetic fibers in the reticulospinal tract and fibers descending from the hypothalamus to the IML. Such lesions are also encountered in multiple sclerosis.

B. Argyll Robertson pupil: This condition occurs in syphilitic patients with CNS complications. In brief, the chief symptoms are that the pupils do not contract in response to light but do show constriction as part of the accommodation reflex.

C. Hirschsprung's disease (megacolon): This is characterized by absence of peristalsis in the distal colon, and, consequently, the proximal part of the colon distends (megacolon), which is prone to impaction of feces.

D. Frey's syndrome: In this condition, the parasympathetic fibers eliciting secretory responses in parotid glands grow erroneously into the facial skin overlying these glands. Therefore, stimulation of the parasympathetic nervous system elicits sweating of this facial region.

THE BRAINSTEM AND CRANIAL NERVES

Lateral medullary syndrome (Wallenberg's syndrome).   Lesions of the lateral aspect of the lower half of the brainstem, due to occlusion of the inferior cerebellar arteries, produce loss of pain and temperature on the same side of the face and opposite side of the body, as well as Horner's syndrome (i.e., myosis, ptosis, and decreased sweating on one side of the face due to disruption of the sympathetic supply to the orbit and pupil, or, as applies in the present context, to disruption of descending sympathetic fibers through the brainstem to the spinal cord).

Medial medullary syndrome.   Lesions of the medial aspect of the medulla typically resulting from occlusion of the anterior spinal artery produce contralateral loss of conscious proprioception, contralateral hemiparesis, and weakness of tongue muscles, which are protruded to the side of the lesion. Body paralysis, which involves the side contralateral to the lesion, coupled with cranial nerve weakness, which involves the side ipsilateral to the lesion, is called *alternating hypoglossal hemiplegia.*

Cranial nerves mediate multiple functions in the nervous system: motor nuclei—general somatic efferent (CN III, CN IV, CN VI, and CN XII), special visceral efferent (CN V, CN VII, CN IX, CN X, and CN XI), general visceral efferent (CN III, CN VII, CN IX, and CN X), general somatic afferent (CN V, CN IX, and CN X), special sensory afferent (CN II and CN VIII), or special visceral afferent (CN I, CN VII, CN IX, and CN X).

A COMPARISON BETWEEN SYMPATHETIC AND PARASYMPATHETIC DIVISIONS OF THE AUTONOMIC NERVOUS SYSTEM

	Parasympathetic	Sympathetic
Preganglionic neurons: location	(Target organ is shown in parentheses.) Nucleus of oculomotor nerve (pupil); superior salivatory nucleus of facial nerve, inferior salivatory nucleus of glossopharyngeal nerve (salivary glands); facial nerve (lacrimal glands); dorsal motor nucleus of vagus (GIT, kidney); nucleus ambiguus (heart); intermediolateral cell column of the sacral spinal cord at S2–S4 level.	Intermediolateral cell column of the spinal cord (T1–L2).
Outflow	Cranial nerves III, VII, IX, X; pelvic splanchnic nerves.	Ventral roots at T1–L2.
Preganglionic fibers	Myelinated. The preganglionic fibers are relatively long because the ganglia receiving them are located within the target organ or close to it.	Myelinated. The preganglionic fibers are relatively short because the ganglia receiving them are located at some distance from the target organ.
Transmitter at their terminals (within ganglia)	Acetylcholine.	Acetylcholine.
Ganglia	Ganglia located close to the organs (ciliary, otic); ganglia located within the organs (heart, bronchial tree, GIT).	Paravertebral ganglia in sympathetic chain (22 pairs); prevertebral ganglia (celiac, renal, superior and inferior mesenteric).
Postganglionic fibers	Short, nonmyelinated.	Long, nonmyelinated.
Transmitter at the terminals of post-ganglionic fibers	Acetylcholine.	Norepinephrine (acetylcholine in sweat glands).

(continued)

SENSORY SYSTEMS

Loss of partial or total aspects of the visual field can be understood in terms of damage to the retinal pathways, including their targets in the lateral geniculate nucleus and visual cortex. The schematic diagram shown here depicts the kinds of field deficits that occur following lesions of different aspects of the visual pathway. Key: (A) optic nerve lesion producing total blindness in the left eye; (B) lesion that disrupts the right retinal nasal fibers that project from the base of the left optic nerve, producing right upper quadrantanopia and left scotoma; (C) lesion of optic chiasm, producing bitemporal hemianopsia; (D) unilateral (left) optic tract lesion, producing a right homonymous hemianopsia; (E) interruption of left visual radiations that pass ventrally through the temporal lobe to the lower bank of the visual cortex (i.e., the loop of Meyer), producing an upper right quadrantanopia; (F) interruption of left visual radiations that pass more dorsally through the occipital lobe to the upper bank of the visual cortex, producing a lower right quadrantanopia; and (G) lesion of the left visual cortex, producing a right homonymous hemianopsia.

The principles of an excitatory focus-and-surround inhibition, as well as those of a somatotropic organization, are present within a given receptor system and form the functional basis for discriminative functions in a number of the sensory systems, including the auditory circuit. The auditory pathways are complex and involve the following synaptic connections: first-order root fibers of the spiral ganglion, which originate in the cochlea (organ of Corti), synapse in the cochlear nuclei of the upper medulla; second-order neurons, which project through lateral lemnisci, terminate bilaterally in the inferior colliculus; third-order neurons project to the medial geniculate nucleus; and fourth-order neurons project to the superior temporal gyrus (primary auditory cortex).

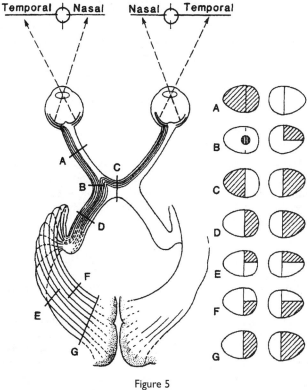

Figure 5
(With permission of Adams et al.)

Vestibular pathway.   First-order neurons originate from vestibular ganglia and have peripheral processes located in specialized receptors in the utricle, saccule, and semicircular canals. The central branches of this neuron reach the brain and terminate in the vestibular nuclei. Second-order neurons may pass to the cerebellar cortex (flocculonodular lobe) or project directly into the medial longitudinal fasciculus, where the fibers may run in a rostral or a caudal direction, terminating in the CN III, CN IV, or CN VI of the midbrain and pons or spinal cord, respectively. Damage to these fibers, especially within the medial longitudinal fasciculus or cerebellum, produces nystagmus (i.e., involuntary movement of the eyes, in the horizontal or vertical plane, first slowly and then followed by a rapid, jerking return).

MOTOR SYSTEMS

Voluntary motor control affecting mainly the flexor system is expressed through the descending pyramidal tracts plus the rubrospinal tract, and control of functions associated with posture is mediated through such descending pathways as the vestibulo- and reticulospinal tracts. Modulation of motor functions is mediated by the basal ganglia and cerebellum. Involuntary motor disturbances at rest (called *dyskinesias*) are associated with the disruption of functions of the basal ganglia, and motor disturbances occurring during attempts at movement are frequently associated with damage to the cerebellum or its afferent or efferent pathways.

I. The basal ganglia consist of the neostriatum (caudate nucleus and putamen), the paleostriatum (globus pallidus), and two additional structures that are anatomically and functionally related to the basal ganglia—the substantia nigra and subthalamic nucleus.

   A. Disorders of the basal ganglia

      1. Parkinson's disease: characterized by "pill rolling" tremor, akinesia (poverty of movement), and rigidity. This disorder is due to a reduction in striatal dopamine following a loss of dopamine neurons in the pars compacta of the substantia nigra, which project to the neostriatum.

      2. Chorea: characterized by short, jerky movements of the distal extremities at rest. It is associated with lesions of the striatum. One form of chorea, called *Huntington's chorea,* is a genetic disorder that is associated with a chromosomal mutation. It results in destruction of GABAergic and cholinergic neurons in the caudate nucleus, and there is concomitant loss of neurons in the prefrontal regions of the neocortex.

      3. Athetosis: characterized by slow, writhing movements of the extremities and muscles of the neck. The lesion may involve the striatum.

      4. Hemiballism: characterized by wild (flailing) movements of the limbs on one side of the body. It is due to damage of the subthalamic nucleus on the contralateral side.

   B. Disorders of the cerebellum

      1. Anterior lobe (paleocerebellum): characterized by a wide, staggering gait ataxia resulting primarily from damage that affects the vermal and paravermal regions of the anterior lobe.

      2. Posterior lobe (neocerebellum): characterized most frequently by loss of coordination while executing voluntary movements.

3. Flocculonodular lobe (archicerebellum): characterized by a loss of equilibrium with the patient displaying a wide, staggering ataxic gait. Lesions of this region also produce eye movement disorders, including nystagmus.

HIGHER AUTONOMIC AND BEHAVIORAL FUNCTIONS

Control of autonomic and endocrine functions as well as emotional behavior are mediated by the limbic system, hypothalamus, and midbrain periaqueductal gray matter. Interrelationships among these three groups of structures are as follows:

1. For the expression of emotional behavior, such as rage and autonomic functions, these are mediated from the medial hypothalamus → midbrain periaqueductal gray → autonomic (i.e., neurons in lower medulla that regulate heart rate, blood pressure, and respiration) and somatomotor neurons (i.e., neurons of the trigeminal nerve that control vocalization) and autonomic and somatomotor neurons of the spinal cord. These processes are further regulated by different groups of neurons within the limbic system (i.e., hippocampal formation, amygdala, septal area), which produce their effects by projecting directly or indirectly to the hypothalamus or midbrain periaqueductal gray.

2. For the regulation of endocrine functions, these are mediated from the supraoptic and paraventricular nuclei of the hypothalamus → posterior lobe of the pituitary, and from the medial hypothalamus → anterior lobe of the pituitary (via the vascular system). Limbic projections to the hypothalamus enable structures such as the hippocampal formation, amygdala, and septal area to modulate endocrine functions of the hypothalamus. Disruption of hypothalamic neurons may alter the mechanism for the expression of rage behavior and, likewise, affect temperature regulation, sexual behavior, feeding, drinking, and endocrine functions. Damage to neurons of the limbic system frequently leads to temporal lobe epilepsy and changes in the threshold for the expression of rage behavior (i.e., when different groups of neurons in the amygdala are damaged, heightened aggressiveness or a reduction in aggression, such as the Klüver-Bucy syndrome, may ensue). Damage to the hippocampal formation can result in temporal lobe epilepsy and short-term memory deficits.

CEREBRAL CORTEX

Dysfunctions associated with cerebrovascular accidents and tumors can be understood in terms of the principles of cortical localization and cerebral dominance. Following is a list of common disorders, their descriptions, and the cortical regions most closely associated with each disorder.

Upper motor neuron paralysis.   Damage to the precentral, premotor, and supplementary motor areas (as well as the internal capsule, crus cerebri, or corticospinal tracts), resulting in a loss of voluntary control of the upper and lower limbs, depending upon the extent of the lesion. This disorder is also associated with hyperreflexia, hypertonicity, and a positive Babinski's sign.

Broca's aphasia.   Damage to the inferior frontal gyrus of the dominant hemisphere. The patient cannot name simple objects but has no difficulty in comprehending spoken language.

Wernicke's aphasia.   Damage to the region of the superior temporal gyrus and/or adjoining regions. The patient has difficulty in comprehending language, but speech appears fluent.

Astereognosia.   Damage to the parietal cortex of the contralateral side results in a failure of tactile recognition of objects (e.g., a blackboard eraser, a pack of cigarettes).

Unilateral sensory neglect.   Damage to the parietal lobe (usually of the right hemisphere) can cause this disorder. The patient typically ignores stimuli on the opposite (i.e., left) side of body space, which includes visual, somatosensory, and auditory stimuli. The individual will neglect the opposite side of the body by, for example, neglecting to shave that side of the face and by denying that there is anything wrong with that side of the body, which may include a motor paralysis. The patient may further draw a picture of flowers or of a clock in which the petals on the flowers or the numbers on the clock are limited to the right side of each of the figures.

Apraxia.   Damage to the posterior parietal cortex can prevent an individual from conceptualizing the sequence of events necessary to carry out a task, even though the basic sensory and motor pathways necessary to produce the required movements are intact. In effect, the patient is thus unable to carry out the task.

Gross Anatomy of the Brain

Questions

DIRECTIONS: Each group of questions below consists of lettered options. For each question, select the one lettered option with which it is **most** closely associated. Each lettered option may be used once, more than once, or not at all.

Questions 1–7

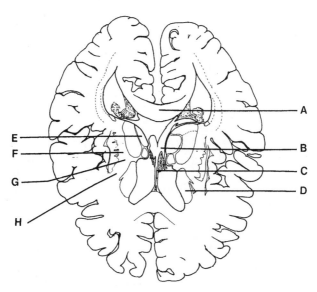

1. Jane was admitted to the emergency room after she was found unconscious by a family member. The 65-year-old woman was diagnosed as having had a cerebrovascular accident. A few days later, she regained consciousness but was unable to move her right leg. An MRI revealed evidence of some brain damage. Select the lettered option on the illustration that most closely corresponds to the affected region.

2. Upon neurological testing, a 55-year-old male who had recovered from a stroke was unable to make smooth, purposeful movements involving mainly his left arm. The movements were jerky and lacked coordination. Select the lettered option on the illustration that most closely corresponds to the affected region. (H

3. A patient admitted to a local hospital presented with difficulties in swallowing, chewing, breathing, and speaking. Further examination revealed significant weakness of the muscles that mediate these functions. Select the lettered option on the illustration that most closely corresponds to the affected region. G

4. A 25-year-old man was involved in a serious automobile accident that resulted in a major head injury. One week following the accident, the patient exhibited significant short-term memory deficit as well as heightened irritibility and aggressiveness. Identify the structure on the illustration that is most closely associated with the affected region. b

5. A 42-year-old woman was diagnosed as having a movement disorder. Further examination suggested that she was suffering from Huntington's disease. Identify the structure on the illustration that is most likely associated with this disorder. D

6. The rostral aspect of the frontal lobe, including the prefrontal cortex, plays a major role in higher-order cognitive functions, and damage to this region of the cortex produces major intellectual impairment. Identify the structure on the illustration that serves as a major afferent source to the frontal region of the cortex. E

7. A 68-year-old man presented with a tremor at rest, slowness of voluntary movement, and upon further examination, increased resistance to passive movement of the limbs. This disorder is associated with a loss of dopamine to a specific region of the forebrain. Identify this region on the illustration.

Questions 8–15

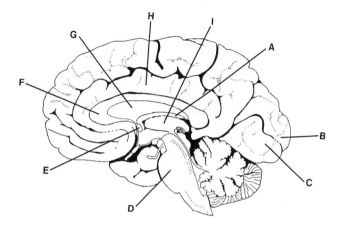

8. A 38-year-old male reported a loss of the ability to smell. Further examination revealed that this patient was suffering from a peripheral neuropathy of the olfactory nerve. Which of the structures shown in the illustration would be most affected in terms of loss of neural transmission?

9. A 67-year-old female was admitted to a hospital after she reported to her primary care physician that she had been having very painful headaches. Further examination revealed the presence of significant increases in intracranial pressure. After viewing an MRI, the neurologist concluded that the woman's condition was due to the presence of a developing tumor along the rostral aspect of the medial wall of the lateral ventricle. Which of the structures in the illustration would be most likely to contain this tumor?

10. A 47-year-old male who had a reputation as a very friendly and quiet individual suddenly displayed marked changes in his personality. In particular, he became short-tempered, impulsive, and threatening to his colleagues in response to what most people would consider innocuous statements. He was referred to the psychiatric ward of the community hospital, and an MRI revealed a cortical tumor. Which of the structures in the illustration is most likely to contain this tumor?

11. An 83-year-old woman was brought to the hospital after having received a routine eye examination, which revealed that she could not see out of the lower half of her left visual field. An MRI revealed evidence that she had experienced a cerebrovascular accident. Which of the regions in the illustration was most likely affected by the stroke?

12. An investigator wishes to determine the effects of stimulation of the output neurons of the hippocampal formation upon excitability levels of the target neurons in the diencephalon. In which of the structures shown in the illustration should he place the stimulating electrode?

13. A 69-year-old woman was admitted to the hospital after being diagnosed with a stroke. After a few days, she presented with difficulty in performing voluntary movements, she lacked coordination, and her movements were clearly jerky in appearance. Which location on the illustration is the most likely locus of the lesion?

14. An elderly man complained of having some difficulty seeing. An ophthalmological examination revealed that he had an upper quadrantanopia. Which location on the illustration is the most likely locus of the lesion?

15. A 48-year-old man had been suffering from epilepsy for a number of years. Drug treatment for this disorder had not been successful and, moreover, in recent months, seizure activity had begun to spread to other regions of the brain, including the opposite side of the brain. For this condition, surgery was indicated in order to reduce the spread of the seizures. Which of the structures on the illustration would most likely be targeted by the neurosurgeon?

Questions 16–24

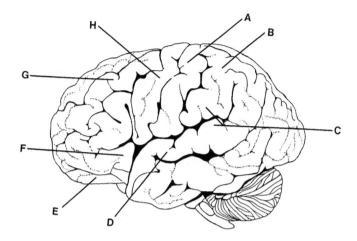

16. A patient brought into surgery for localization of a brain tumor was given an MRI and asked to move the fingers of his right hand. Which is the most likely site on the illustration where the MRI would display a population response of neuronal activation?

17. A patient presented with loss of capacity to experience the feeling of a tuning fork when applied to the right leg. Which region on the illustration is most likely to be affected by a cortical lesion?

18. A patient experienced great difficulty in appreciating the meaning of spoken or written words. Which place on the illustration is the most likely locus of a lesion that would cause such a deficit?

19. After having received a head injury, a 23-year-old male complained of a partial loss of hearing. An MRI revealed evidence of brain injury. Which place on the illustration is the most likely locus of such damage?

20. An elderly patient who had been diagnosed with a brain tumor found that he was unable to verbally express his thoughts in a meaningful way. Which place on the illustration is the most likely location of such a lesion?

21. Following an automobile accident in which a 23-year-old male received severe injuries to his head and parts of his body, he was admitted to the emergency room and then transferred to a rehabilitation center. Approximately a week after the accident, the patient became quite irritable and scored poorly on card sorting, delayed alternation, and measures of intellectual skills. Which region of the brain in the illustration was most clearly affected by the accident and whose injury could most readily account for these deficits?

22. A patient was unable to voluntarily move his eyes to the right. An MRI revealed a small tumor located in the cerebral cortex. Which region of the illustration is the most likely location of this tumor?

23. A 66-year-old male suffered a stroke that produced the following deficits: negligence of the opposite body half and visual space and contralateral paralysis of the upper limb. Which of the regions on the illustration is most closely associated with the deficit producing contralateral negligence?

24. In the case of the aforementioned individual, damage to which of the regions on the illustration is the cause of the contralateral limb paralysis?

Questions 25–35

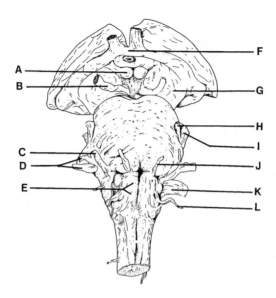

25. A 48-year-old woman complained of stomach pains. The diagnosis revealed an ulceration of the stomach wall due to overactivity of the parasympathetic input to the stomach. It was recommended that the patient have the cranial nerve partially severed, which innervates the stomach wall. On the illustration, identify the cranial nerve in question.

26. An MRI administered to a patient revealed the presence of a tumor situated in the region of the cerebellopontine angle. The patient noted considerable weakness when attempting to bite. On the illustration identify the affected cranial nerve.

27. Damage to which region(s) shown in the illustration will likely affect the integrity of the Papez circuit, causing disruption of memory and emotional processes?

28. A 28-year-old man was exposed to very cold temperatures for several days and noted sometime afterward that he was unable to smile and display other aspects of facial expression. On the illustration identify the affected cranial nerve.

29. A 78-year-old woman was admitted to a local hospital after finding that she was unable to move her right arm and leg. In addition, she displayed diminution in strength of chewing, facial expression, and speech. An MRI revealed the presence of a tumor situated in the brainstem. Which structures shown on the illustration would most likely be affected by the tumor?

30. A 63-year-old man was admitted to the emergency room and received an MRI, which indicated the presence of a vascular occlusion of a part of the brainstem. The patient was unable to feel any sensation on the left side of his face, chin, and forehead. Which of the cranial nerves shown on the illustration was most closely affected by the stroke?

31. A 30-year-old man complained that he was having difficulty seeing properly and, in particular, was experiencing double vision. The ophthalamologist noted that the patient's right eye was normally abducted downward and the pupil was dilated. A subsequent MRI indicated the presence of a tumor impinging upon a cranial nerve. On the illustration, identify the affected cranial nerve.

32. A neurological examination was given to a 60-year-old female because she was experiencing double vision and was unable to abduct the left eye. The examination revealed the likely presence of a small lesion of the brainstem. Which of the cranial nerves shown on the illustration was affected by this lesion?

33. An individual complained about having headaches and experiencing partial blindness, which were later identified as a bitemporal hemianopsia. A neurological examination, including an MRI, indicated that the patient had a brain tumor. Which of the structures shown on the illustration is affected by the tumor?

34. A 43-year-old female experienced dizziness, loss of balance, some nystagmus, and ringing in the ear. A neurological exam suggested damage to a cranial nerve, perhaps associated with a small peripheral tumor. On the illustration, indicate the affected cranial nerve.

35. Following her admission to the emergency room of a local hospital, a 71-year-old female received a diagnosis of having had a small brainstem stroke. After two weeks, the patient appeared normal, with the exception that her tongue deviated to the left side when she was asked to protrude it. Which structures shown on the illustration was most clearly affected by the stroke?

DIRECTIONS: Each item below contains a question or incomplete statement followed by suggested responses. Select the **one best** response.

36. A young boy was admitted to the emergency room after having experienced severe nausea, headache, and fever. The neurologist concluded that he was suffering from a form of bacterial meningitis. His cerebrospinal fluid (CSF) would most likely indicate which of the following?

a. Increased protein, decreased glucose, decreased neutrophils
b. Increased protein, decreased glucose, increased neurophils
c. Increased protein, normal glucose, normal neutrophils
d. Decreased CSF pressure, decreased protein, decreased glucose
e. Decreased protein, normal CSF pressure, increased glucose

37. Following an automobile accident, a teenage boy was admitted to the emergency room and diagnosed as having a subarachnoid hemorrhage. Which of the following cerebrospinal fluid findings would be expected in this individual?

a. Increased CSF pressure, bloody appearance of CSF, increased red cells, increased protein, decreased glucose
b. Decreased CSF pressure, bloody appearance of CSF, decreased red cells, decreased protein, decreased glucose
c. Normal pressure, normal red cells, increased protein, increased glucose, normal color of CSF
d. Clear CSF, normal pressure, decreased protein, increased red cells, increased glucose
e. Cloudy CSF, increased CSF, increased neutrophils, normal protein, normal glucose

38. A 70-year-old male was brought to the emergency room after experiencing headaches, nausea, and dizziness. An MRI revealed the presence of a brain tumor, which had produced a noncommunicating hydrocephalus. Which of the following is the most likely location of the tumor?

a. White matter of the cerebral cortex
b. Medial thalamus
c. Interventricular foramen
d. Pontine cistern
e. Cisterna magna

39. Which of the following statements about the blood-brain barrier is correct?

a. It has well-developed capillary pores that allow for selective diffusion of substances
b. It is selectively permeable to certain compounds such as biogenic amines
c. It is found within all structures enclosed by the meninges, including the pineal gland
d. Tight junctions associated with the blood-brain barrier are formed exclusively by neuronal or glial processes
e. The blood-brain barrier is generally limited to highly vascular regions of the brain, such as those present at the level of the ventromedial hypothalamus

Gross Anatomy
of the Brain

Answers

1–7. The answers are 1-F, 2-H, 3-G, 4-B, 5-D, 6-E, 7-D. (*Nolte, pp 65–69, 375–390, 451–453, 513–524, 559–561, 565–582.*) This figure is a horizontal view of the brain at the level of the head of the caudate nucleus and the internal capsule. The posterior limb of the internal capsule (F) contains fibers that arise from the leg region of the cerebral cortex and project to lumbar levels of the spinal cord, thus serving as UMNs for the elicitation of voluntary movement of the contralateral leg. Fibers in the anterior limb of the internal capsule (H) project in large numbers to deep pontine nuclei and represent first-order neurons in a pathway linking the cerebral cortex with the cerebellum. These fibers comprise a part of the reciprocal feedback circuit linking the cerebellar and cerebral cortices. Disruption of a part of this circuit can result in the ability to produce smooth, coordinated, purposeful movements. Pseudobulbar palsy is characterized in part by a weakness of the muscles controlling swallowing, chewing, breathing, and speaking. It results from a lesion of the UMNs associated with the head region of the cortex, which pass through the genu of the internal capsule (G) en route to brainstem cranial nerve nuclei upon which they synapse. The descending column of the fornix (B), situated along the midline of the brain, contains fibers that arise from the hippocampal formation and project to the septal area and to the medial hypothalamus, including the mammillary bodies. This pathway plays an important role in the regulation of emotional behavior and short-term memory functions. Disruption of the hippocampal formation or its output pathway, the fornix, would affect levels of emotionality and short-term memory.

The head of the caudate nucleus (D) is part of an important element of the motor systems called the *basal ganglia*. It receives significant inputs from several regions associated with motor functions. These include the cerebral cortex and the dopamine-containing region of the substantia nigra (i.e., the pars compacta). Huntington's disease is associated with a loss of GABA levels within the neostriatum and, in particular, the caudate nucleus. The mediodorsal thalamic nucleus (E) projects large quantities of axons to extensive regions of the rostral half of the frontal lobe, including the pre-frontal cortex. It also receives significant projections from the prefrontal region of the cortex.

8–15. The answers are 8-E, 9-G, 10-H, 11-B, 12-A, 13-D, 14-C, 15-F.
(Afifi, pp 47–58, 422–424, 426–430, 476–477.) This figure is a midsagittal section of the brain. A major portion of the anterior commissure (E) contains fibers mediating olfactory signals that arise from the olfactory bulb and decussate to the contralateral olfactory bulb. The septum pellucidum (G) forms the medial wall of the lateral ventricle, which in fact separates the lateral ventricle on one side from that on the opposite side. The cingulate gyrus (H) is a prominent structure on the medial aspect of the cerebral cortex and constitutes a component of the limbic lobe. As part of the limbic system, its functions relate in part to the regulation of emotional behavior. Accordingly, tumors of this region have resulted in marked changes in emotionality. The primary visual cortex lies on both banks of the calcarine fissure. Cells located on the upper bank of this fissure (B) receive inputs from the lateral geniculate nucleus that relate to the lower visual field. Therefore, a lesion of this region would result in a lower visual field deficit.

The major output pathway of the hippocampal formation is the fornix system of fibers (A), which arises from cells in its subicular cortex and adjoining regions of the hippocampus. These fibers are then distributed to the anterior thalamic nucleus, mammillary bodies, and septal area. Accordingly, the most effective way of activating the output pathways of the hippocampal formation would be to stimulate these fibers of the fornix. The basilar portion of the pons (D) lies in the ventral half of this region of the brainstem. It receives inputs from each of the lobes of the cerebral cortex, which it then relays to the cerebellar cortex. As noted in the answer to question 2, this circuit mediates functions associated with the regulation of voluntary movements of the limbs. Disruption of any part of this circuit, whether at the level of the internal capsule or basilar pons, would affect inputs from the cerebral cortex to the hemispheres of the cerebellar cortex, thus eliminating key inputs necessary for the expression of smooth, coordinated movements. With respect to the neurons located on the lower bank of the calcarine fissure (C), they receive inputs from the lateral geniculate nucleus that relate to the upper retinal (or temporal) visual fields. Therefore, a lesion of this region would produce an upper quadrantanopia (i.e., loss of one-quarter of the visual field). The corpus callosum (F) constitutes the major channel by which the cerebral cortex on one side can communicate with the cortex of the opposite side. In order to stop the spread of seizures from one hemisphere to the other (when the seizures are severe), cutting of the corpus callosum is carried out.

16–24. The answers are 16-H, 17-A, 18-C, 19-D, 20-F, 21-E, 22-G, 23-B, 24-H. (*Nolte, pp 52–60, 62–69, 375–394, 440–445, 507–524.*) This figure is a lateral view of the cerebral cortex. Cells in the "arm" area of the primary motor cortex (H) project their axons to the cervical level of the spinal cord and are activated at the time when a response of this limb occurs. The leg region of the left primary somatosensory cortex (A) lies immediately caudal to the central sulcus, is almost devoid of pyramidal cells, is referred to as a *granulous cortex,* and receives inputs from the right leg. Damage to this region would result in loss of vibration sensibility (as well as tactile sensation and two-point discrimination) from the right leg. Damage to the cells situated in the region of the dorsal border of the superior temporal gyrus and the adjoining area of the inferior parietal lobule (Wernicke's area; C) causes impairment in the appreciation of the meanings of written or spoken words.

The primary, secondary, and tertiary auditory receiving areas in the cortex are located mainly in the superior temporal gyrus (D). It is the final receiving area for inputs from the medial geniculate nucleus, which represents an important relay in the transmission of auditory signals to the cortex. Damage to this region of the cortex would result in some hearing loss. An additional area of the cortex governing speech (F) is called the *motor speech area,* or *Broca's area.* It is situated in the inferior aspect of the frontal lobe immediately rostral and slightly ventral to the precentral gyrus. Lesions of this region produce impairment of the ability to express words in a meaningful way or to use words correctly. The orbital frontal cortex (E) lies in a position inferior and rostral to Broca's motor speech area. This region governs higher-order intellectual functions and some aspects of emotional behavior. Damage to this region often results in personality changes and emotionality. The caudal aspect of the middle frontal gyrus (G) contains cells that, when activated, produce conjugate deviation of the eyes. This action is believed to be accomplished, in part, by virtue of descending projections to the superior colliculus, pretectal region, and horizontal gaze center of the pons. A lesion of this region would result in loss of capacity to produce voluntary horizontal movement of the eyes in one direction. Lesions of the posterior parietal lobe (B) of the nondominant hemisphere will produce a disorder of body image, referred to as *sensory neglect*. The patient will frequently fail to recognize or neglect to shave or wash those body parts. The patient may even fail to recognize the presence of a hemiparesis involving that part of the body as well. The precentral gyrus (H) constitutes the primary motor cortex. Lesions of this region produce a UMN paralysis involving a contralateral limb.

25–35. The answers are 25-K, 26-H, 27-A, 28-C, 29-G, 30-I, 31-B, 32-J, 33-F, 34-D, 35-L. (*Nolte, pp 255–280, 284–287.*) This figure is a ventral view of the brainstem. Fibers that arise from the dorsal motor nucleus and nucleus ambiguus (in part) exit the brain on the lateral side of the medulla as part of the vagus nerve (K) and innervate the myenteric plexus and smooth muscles of the stomach, which normally function to produce gastric secretions. Cutting some of these fibers would result in a reduction in gastric secretions. The tumor affected the motor component of the trigeminal nerve. The motor root (H) lies medial to the sensory root and innervates the muscles of mastication. The mammillary bodies (A), which lie on the ventral surface of the brain at the caudal aspect of the hypothalamus, receive many of their inputs from the hippocampal formation and project to the anteroventral thalamic nucleus as the mammillothalamic tract, which in turn send their axons to the cingulate gyrus and then back to the hippocampal formation, forming what is referred to as the *Papez circuit*. This circuit has been associated with memory functions and the regulation of emotional behavior. The facial nerve (C) exits the brain at the level of the ventrolateral aspect of the caudal pons, and its special visceral efferent component innervates the muscles of facial expression. Damage to this nerve causes loss of facial expression on the side of the face ipsilateral to the affected nerve.

The cerebral peduncle (G) is situated in the ventrolateral aspect of the midbrain and contains fibers of cortical origin that project to all levels of the neuraxis of the brainstem and spinal cord. A lesion in this region would affect upper motor neurons that control motor functions associated with both the body and the head region, producing diminution in strength of the muscles of the head and paralysis of the leg and arm. Note that the selection of choice E, the pyramids, would not have been correct, since the fibers present at this level can only terminate within the medulla or spinal cord, and therefore could not account for the loss of muscle strength associated with the head. First-order somatosensory fibers from the region of the face (I) enter the brain laterally at the level of the middle of the pons as the sensory root of the trigeminal nerve. Damage to this nerve would cause loss of sensation associated with the face. The oculomotor nerve (B) exits the brain at the level of the ventromedial aspect of the midbrain, and some fibers of the general somatic efferent component of this nerve innervate the medial rectus. Damage to this component results in a loss of ability for medial gaze, and the eye will additionally be directed downward because of the unopposed action of cranial nerve IV. Another component of the oculomotor nerve, the GVE component, constitutes the preganglionic parasympathetic neuron in a disynaptic pathway whose postganglionic division innervates the pupillary constrictor muscles. Accordingly, damage to the preganglionic division results in loss of pupillary constriction, which normally occurs in the presence of light as well as in accommodation, and the eye will dilate because of the unopposed action of the sympathetic fibers. The abducens nerve (J) exits the brain at a ventromedial position at the level of the medulla-pontine border, and its fibers innervate the lateral rectus muscle. Damage to this nerve results in a lateral gaze paralysis.

The optic chiasm (F) contains fibers that cross over to reach the lateral geniculate nucleus on the side contralateral to the retina from which they originated. Such fibers are associated with the temporal (i.e., lateral) visual fields. Therefore, damage to the optic chiasm will cause blindness in the lateral half of each of the visual fields. Such a deficit is referred to as *bitemporal hemianopsia*. First-order neurons from the labyrinth organs (D) (i.e., semicircular canals, saccule, and utricle) convey information concerning the position of the head in space along the vestibular component of the eighth nerve into the CNS. This nerve enters the brain laterally at the level of the upper medulla. Damage to this nerve could result in symptoms such as ringing in the ear, nystagmus, loss of balance, and dizziness. The hypoglossal nerve (L) exits the brain at the level of the middle of the medulla between the pyramid and the olive. These fibers innervate muscles that move the tongue toward the opposite side. For this reason, a lesion of the hypoglossal nucleus or its nerve will result in a deviation of the tongue to the side of the lesion because of the unopposed action of the contralateral hypoglossal nerve, which remains intact.

36. The answer is b. (*Greenberg, 5/e, pp 33–35. Afifi, p 574.*) In individuals suffering from bacterial meningitis, the CSF is under increased pressure.

Glucose levels are low because of glucose utilization by the bacteria; neutrophils are increased in response to the bacteria, and protein is also increased, possibly because of a subarachnoid block.

37. The answer is a. (*Afifi, pp 574–575.*) As a result of a subarachnoid hemorrhage, the CSF is bloody. Due to bleeding into the subarachnoid space, there is an increase in CSF pressure as a result of a rupture of an intracranial artery. The presence of blood will increase protein levels and red cells, while glucose levels will be reduced.

38. The answer is c. (*Waxman, 2/e, pp 162–163.*) A noncommunicating hydrocephalus is the result of an obstruction of one of the channels connecting one ventricle to the next, or the outflow of the fourth ventricle through its foramina, resulting in an enlargement of one or more of the ventricles. In the choices given for this question, the interventricular foramen, connecting the lateral with the third ventricle, is the only possible correct answer. A blockade of the interventricular foramen would lead to an enlargement of the lateral ventricle.

39. The answer is b. (*Kandel, pp 1288–1294. Nolte, 3/e, pp 136–139.*) The blood-brain barrier is selectively permeable to certain types of substances, such as biogenic amines, and not to others. The barrier is formed by tight junctions consisting of capillary endothelial cells that are frequently in contact with the glial end-feet of astrocytes. The barrier does not contain well-developed capillary pores. It is not found within circumventricular organs such as the subfornical organ and the pineal gland, but it is applied to all other brain tissues.

Development

Questions

DIRECTIONS: Each item below contains a question or incomplete statement followed by suggested responses. Select the **one best** response to each question.

Item 40–41

After an examination of an infant of approximately three months, it was discovered that the anterior neuropore had failed to close.

40. Which of the following deficits is most likely to appear?

a. Mental retardation
b. Loss of tactile sensation
c. Problems in ability to swallow
d. Loss of reflex activity
e. Respiratory difficulties

41. At approximately four years of age, a child had an MRI that revealed the presence of brain damage. Which of the following regions would most likely be affected by this disorder?

a. Medulla
b. Pons
c. Midbrain
d. Diencephalon
e. Cerebral cortex

42. A parent brought her child to a pediatric neurologist because the boy exhibited a number of serious neurologic signs. These included lack of coordination, especially around the region of the trunk, vomiting, lack of ability to develop new motor skills, headaches, and an enlarged cranium. Which of the following is the most likely diagnosis?

a. Pyramidal tract syndrome
b. Spina bifida
c. Anencephaly
d. Dandy-Walker syndrome
e. Meningomyelocele

43. In the course of development, an abnormality appears in which neural crest cells fail to develop. Which of the following cell types is most clearly affected by this abnormality?

a. Dorsal horn cells
b. Ventral horn cells
c. Dorsal root ganglion cells
d. Hypoglossal neurons
e. Intermediolateral cell column neurons

44. A developmental abnormality occurred that selectively affected neurons derived from the basal plate. Which of the following cell groups would be preserved from such an abnormality?

a. Hypoglossal nucleus
b. Alpha motor neurons
c. Gamma motor neurons
d. Proper sensory nucleus
e. Abducens nucleus

45. A teenage girl complained about a loss of pain and temperature sensation around the region of her waist on both sides. A further analysis revealed that this dysfunction represented a congenital defect. This defect could be described as

a. Arnold-Chiari malformation
b. Syringomyelia
c. Dandy-Walker syndrome
d. Anencephaly
e. Spina bifida

46. A developmental malformation was discovered in a 3-year-old boy. It presented as sensory and motor deficits of lower extremities as well as some back pain and bladder difficulties. What was the diagnosis provided by the neurologist?

a. Dandy-Walker syndrome
b. Tethered cord
c. Spina bifida
d. Syringomyelia
e. Encephalocele

47. A 9-year-old girl was seen by an endocrinologist after it became apparent that her weight and height were below average and that her growth rate was also quite slow. Further analysis revealed the likelihood of the presence of a congenital malformation involving incomplete growth of the anterior pituitary. Which of the following is the probable source of the developmental defect?

a. Basal plate
b. Alar plate
c. Sulcus limitans
d. Rhombic lips
e. Rathke's pouch

48. A developmental abnormality results in reduced production of CSF. Which of the following developmental zones is most likely associated with this dysfunction?

a. Basal plate
b. Alar plate
c. Neural crest
d. Roof plate
e. Floor plate

49. The cerebellum is derived from which of the following cell groups or vesicles?

a. Neural crest cells
b. Rhombic lips
c. Mesencephalon
d. Sulcus limitans
e. Telencephalon

50. A young child was brought into the hospital emergency room because he had episodes of vomiting, headaches, problems in acquisition of motor skills, cranial nerve dysfunction, and problems in breathing. To which of the following disorders does this combination of syndromes most closely relate?

a. Cleft palate
b. Hydrocephalus
c. Anencephaly
d. Syringomyelia
e. Congenital aneurysm

51. A brain MRI scan taken from a 6-month-old baby revealed that while the overall size of the cerebral cortex was normal, the size of the pyramidal tracts was considerably smaller than normal. What is the most likely explanation for this defect?

a. Reduction in the numbers of cortical neurons giving rise to pyramidal tract fibers
b. Reduction in the numbers of synaptic contacts made by pyramidal tract neurons
c. Reduction in the extent of myelin found on pyramidal tract neurons
d. Reduction in the amount of neurotransmitter released by pyramidal tract neurons
e. Reduction in the numbers of glial cells attached to pyramidal tract neurons

52. In the process of histogenesis, neuronal death can occur as a function of apoptosis. What is the most likely basis for apoptosis?

a. Excessive stimulation of an afferent nerve fiber
b. Loss of acetylcholine released at nerve endings
c. The beginning of myelin formation
d. Elimination of nerve growth factor
e. Reduction in brain serotonin levels

Development

Answers

40–41. The answers are 40-a, 41-e. *(Afifi, pp 513–519. Nolte, 5/e, pp 46–51.)* When the anterior neuropore fails to close, there is protrusion of CSF, glia, meninges, and neighboring brain tissue. This results in damage to the cerebral hemispheres and cerebellum. Accordingly, the damage to the cerebral hemispheres is directly related to the onset of mental retardation. The other choices are more closely related to processes associated with the lower brainstem and spinal cord.

42. The answer is d. *(Afifi, pp 513–519. Nolte, 5/e, pp 46–51.)* The constellation of neurological signs seen in this child is characteristic of the Dandy-Walker syndrome. It involves the presence of hydrocephalus and damage to the cerebellar vermis. The other choices constitute developmental disorders affecting other regions of the CNS, such as the spinal cord or cerebral cortex, which do not produce the syndromes in this case.

43. The answer is c. *(Nolte, pp 37–39.)* A number of structures, such as the dorsal root ganglia, sympathetic ganglia, and chromaffin cells of the adrenal medulla, are derived from neural crest cells.

44. The answer is d. *(Nolte, pp 37–39.)* Structures associated with sensory functions, such as the proper sensory nucleus of the dorsal horn of the spinal cord, are derived from the alar plate. In contrast, structures related to motor functions, including the hypoglossal and abducens nuclei and alpha and gamma motor neurons, are derived from the basal plate.

45. The answer is b. *(Nolte, pp 517–518.)* Syringo(hydro)myelia is a cavitation around the central canal of the spinal cord and is filled with CSF. Damage to this region is usually segmental in nature and would affect those fibers that cross in the spinal cord and include principally the spinothalamic tracts. Damage to these tracts because of the cavitation around the central canal would result in segmental loss of pain and temperature sensations.

46. The answer is b. *(Afifi, pp 519–520.)* A tethered cord syndrome is characterized by a shortened and/or thickened filum terminale, resulting in the spinal cord becoming anchored to the subcutaneous tissue. This results in sensory and motor deficits in the lower extremities as well as bladder difficulties, back pain, and scoliosis.

47. The answer is e. (*Martin, p 423.*) The anterior lobe of the pituitary is formed as an in-pocket derivative of the ectodermal stomodeum, called Rathke's pouch.

48. The answer is d. (*Nolte, pp 43–46.*) The choroid plexus is attached to the roof of the ventricles and is thus derived from the roof plate.

49. The answer is b. (*Nolte, pp 38–43.*) The cerebellum is formed from the dorsolateral aspects of the alar plates, which bend medially and posteriorly to form the rhombic lips.

50. The answer is b. (*Afifi, pp 513–521.*) The symptoms described are characteristic of hydrocephalus. Hydrocephalus may come about as a result of defects such as the failure of formation of the cerebellar vermis, the foramens of Magendie and Luschka, or the corpus callosum. There is an enlarged cranium as a result of the buildup of CSF, causing brain damage. Several of the symptoms may also be caused by a compression of the posterior fossa and the absence of a cerebellar vermis. Cleft palate is a fissure of the medial aspect of the lip and would not result in the symptoms described previously. Anencephaly is the complete or partial absence of the brain and is not compatible with life. Syringomyelia is associated with bilateral segmental loss of pain and temperature. A congenital aneurysm can occur in a variety of places within the CNS and is typically associated with stroke in the adult.

51. The answer is c. (*Afifi, pp 505–508.*) Extensive myelination occurs in postnatal development. The failure of the pyramidal tracts to form myelin would account for the reduction in their size. In this particular situation, the size of the cerebral cortex was approximately normal, suggesting that there was no significant decrease in cortical cells. Variation in the numbers of synaptic contacts, transmitter formation, and glial cells would not account for a reduction in the size of the pyramidal tract.

52. The answer is d. (*Purves, pp 503–506.*) When nerve growth factor is eliminated, cell death results and involves fragmentation, shrinkage, and ultimate phagocytosis of the cell. Apoptosis is believed to be triggered by a biochemical process that causes transcription of a variety of genes. Nerve growth factor blocks the activation of this process. It should also be noted that this form of cell death differs from that occurring after nerve injury or trauma to the nerve. The other choices listed are unrelated to the process of apoptosis.

The Neuron

Questions

DIRECTIONS: Each item below contains a question or incomplete statement followed by suggested responses. Select the **one best** response to each question.

Item 53–54

The methods involving microinjections of Fluoro-Gold or horseradish peroxidase (HRP) have been employed over the past few decades by many investigators.

53. What can these methods identify?

a. Cell bodies
b. Metabolic activity of neurons
c. Sensory endings of nerve fibers
d. CNS receptors
e. Degenerating axons

54. What is the principle that these methods utilize?

a. Metabolic mapping of CNS pathways
b. Anterograde labeling of degenerating axons
c. Retrograde transport
d. Anterograde transport
e. Visualization of demyelinating peripheral nerves

Item 55–56

Substances such as tritiated amino acids and phaseolus vulgaris agglutinin microinjected into specific regions of the brain have also been employed by many investigators for the study of the nervous system.

55. What do these methods specifically label?

a. Cell bodies
b. Glial cells
c. Sensory receptors
d. Motor end plates
e. Axons and axon preterminals

56. What is the principle that these methods utilize?
a. Metabolic mapping of CNS pathways
b. Staining of degenerating axons
c. Retrograde transport
d. Anterograde transport
e. Retrograde degeneration

57. What is the objective of the use of the methods of MRI and 2-deoxyglucose (2-DG) autoradiography?
a. Label dopamine receptors
b. Label serotonin receptors
c. Label metabolically active structures
d. Stain individual cell bodies, dendrites, and axons
e. Stain astrocytes

58. Which of the following procedures would be utilized in order to show positive staining of groups of serotonin neurons?
a. Electrical brain stimulation
b. Glutamate stimulation of the brain
c. HRP staining of neurons
d. Immunocytochemical labeling
e. Metabolic staining of neurons

59. An individual sustained a severe knife wound, damaging a spinal nerve adjoining its entry to the spinal cord. If one could examine this peripheral nerve and its cell body, which of the following events would he or she most likely observe?
a. A displacement of the nucleus toward the periphery of the cell
b. A mitotic division of the neuronal cell body
c. A more intense staining of the cell body
d. Degeneration of processes along the axon proximal but not distal to the lesion
e. An initial loss of mitochondria in the axoplasm at Ranvier's node

60. A 65-year-old man is diagnosed with a form of a peripheral neuropathy. What effect will this disorder have upon the patient?
a. A loss in motor function, but sensory functions will remain largely intact
b. A reduction in conduction velocity of the affected nerve
c. An increase in the number of Ranvier's nodes
d. Degeneration of myelin but the axon will typically remain intact
e. Signs of a UMN paralysis

61. Which of the following statements about nerve cells is correct?

a. Typically, one copy of the same peptide is cut from the same precursor molecule
b. It is generally recognized that the cytosol provides the source of selective protein synthesis limited to neurotransmitters
c. Cytosolic proteins show significant modification or processing following their translation
d. Nuclear and mitochondrial proteins that are encoded by the cell's nucleus are targeted to their proper organelle by a process called *posttranslational importation*
e. Secretory proteins undergo little or no modification or processing after translation

62. Which of the following statements concerning axoplasmic transport is correct?

a. Large membranous organelles are transported by slow axonal transport
b. Cytosolic proteins are transported by fast transport
c. Retrograde transport is generally limited to a fixed rate of movement of particles
d. Anterograde transport is dependent upon microtubules

63. Which of the following statements correctly characterizes ion channels?

a. The passage of ions through ion channels typically requires an active mechanism
b. A common stimulus serves as the basis for opening ion channels
c. Exposure of a ligand-gated channel to continuous high concentrations of its ligand is the necessary and sufficient stimulus for opening that channel
d. The opening or closing of an ion channel may be affected by the use of drugs

64. Which of the following statements concerning the resting membrane potential is correct?

a. Passive fluxes of Na^+ and K^+ are balanced by an active pump that derives energy from enzymatic hydrolysis of adenosine 5'-triphosphate (ATP)
b. A membrane is depolarized when the differences between the charges across the membrane are increased
c. As the inside of the cell is made more negative with respect to the outside, the cell becomes depolarized
d. In a cell whose membrane possesses only K^+ channels, the membrane potential cannot be determined
e. The resting membrane potential is unrelated to the separation of the charge across the membrane

65. Which of the following statements concerning the length constant is correct?

a. The length constant is the distance along a dendrite where the change in membrane potential produced by a current becomes stable
b. The length constant increases as the membrane resistance increases
c. The length constant increases as the axial resistance increases
d. The length constant is greater in unmyelinated than in myelinated fibers
e. As the length constant increases in a postsynaptic neuron, the efficiency of electronic conduction of synaptic potentials (at that synapse) decreases

66. Which of the following statements concerning ligand gating of neuronal membrane channels is true?

a. The normal triggering mechanism for gating involves nonspecific binding by large classes of molecules
b. Channels are opened when a given molecule selectively binds with the gating molecule
c. Ligand gating is triggered by changes in the electrical potential across the membrane
d. The channels are constructed of a mixture of proteins and lipids
e. The gating molecule shows no conformational change during the gating process

67. After the occurrence of an action potential, there is a repolarization of the membrane. What is the principal explanation for this event?

a. Potassium channels have been opened
b. Sodium channels have been opened
c. Potassium channels have been inactivated
d. The membrane becomes impermeable to all ions
e. There has been a sudden influx of calcium

68. During an in vitro experiment, the membrane potential of a nerve cell is hyperpolarized to −120 mV. At that time, a transmitter, known to be inhibitory in function, is applied to the preparation and results in a depolarization of the membrane. What is the most likely reason for this occurrence?

a. Inhibitory transmitters normally depolarize the postsynaptic membrane
b. The normal response of the postsynaptic membrane to any transmitter is depolarization
c. The inhibitory transmitter activates ligand-gated potassium channels
d. Sodium channels become inactivated
e. Calcium channels become activated

Item 69–70

The neurophysiologist Kuffler studied the electrophysiology of glial cells, using the optic nerve and its surrounding glial sheath. He found that the mean value of the resting potential of these cells, as recorded by intracellular microelectrodes, was 89.6 mV. The potassium concentration in the bathing solution was 3 meq/L. Assume that $RT/F = 61$.

69. Assuming that the resting potential is equivalent to the potassium equilibrium potential, calculate the approximate intracellular potassium concentration (in meq/L).

a. 11
b. 33
c. 88
d. 140
e. 155

70. What would be the concentration of potassium (meq/L) in the bathing fluid in order to depolarize the membrane potential to zero?

a. 11
b. 33
c. 88
d. 140
e. 155

71. What is the probable explanation for the depolarization of glial cells following stimulation of nerve fibers?

a. A delayed increase in potassium conductance
b. An early sodium influx
c. A large efflux of sodium ions
d. A temporal summation that results in a long-lasting depolarization
e. An influx of chloride ions

72. Stimulation of the optic nerve with a volley of impulses caused a slow and long-lasting depolarization of the associated glial cells. The mean value of the depolarization was 12.1 mV. If this depolarization was due solely to an increase in potassium ion concentration in the intracellular clefts, calculate the change in the concentration of potassium in the extracellular environment (in meq/L).

a. 1.79
b. 36.30
c. 137.00
d. 140.50
e. 5.35×10^{-6}

73. Where is the trigger zone that integrates incoming signals from other cells and initiates the signal that the neuron sends to another neuron or muscle cell?

a. Cell body
b. Dendritic trunk
c. Dendritic spines
d. Axon hillock and initial segment
e. Axon trunk

74. Which of the following statements concerning the membrane time constant is correct?

a. The time constant is a function of the membrane's resistance and capacitance
b. The time constant is unrelated to the membrane's capacitance
c. The time course of the rising phase of a synaptic potential is specifically dependent upon the time constant for that cell
d. The falling phase of a synaptic potential is dependent upon active and passive membrane properties
e. The integration of synaptic potentials is unrelated to the length of the time constant

75. Which of the following statements concerning sodium channels is true?

a. They are opened when the membrane is hyperpolarized
b. They display a high conductance in the resting membrane
c. They open rapidly following depolarization of the membrane
d. They are rapidly inactivated by tetraethylammonium
e. They are rapidly activated by tetrodotoxin

76. The equilibrium potential for potassium, as determined by the Nernst equation, differs from the resting potential of the neuron. Which of the following best accounts for this difference?

a. An active sodium-potassium pump makes an important contribution to the regulation of the resting potential
b. The membrane is permeable to ions other than potassium
c. The Nernst equation basically considers only the relative distribution of potassium ions across the membrane
d. The resting potential is basically dependent upon the concentration of sodium but not potassium ions across the membrane
e. The Nernst equation fails to account for local changes in temperature that influence the resting membrane potential

77. Based upon one's knowledge of the typical distribution of ions across a cell membrane, which value would represent the appropriate resting membrane potential?

a. +70 mV
b. +30 mV
c. 0 mV
d. −70 mV
e. −100 V

78. If a membrane is permeable only to sodium ions and the concentration of sodium ions on one side of the membrane is the same as that on the other side, then which of the following statements would best characterize the resting membrane potential for that cell?

a. A pump mechanism will cause the cell to become hyperpolarized
b. The membrane potential would be zero
c. The tendency would be for current to be directed inwardly
d. The membrane potential could not be predicted from the Nernst equation
e. There would be an initial decrease followed by an increase in membrane potential

79. Which of the following items best characterizes this description: A graded, fast potential, lasting from several milliseconds to seconds, resulting from a chemical transmitter binding to a receptor to produce either an excitatory postsynaptic potential (EPSP) that depends upon a single class of channels for sodium and potassium or an inhibitory postsynaptic potential (IPSP) that is dependent upon chloride or potassium conductance.

a. Receptor potentials
b. Electrical postsynaptic potentials
c. Increased-conductance postsynaptic potentials
d. Decreased-conductance postsynaptic potentials

80. To which of the following does the term *all-or-none response* most closely relate?

a. The resting potential
b. Increased-conductance presynaptic potentials
c. Increased-conductance postsynaptic potentials
d. The generator potential
e. The action potential

81. To which of the following does the passive spread of a presynaptic current across a gap junction that is activated by changes in voltage, pH, or calcium ion levels most closely relate?

a. The resting potential
b. The action potential
c. Electrical presynaptic potentials
d. Electrical postsynaptic potentials
e. Receptor potentials

82. A young woman in her early twenties experiences loss of sensation in her legs and weakness in her limbs. A neurological examination further indicated some spasticity of the limbs as well. The neurologist provided a preliminary diagnosis of onset of multiple sclerosis. Assuming that this diagnosis is correct, which of the following can best account for the diminution of sensory and motor functions?

a. Loss of Schwann cells in peripheral neurons
b. An overall loss of dopaminergic release throughout the brain and spinal cord
c. Loss of peripheral cholinergic neurons
d. Demyelination of CNS neurons
e. Proliferation of oligodendrocytes

The Neuron

Answers

53–54. The answers are 53-a, 54-c. *(Martin, pp 23–27.)* With HRP histochemistry, the glycoprotein enzyme HRP is injected into the region of the terminal endings of the neuronal pathway under examination and is incorporated into the axons through a process of micropinocytosis. HRP is then retrogradely transported back to the cell bodies of origin of that pathway, where it is then degraded. By reacting the tissue with an appropriate substrate, the labeled cells can be visualized under light microscopy.

55–56. The answers are 55-e, 56-d. *(Martin, pp 23–27.)* The mapping of pathways utilizing anterograde tracing of fibers depends upon the process of axonal transport. For example, if a tritiated amino acid such as ^{3}H-leucine is microinjected into a region of the brain, it gets synthesized into protein in the cell bodies and transported down the respective axons to their terminals. By utilizing autoradiographic methods, one can identify the loci of the label contained in the protein that has been transported to the axon terminals. The application of phaseolus vulgaris agglutinin also utilizes the principle of anterograde transport to map the distribution of pathways from cell bodies injected with this substance.

57. The answer is c. *(Martin, pp 23–27.)* MRI permits the visualization of the degenerative process that results in demyelination of axons. 2-deoxyglucose autoradiography is used to metabolically map pathways and structures that are functionally active as a result of sensory, chemical, or electrical stimulation of nervous tissue. Local variations in energy metabolism can be visualized because the glucose analog ^{14}C-2-deoxyglucose (2-DG) is phosphorylated to 2-DG-6-phosphate, where it is not further metabolized and is retained in the neuron. The rate of incorporation into neurons is related to the rate of glucose utilization, which is, itself, a function of energy metabolism.

58. The answer is d. *(Martin, pp 23–27. Kandel, pp 891–895.)* Immunocytochemical methods, including in situ hybridization, have been used to identify the presence and localization of specific neurotransmitters and receptors, such as serotonin.

59. The answer is a. *(Afifi, pp 30–34. Nolte, pp 18–21.)* Damage to a nerve fiber proximal to its cell body will cause, among other changes, retrograde degeneration of the cell body. A number of changes occur in the neuron during the process of retrograde degeneration. The cell body initially shows some swelling and becomes distended. At the beginning of the degenerative process, there is an accumulation of mitochondria in the axoplasm at Ranvier's nodes. The nucleus is then displaced toward the periphery of the cell. The Nissl granules break down, first in the center of the cell; later, the breakdown spreads outward. In addition, the axonal process distal to the site of the lesion will undergo degeneration. It should be noted that retrograde degeneration procedures were used experimentally prior to the advent of histochemical methods for identifying cell bodies of origin of given pathways in the CNS.

60. The answer is b. *(Kandel, pp 82–83, 700–704.)* In a peripheral neuropathy, there may be damage to either the myelin or the axon directly, although more often there is damage to the myelin. Because of myelin (or axonal) damage, there is a reduction (or loss) of conduction velocity. The disorder may affect both sensory and motor components of the peripheral nerve, thereby causing dysfunction in both the sensory and the motor processes associated with that nerve. Because there is peripheral neuronal damage, the motor loss will be reflected in a weakness, paralysis, or reflex activity associated with the affected muscle, as well as impairment of sensation.

61. The answer is d. *(Kandel, pp 88–98.)* Nuclear and mitochondrial proteins are encoded by the nucleus and are formed on free polysomes. The mechanism by which they are targeted to their proper organelle is called *posttranslational importation.* Specific receptors bind and translocate these proteins, and it is the recognition of the structural features of these proteins that allows for transport into the nucleus from the cytoplasm. In the processing of large proteins such as opioid peptides, more than one copy and different peptides are produced from the same precursor molecule. This precursor is referred to as a *polyprotein* because more than one active peptide is present. All protein synthesis begins in the cytosol. Cytosolic proteins are the most extensive type of protein in the cell and include those that make up the cytoskeleton and enzymes that catalyze the different metabolic reactions of the cell. Messenger RNAs (mRNAs) for these proteins pass through nuclear pores, become associated with ribosomes, and ultimately form free polysomes in the cytoplasm of the cell. Cytosolic proteins display little modification or processing compared with proteins that remain attached to the membranes of the endoplasmic reticulum or the Golgi apparatus. Messenger RNA that encodes proteins that will become a constituent of organelles or secretory products is formed on polysomes that are attached to the endoplasmic reticulum. Such sheets of membrane in association with ribosomes are called *rough endoplasmic reticulum*. Secretory products typically undergo significant modification after translation. For example, neuropeptide transmitters are cleaved from polypeptide chains, in part, in the endoplasmic reticulum and the Golgi apparatus.

62. The answer is d. *(Kandel, pp 100–104.)* Transport in either direction utilizes microtubules as a vehicle or track by which the particles are transported. Among the particles transported down the axon from the cell body are newly synthesized membranous organelles, including synaptic vesicles or their precursors, which ultimately reach the axon terminals. In retrograde transport, the particles transported include endosomes generated from the nerve terminal, mitochondria, and components of the endoplasmic reticulum. Large membranous organelles are transported along the axon both anterogradely and retrogradely by fast axonal transport. In contrast, cytosolic proteins and components of the matrix of the cytoskeleton are transported by slow axonal transport. There are different rates of retrograde transport in which the faster component is approximately twice as fast as the slow component.

63. The answer is d. *(Kandel, pp 107–116.)* Ion flux through ion channels is considered to be passive in nature and functions in the absence of any mechanism that requires energy metabolism. Cation channels are generally associated with membranes that are semipermeable to selective ions such as Na^+, K^+, or Cl^-. The electrochemical gradient is a function of two forces: (1) the chemical concentration gradient, which is derived from the relative differences in the distributions of ions across the membrane, and (2) the electrical potential difference between the two sides of the membrane as a function of the distribution of the ionic charges. When ions may flow through channels, current varies as a function of concentration. However, at high ionic concentration differences, a saturation phenomenon is observed that is due to resistance to flow through the channels. It is believed that different kinds of stimuli can function to open or close channels. For example, mechanical activation may lead to the opening of channels. Some channels (ligand-gated) are regulated by the noncovalent binding of chemical ligands such as neurotransmitters; others (electrically gated) are affected by changes in membrane voltage that cause a change in the conformation of the channel. Alternatively, relatively long-lasting changes may result when second messengers bind to the channel, at which time there is protein phosphorylation mediated by protein kinases. Such modification of the channel can be reversed by dephosphorylation. In contrast, when a ligand-gated channel is exposed to prolonged, high concentrations of its ligand, it tends to become refractory (i.e., desensitized to the presence of that ligand).

64. The answer is a. *(Kandel, pp 125–138.)* The potential difference across the membrane is a result of the separation of charge and is called the *resting membrane potential*. Accordingly, the potential difference across the membrane is a direct function of the numbers of positive and negative charges on either side of the membrane. As the separation of charge (i.e., differences between the charges) across the membrane is reduced, the membrane is said to be depolarized. Conversely, as the difference between the charges is increased, the membrane becomes hyperpolarized. In the latter case, the inside of the cell is made more negative with respect to the outside. If a cell has only a single channel in its membrane (such as for K^+), the gradients for the other ions become irrelevant and the membrane potential will approach the equilibrium potential for the single ion (K^+ in this example). There is a tendency for ions to leak down their electrochemical gradients from one side of the membrane to the other. For there to be a steady resting membrane potential, the gradients across the membrane must be held constant. Changes in ionic gradients are avoided, in spite of the leak, by the presence of an active Na^+, K^+ pump (a membrane protein) that moves Na^+ out of the cell and at the same time brings K^+ into the cell. Such a pumping mechanism requires energy because it is working against the electrochemical gradients of the two ions. The energy is derived from the hydrolysis of ATP.

65. The answer is b. *(Kandel, pp 222–223.)* The length constant is defined as R_m/R_a, where R_m equals membrane resistance and R_a equals axial resistance. It is the distance along a fiber where a change in membrane potential produced by a given current decays to a value of approximately one-third of its original value. As can be seen from the definition, the length constant is directly proportional to the membrane resistance and inversely related to the axial resistance (i.e., the resistance of the cytoplasm within the fiber). The membrane resistance is increased significantly through the process of myelination, which thus produces an increase in the value of the length constant. When the length constant along a dendrite is relatively large, it has the effect of increasing the efficiency of electrotonic conduction along the dendritic process as compared with a similar dendrite with a smaller-length constant. In this manner, the synaptic potential along the dendrite distal to the synapse will be relatively larger in a dendrite that has a larger-length constant than one that has a smaller-length constant.

66. The answer is b. *(Kandel, pp 105–119, 185, 196, 240.)* The triggering mechanism for ligand gating involves the selective binding of a particular molecule with the protein channel. This binding causes a conformational change of the channel protein that results in the movement of the channel back and forth, which, in effect, opens or closes the channel. Neurotransmitters can regulate channels as a result of their binding properties. An example is the action of acetylcholine at the neuromuscular junction, which is capable of activating channels in the membrane of skeletal muscle. Most cation channels are selective for sodium, potassium, or calcium. Ion channels are composed of large-membrane glycoproteins that vary widely in their molecular weights. In contrast to ligand gating, other types of channels may be activated by changes in the electrical potential across the cell membrane, a process referred to as *voltage gating*.

67. The answer is a. *(Kandel, pp 150–164.)* In the late phase of the action potential, potassium channels become opened and potassium efflux produces a hyperpolarization of the membrane. During the repolarization of the membrane, sodium channels are closed (sodium inactivation). Recall that activation of sodium channels is associated with the generation of the action potential. Calcium has a strong electrochemical gradient that drives it into the cell; this coincides with the upstroke of the action potential. A number of different types of calcium-gated potassium channels have been described that are activated during the action potential. Thus, it would appear that calcium influx during the action potential could generate opposing effects. On the one hand, calcium influx carries a positive charge into the cell, which contributes to the depolarization of the membrane. On the other hand, calcium influx may help to open up more potassium channels, which contributes to an outward ionic flow of potassium that causes repolarization of the membrane.

68. The answer is c. *(Kandel, pp 125–138.)* To understand how an inhibitory transmitter can actually cause a partial depolarization of the membrane, refer to the Goldman equation. The release (or application) of an inhibitory transmitter will serve to open specific ion channels, notably those of potassium. If the membrane is artificially hyperpolarized to −120 mV, the opening of the potassium channel will lead to a redistribution of the ions across the membrane to a normal level. If the normal equilibrium potential for potassium is approximately −75 mV, then application of an inhibitory transmitter (that typically functions by opening potassium channels) will result in a redistribution of potassium ions toward the potassium equilibrium potential (i.e., −75 mV). Consequently, the membrane potential will be reduced (i.e., depolarized) from −120 mV to a value close to −75 mV. Other possible answers are clearly incorrect. Inhibitory transmitters normally function to hyperpolarize the membrane. Postsynaptic membranes may either be depolarized or hyperpolarized, depending upon the nature of the transmitter and receptor complex present at the synapse. Since the influx of calcium during the depolarization phase of the action potential leads to opposing effects, activation of this channel cannot account for the observed effects. Inactivation of sodium channels would not result in a depolarization of the membrane, but, instead, may contribute to the hyperpolarization of the membrane.

69. The answer is c. (*Kandel, pp 132–138.*) To solve the problem, use the Goldman equation, which reduces to the Nernst equation:

$$\text{Equilibrium potential} = (RT/F) \propto \ln (K_i)/(K_o)$$
$$-89.6 = 61 \, [\ln (K_i) - \ln (3)]$$
$$-89.6/61 = \ln (K_i) - 0.48$$
$$1.47 = \ln (K_i) - 0.48$$
$$1.95 = \ln (K_i)$$
$$88.54 = K_i$$

70. The answer is c. (*Kandel, pp 132–138.*) If the bathing solution is brought to 88 meq/L, the ionic concentrations outside and inside the membrane would be equal and, therefore, the membrane potential would be depolarized to zero.

71. The answer is a. (*Kandel, pp 132–138.*) In this situation, the roles of sodium and chloride ions were not of central importance. Temporal summation also cannot account for these findings and is thus irrelevant to the question at hand. The depolarization of 12.1 mV can be attributed to an increase in the concentration of potassium in the intracellular cleft.

72. The answer is a. *(Kandel, pp 132–138.)* Use the Goldman equation reduced to the Nernst equation. The resting membrane potential is −89.6 mV, $RT/F = 51$, the potassium concentration is 3 meq/L, and K_i is calculated to be 88.54 mV.

$$\text{Equilibrium potential} = (RT/F) \infty\ 61\ \ln\ (K_o/K_i)$$
$$-89.6 - 12.1 = 61\ \infty\ \ln\ (K_o - 88.54)$$
$$-77.5 = 61\ \infty\ (\ln K_o - \ln 88.54)$$
$$-1.27 = \ln K_o - \ln 88.54$$
$$-1.27 - (-1.95) = \ln K_o$$
$$+0.68 = \ln K_o$$
$$4.79\ \text{meq/L} = K_o$$

Therefore, the change in extracellular potassium would be
$$4.79 - 3.00 = 1.79\ \text{meq/L}$$

73. The answer is d. *(Kandel, pp 222–223.)* The trigger zone for the initiation of impulses from a neuron includes a specialized region of the cell body—the *axon hillock*—together with the section of the axon that adjoins this region—the *initial segment*. Other components of the neuron, such as the dendrites and cell body, receive inputs from afferent sources but are not capable of initiating impulses at these sites. The same is true concerning more distal aspects of the axon over which the impulse is conducted.

74. The answer is a. *(Kandel, pp 140–149.)* The time and space constants represent passive properties of a neuron. The electrical equivalent circuit utilizes the concept that a membrane has both capacitive and resistive properties in parallel, in which case, the rising phase of a potential change is governed in part by the product of the resistance and capacitance of the membrane. The rising phase of a synaptic potential is governed by both active and passive properties of the membrane; however, the falling phase is regulated solely by the passive properties. As the time constant is increased, the probability of integration of converging synaptic signals is increased because such signals will be more likely to overlap in time (temporal summation).

75. The answer is c. *(Kandel, pp 105–123, 154–169.)* Sodium channels are rapidly opened following depolarization of the membrane. The rapid influx of ions results in a further depolarization of the membrane, which, in turn, can lead to an action potential. When the membrane is hyperpolarized, sodium channels are closed. Moreover, in the resting membrane, sodium channels are not activated. Tetraethylammonium is a drug that selectively blocks only potassium channels. Tetrodotoxin blocks sodium channels.

76. The answer is b. (*Kandel, pp 125–148.*) Because the membrane is a leaky one, the sodium-potassium pump serves an important function in actively transporting ions from one side of the membrane to the other. The membrane is permeable to ions other than potassium, such as sodium and chloride. This fact is taken into consideration in the Goldman equation. This equation includes the distribution of all of these other ions in its formula for determining the value of membrane potential. Accordingly, the resting membrane potential is dependent upon the concentration of these other ions as well as potassium. While it is true that the Nernst equation considers the relative distribution of potassium ions across the membrane, this statement in itself does not explain why the equilibrium potential for potassium differs from the resting potential of the neuron. The statement that the Nernst equation does not take into account differences in temperature is false. But, again, even if that statement were true, it would nevertheless not account for the differences between the equilibrium potential for potassium and the resting potential of the neuron.

77. The answer is d. (*Purves, pp 42–46.*) At rest, the cell typically generates a constant voltage across the membrane. The voltage is negative (inside), varying from approximately −40 to −90 mV, which is determined by the relative concentrations of the different ions inside and outside the membrane.

78. The answer is b. (*Kandel, pp 175–295. Purves, pp 44–45, 99–114.*) If the cell membrane is permeable to only one ion such as sodium, and the concentration of this ion is equal on both sides of the membrane, then there will be no membrane potential recorded across the membrane. This is intuitively so, as determined from the Nernst equation, where both the numerator and denominator are the same, therefore generating the logarithm of 1, whose value is 0.

79. The answer is c. (*Kandel, pp 175–295; Purves, pp 44–45, 85–97, 99–114.*) Increased-conductance postsynaptic potentials are fast, graded potentials, lasting from several milliseconds to several seconds. If the potential is an EPSP, it depends upon a single class of ligand-gated channels for sodium and potassium. If the response is an IPSP, then it depends upon ligand-gated channels for potassium and chloride. Decreased-conductance postsynaptic potentials are mediated by a chemical transmitter or intracellular messenger to produce a graded, slow potential, lasting from seconds to minutes. This response is related to a closure of sodium, potassium, or chloride channels. Receptor potentials result from the application of a sensory stimulus that produces a fast, graded potential that involves a single class of channels for both sodium and potassium.

80. The answer is e. *(Purves, pp 43–74.)* The action potential is characterized by an all-or-none response in which the overshoot may reach an amplitude of up to 100 mV. The mechanism involves separate ion channels for sodium and potassium. The resting potential is characterized by a relatively steady potential, usually in the region of 270 mV, but which may range from 235 to 270 mV. This potential is mainly dependent upon potassium and chloride channels.

81. The answer is d. *(Kandel, pp 140–148.)* Electrical postsynaptic potentials involve the passive spread of current across a gap junction that is permeable to a variety of small ions. The stimulus for such activation may be a change in either voltage, pH, or intracellular calcium. Answers and explanations for questions 74 to 77 relate to the other choices presented.

82. The answer is d. *(Greenberg, pp 167–170.)* Multiple sclerosis is a demyelinating disease. The lesions may also involve some reactive gliosis and axonal degeneration as well. It occurs mainly in the white matter of the spinal cord and brain as well as in the optic nerve.

The Synapse

Questions

DIRECTIONS: Each item below contains a question or incomplete statement followed by suggested responses. Select the **one best** response to each question.

83. Which of the following characteristically include *gap junctions?*

a. Axodendritic synapses
b. Axoaxonic synapses
c. Axosomatic synapses
d. Dendrodendritic synapses
e. Electrical synapses

84. Which of the following characterizes a principal feature of axosomatic synapses?

a. It is referred to as a type I synapse
b. They have an electrical continuity linking the pre- and postsynaptic cells
c. They are typically inhibitory
d. Synaptic transmission is mediated by glutamate
e. They form the predominant synapse of cortical projections to the neostriatum

85. In a typical chemical synapse, which of the following constitutes the correct sequence of events involved in neurotransmission?

a. The action potential stimulates the presynaptic terminal → the presynaptic terminal is depolarized, opening voltage-gated Ca^{2+} ion channels, causing an influx of these ions into the presynaptic terminal → release of the transmitter into the synaptic cleft by exocytosis → a postsynaptic current produces an excitatory postsynaptic potential (EPSP) or an inhibitory postsynaptic potential (IPSP), changing the excitability of the postsynaptic cell

b. Release of the transmitter into the synaptic cleft by exocytosis → an influx of Ca^{2+} through channels, causing the vesicles to fuse with the presynaptic membrane → opening of the postsynaptic channels → binding of the transmitter to the receptor molecules in the postsynaptic membrane

c. The vesicular membrane is retrieved from the plasma membrane → release of the transmitter into the synaptic cleft by exocytosis → the action potential stimulates the presynaptic terminal → binding of the transmitter to the receptor molecules in the postsynaptic membrane

d. Opening or closing of the postsynaptic channels → depolarization of the presynaptic terminal causing an opening of Ca^{2+} ion channels → release of the transmitter into the synaptic cleft by exocytosis → synthesis and storage of the transmitter in the presynaptic terminal

e. The presynaptic terminal is depolarized, opening voltage-gated Ca^{2+} ion channels, causing an influx of these ions into the presynaptic terminal → opening or closing of the postsynaptic channels → release of the transmitter into the synaptic cleft by exocytosis → the vesicular membrane is retrieved from the plasma membrane

86. Which of the following statements correctly characterizes synapses?

a. Synaptic vesicles constitute important features for transmission in both chemical and electrical synapses

b. A postsynaptic neuron typically receives input from different presynaptic axons that are either excitatory or inhibitory, but it cannot receive inputs from both types

c. Synaptic delay is approximately the same for both chemical and electrical synapses

d. Receptors can provide a gating function with respect to a given ion channel

e. The mechanism of indirect gating of ions normally does not involve the activation of G-proteins

87. Which of the following properties or characteristics are correct in comparing γ-aminobutyric acid (GABA) with glycine?

a. Both are known to have inhibitory as well as excitatory properties
b. Both utilize a similar mechanism of gating of the chloride channel
c. GABA but not glycine utilizes receptors that are transmembrane proteins
d. Glycine is associated with the generation of seizure activity, but the effects of GABA are to block such activity
e. Glycine generates its most significant effects in the cerebral cortex, while the effects of GABA are more restricted to the basal ganglia, brainstem, and spinal cord

88. Which of the following correctly describes the N-methyl-D-aspartate (NMDA) receptor?

a. It controls a high-conductance anion channel
b. The NMDA channel is easily blocked by the presence of magnesium
c. NMDA is selective for ionotropic receptors
d. Insufficient amounts of glutamate, acting through NMDA receptors, may cause neuronal cell death
e. Current flow is blocked in the presence of glutamate, leading to hyperpolarization of the cell

89. Which of the following is a second messenger system directly activated by the binding of norepinephrine to a β-adrenergic receptor?

a. Inositol 1,4,5-triphosphate (IP_3)
b. Adenosine 3′,5′-cyclic phosphate (cAMP)
c. Diacylglycerol (DAG)
d. Arachidonic acid
e. Prostaglandins

90. Which of the following governs hyperpolarization of a neuron?

a. Chloride and sodium
b. Chloride and potassium
c. Potassium and sodium
d. Sodium and calcium
e. Sodium only

91. Which of the following governs the direct release of a neurotransmitter?

a. Sodium influx
b. Sodium efflux
c. Potassium influx
d. Potassium efflux
e. Calcium influx

92. Which of the following statements is appropriate to second messengers within neurons?

a. They have little effect upon receptors
b. They regulate gene expression that leads to neuronal growth and synthesis of new proteins
c. They generally do not interact in the opening or closing of ion channels
d. Glutamate always has excitatory effects upon metabotropic receptors
e. They are directly involved in the gating of sodium channels by NMDA receptors

93. NMDA, kainate, and quisqualate all act on which of the following receptors?

a. GABA receptors
b. Excitatory amino acid receptors
c. Adrenergic receptors
d. Opioid receptors
e. Dopamine receptors

The Synapse

Answers

83. The answer is e. *(Kandel, pp 178–180. Purves, pp 99–101.)* Electrical synapses are less common than chemical synapses but can be found in the nervous systems of different species. A unique feature of electrical synapses is that two neurons communicate with each other by having the membranes of each neuron lie very close together. The contact between the neurons is called a *gap junction*. These junctions contain aligned paired channels so that each paired channel forms a pore larger than those observed in ligand-gated channels and which allows for the bidirectional transmission.

84. The answer is c. *(Kandel, pp 209–217. Purves, pp 1–8, 415–417.)* Axon terminals that make synaptic contact with the soma of postsynaptic cells are frequently observed to be inhibitory and are referred to as *type II synapses*. A classic example of this is in the cerebellar cortex, where an interneuron (basket cell) makes synaptic contact with the soma of the Purkinje cell. These are chemical and not electrical synapses, and their actions are frequently mediated by GABA. Activation of the basket cell results in subsequent inhibition of the Purkinje cell. The overwhelming number of excitatory synapses are observed to be axodendritic. They are referred to as *type I synapses* and are frequently characterized by specialized extensions of the dendrites called *spines*. These synapses also display a dense basement membrane and a prominent presynaptic density. Cortical projections to the neostriatum have been shown to be excitatory and their functions mediated by glutamate.

85. The answer is a. *(Purves, pp 101–104.)* The sequence of events that occur in the transmission of a chemical synapse is as follows: The transmitter is synthesized and stored in the presynaptic vesicles. The action potential is propagated down the presynaptic axon to its presynaptic terminal. The presynaptic terminal is then depolarized, which causes the opening of voltage-gated Ca^{2+} channels. Then there is Ca^{2+} through these channels, causing the vesicles to fuse with the presynaptic membrane. The transmitter is then released into the presynaptic cleft (by exocytosis) and binds to receptor molecules in the postsynaptic membrane. This leads to the opening or closing of postsynaptic channels. The resultant current results in an EPSP or IPSP, which causes a change in excitability of the post-synaptic cell. The vesicular membrane is then retrieved from the plasma membrane.

86. The answer is d. *(Kandel, pp 207–219. Purves, pp 99–114.)* Perhaps the most significant feature of the receptor is that it serves a gating function for particular ions. It can do this either directly, if it is part of the ion channel, or indirectly, by activating a G protein that, in turn, activates a second messenger system. This process results in a modulation of the ion channel's activity. In particular, the G protein stimulates adenylate cyclase, converting ATP to cAMP. In turn, cAMP induces activation of cAMP-dependent protein kinase, which modulates channels by phosphorylating the channel protein or some other protein that works on that channel. The synaptic vesicles may be round or flat, and filled or empty. They are typically filled with a neurotransmitter that is released onto the synaptic cleft. The receptive process on the postsynaptic region (i.e., the postsynaptic receptor) takes on a very important function. The binding of the transmitter to the receptor molecule is determined by this receptor, which is a membrane-spanning protein. When the transmitter is released onto the postsynaptic membrane, it leads to an action potential in the postsynaptic neuron (see the answer to question 81 for further details). In contrast, transmission at electrical synapses are mediated through gap junctions. Because the pre-synaptic and postsynaptic membranes of (gap junctions of) electrical synapses are connected by gap junction channels, electrical synapses function by means of the passive flow of ionic current through the gap junction from one neuron to the next. Postsynaptic neurons can receive both excitatory and inhibitory inputs. A classic example is a ventral horn motor neuron, which may receive an excitatory sensory input emanating from the same side of the body and an inhibitory input from the contralateral side. (See the chapter entitled "The Spinal Cord" for further discussion of this point.) Because of the nature of the difference in mechanisms for synaptic transmission and the relative sizes of the synaptic gaps, which are much smaller for electrical synapses, the synaptic delay for electrical synapses is much shorter than that for chemical synapses.

87. The answer is b. *(Kandel, pp 214–221. Purves, pp 128–131.)* Both GABA and glycine are inhibitory transmitters found in the spinal cord and elsewhere in the CNS. Glycine was originally shown to be present in the spinal cord, but more recent studies have shown it to be present in the brain as well. However, its effects in the brain are believed to be much weaker than in the spinal cord. Both are inhibitory and act on a similar chloride channel, which, when activated, permits this ion to enter the cell and make it more negative (i.e., hyperpolarize the cell). Since both transmitters are inhibitory, it is assumed that their actions would be to inhibit seizure activity, although this has only been shown for GABA. Each of the channels is formed from a transmembrane protein. It contains a transmitter-binding site on the outer side of the membrane, and its conducting pore is embedded in the cell membrane. Another feature—that both channels produce electrical signals as a result of the movement of ions down their electrochemical gradients within their channels—is common to excitatory and inhibitory transmitters.

88. The answer is b. *(Kandel, pp 212–215. Purves, pp 127–129.)* The NMDA receptor regulates a channel permeable to several cations, which include calcium, sodium, and potassium. This channel, however, is easily blocked by magnesium. In fact, it requires a significant depolarization of the membrane in order for magnesium to be exuded from the channel so that sodium and calcium can enter the cell. Glutamate receptors can be divided into two categories: (1) metabotropic receptors that gate channels indirectly through second messengers and (2) ionotropic receptors that gate channels directly. One of the unusual features of this transmitter-gated channel is that it is also gated by voltage. Thus, conductance reaches its peak when both glutamate is present and the cell is depolarized. High concentrations of glutamate could result in death of the cell. This may be due to an unusually large influx of calcium through NMDA-activated channels. The calcium might activate proteases, resulting in the formation of free radicals that could be toxic to the cell. (See below for further discussion of NMDA receptors.)

89. The answer is b. *(Kandel, pp 181–185, 281–294. Purves, pp 103–111, 117–137.)* When norepinephrine reaches a β-adrenergic receptor, a G-protein activates adenyl cyclase, which generates a second messenger, cAMP, from ATP. cAMP activates a cAMP-dependent kinase that alters the conformation of regulatory subunits of other kinases. This frees catalytic subunits to phosphorylate-specific proteins, which in turn leads to the cellular response. IP$_3$ and DAG are associated with the transmitter acetylcholine, which binds to muscarinic receptors, and arachidonic acid is linked to histamine, which binds to histamine receptors. Prostaglandins are metabolites of arachidonic acid.

90. The answer is b. *(Kandel, pp 181–185, 281–294. Purves, pp 103–111, 117–137.)* In neurons within the CNS, an inhibitory transmitter will open chloride channels. In addition, second messengers may also mediate inhibition. It is likely that they do so by opening potassium channels. When a chloride channel is opened, it will lead to movement of this ion down its concentration gradient and into the cell. This will make the cell more negative (i.e., hyperpolarized). At the same time, there will be an efflux of potassium, which will also produce hyperpolarization of the cell because positive charges are now being removed. On the other hand, sodium and calcium influx are associated with depolarization of the cell.

91. The answer is e. *(Kandel, pp 208–226, 253–276. Purves, pp 103–111.)* Experimental methods permit evaluation of the relative contributions of different ions in the regulation of transmitter release. Neither tetrodotoxin, which blocks voltage-gated sodium channels, nor tetraethylammonium, which blocks voltage-gated potassium channels, will block the generation of a postsynaptic potential when the presynaptic cell is artificially depolarized. In contrast, presynaptic calcium influx triggers the release of the transmitter and results in a postsynaptic potential. Moreover, when presynaptic calcium influx is blocked, no postsynaptic potential is produced. Action potentials at the presynaptic axon terminals open up calcium channels, permitting calcium influx. This event helps move synaptic vesicles to active sites as actin filaments (which anchor the vesicles) are dissolved.

92. The answer is b. *(Kandel, pp 182–185, 208–226, 253–276.)* Second messenger kinases can lead to the phosphorylation of ion channel proteins. Such a process can lead to either the closing of a previously open ion channel or the opening of a previously closed channel. For example, norepinephrine acts through cAMP to close the potassium channel, resulting in an increase in excitability. Second messengers can phosphorylate transcriptional regulatory proteins and thus alter gene expression. In particular, existing proteins may be altered and new proteins may be synthesized. Moreover, such effects may generate other alterations, such as the induction of neuronal growth. Second messengers can also interact directly with an ion channel to cause it to open or close (in the absence of a protein kinase). They also can produce a level of desensitization in receptors, which is a function of the extent of phosphorylation. While glutamate excites ionotropic receptors, it has a more diverse modulatory effect upon metabotropic receptors, which could be expressed in either receptor excitation or inhibition. The direct gating of ion channels by NMDA receptors is an example of a process that does not immediately involve a second messenger.

93. The answer is b. (*Kandel, pp 212–214. Purves, pp 153–159.*) NMDA, kainate, and quisqualate act upon excitatory amino acid receptors. The NMDA receptor differs from the other types of receptors in that it is blocked by Mg^{2+} and controls a cation channel permeable to calcium, sodium, and potassium. Pharmacologically, NMDA receptors can be blocked by 2-amino-5-phosphonovaleric acid. The quisqualate receptor is activated by quisqualic acid; it has a high affinity for L-glutamate and α-amino-hydroxy-5-methyl-4-isoxazolepropionic acid (AMPA). The kainate receptor is activated by kainic acid. It regulates a channel that is permeable to sodium and potassium, binds AMPA, and is important in the process of excitotoxicity.

Neurochemistry/ Neurotransmitters

Questions

DIRECTIONS: Each item below contains a question or incomplete statement followed by suggested responses. Select the **one best** response to each question.

Item 94–95

A middle-aged man was brought into the hospital for a neurological examination after displaying uncontrollable movements of his upper limbs. The diagnosis given for this individual was that he had a rare genetic disorder affecting dopamine synthesis in brainstem neurons. However, there was some controversy concerning at what step in the biosynthesis of dopamine this failure took place.

94. One group of neurologists argued that the failure lay in the immediate precursor stage in the biosynthesis of dopamine. If this was the correct conclusion, what was the precursor?

a. Tyrosine
b. Tyrosine hydroxylase
c. Tryptophan
d. L-dihydroxyphenylalanine (L-dopa)
e. Dopamine β-hydroxylase

95. However, another group of physicians argued that this disorder was associated with the rate-limiting step in the biosynthesis of dopamine. If this was the correct analysis, what was the rate-limiting step?

a. Tryptophan hydroxylase
b. Tyrosine hydroxylase
c. Dopamine β-hydroxylase
d. Phenylethanolamine-N-methyltransferase
e. Choline acetyltransferase

96. A baby was born with an inherited autosomal recessive trait in which there was a delay in development, resulting in the occurrence of seizures and mental retardation. The child was diagnosed as having phenylketonuria (PKU). What is the likely neurochemical locus of this genetic defect?

a. Tyrosine
b. Tryptophan
c. Tryptophan hydroxylase
d. Dopamine
e. Phenylalanine (Phe) hydroxylase

97. Which of the following statements concerning the end plate potential is correct?

a. It is dependent upon the release of dopamine from the nerve ending
b. The amplitude of this potential is much higher than CNS postsynaptic potentials
c. It is an all-or-none response
d. It is unrelated to the concentration of transmitter released from the presynaptic terminals
e. It is selectively associated with the opening of chloride channels

98. What best characterizes the channel at the neuromuscular junction associated with the end plate potential?

a. Blocked by a noradrenergic β-receptor antagonist
b. Blocked by an N-methyl-D-aspartate- (NMDA-) receptor antagonist
c. Blocked by an α-amino-hydroxy-5-methyl-4-isoxazolepropionic acid- (AMPA-) receptor antagonist
d. Nicotinic gated
e. Muscarinic gated

Item 99–100

The following case relates to the next two questions. After an individual was admitted to the hospital, it was determined that he displayed a variable weakness of cranial nerve and limb muscles but showed no clinical signs of denervation from tests, which included electromyogram (EMG) recordings. This disorder was partially reversed by the administration of drugs that inhibit acetylcholinesterase.

99. From which of the following was the individual likely suffering?

a. Multiple sclerosis (MS)
b. Amyotrophic lateral sclerosis (ALS)
c. Myasthenia gravis
d. Combined system disease
e. Muscular dystrophy (MD)

100. Which of the following can constitute the likely basis for this disorder?

a. The production of excessive quantities of acetylcholine (ACh)
b. The production of antibodies that act against nicotinic ACh receptors
c. A minor stroke involving the motor strip of the cerebral cortex
d. A vitamin B deficiency
e. Viral encephalitis

101. A 10-year-old boy accidentally swallowed a toxic substance that contained a neurotoxin, whose actions mimic those of curare. This resulted in a neuromuscular blockade, partial respiratory failure, and paralysis. Which of the following is the most likely receptor to which this toxin binds?

a. $GABA_A$ receptor
b. $GABA_B$ receptor
c. Nicotinic receptor
d. NMDA receptor
e. Histamine receptor

Item 102–103

The following case relates to the next two questions. An individual who complains about disruption in limb muscle function was diagnosed with a disorder in which the transmitter released at the neuromuscular junction was not removed from the synaptic cleft.

102. What is the primary mechanism involved in removal of the transmitter at the neuromuscular junction?

a. Enzymatic degradation
b. Diffusion
c. Reuptake
d. Actions of antibodies
e. Distribution of sodium and potassium ions along muscle membrane

103. What is the enzyme required for the metabolism of the transmitter at the neuromuscular junction?

a. Choline acetyltransferase
b. Glutaminase
c. Glutamine synthetase
d. Acetylcholinesterase
e. Serine hydroxymethyltransferase

Item 104–106

The following case relates to the next three questions. An individual was admitted to the emergency room of a hospital after taking a drug of abuse that destroyed selective groups of neurons in the brainstem. After the individual became ambulatory, he was chronically depressed.

104. Which of the following neuronal groups in the brainstem might be related, either directly or indirectly, to this person's condition?

a. Vestibular nuclei
b. Nucleus ambiguus
c. Trigeminal spinal nucleus
d. Dorsal column nuclei
e. Raphe nuclei

105. What is the neurotransmitter loss most likely linked to these symptoms?
a. Enkephalin
b. Dopamine
c. Norepinephrine
d. Serotonin
e. Glycine

106. Which of the following would constitute an accepted approach toward the treatment of this disorder?
a. A serotonin reuptake inhibitor (SSRI)
b. A CNS depressant
c. A dopaminergic antagonist
d. A noradrenergic antagonist
e. An NMDA blocker

107. A functional relationship was recently suggested between excess epinephrine in the brain and manic states. If one were to develop a drug that controls mania by reducing brain epinephrine levels, at what step would such a drug act to *selectively* block the synthesis of epinephrine?
a. Tyrosine hydroxylase
b. Dopamine β-hydroxylase
c. Phenylethanolamine-N-methyltransferase
d. 5-hydroxy-indole-O-methyltransferase
e. Tryptophan hydroxylase

108. In response to a form of sleep disorder in which individuals tend to suffer from excessive sleep, a pharmaceutical company undertakes to develop a drug that selectively alleviates this problem by blocking the rate-limiting step in the biosynthesis of serotonin. Which of the following would represent the rate-limiting step?
a. Tyrosine hydroxylase
b. Tryptophan hydroxylase
c. Phenylethanolamine-N-methyltransferase
d. Dopamine β-hydroxylase
e. Glutamic acid decarboxylase

Item 109–112

The following case relates to the next four questions. An elderly individual was admitted to a hospital after a long period in which the family had complained that he showed increasing incidences of disorientation coupled with memory loss. The patient was diagnosed with Alzheimer's disease and a few years later, after further physical and mental deterioration, the patient died. An autopsy was taken of his brain and regional brain chemistry and neuropathology identified.

109. Which of the following would represent likely sites where the neuropathology could be identified?

a. Cerebellar cortex, hypothalamus, red nucleus
b. Substantia nigra, midbrain periaqueductal gray, ventrolateral thalamus
c. Nucleus gracilis, deep pontine nuclei, vestibular nuclei
d. Cerebral cortex, basal nucleus of Meynert, hippocampus
e. Fastigial nucleus, subthalamic nucleus, superior colliculus

110. Which of the following neurotransmitters is most often implicated in this disorder with respect to the affected brain regions?

a. Histamine
b. Substance P
c. ACh
d. Enkephalin
e. Dopamine

111. Which of the following would likely be shown in the affected regions upon examination of the brain?

a. A decrease in substance P in the hypothalamus and brainstem reticular formation
b. Marked degeneration of most myelinated pathways
c. Amyloid deposits and neurofibrillary tangles
d. Marked retrograde degeneration in sensory neurons of the brainstem
e. Glial loss associated with the medial lemniscus and spinothalamic pathways

112. Which of the following would constitute a promising therapeutic strategy for treatment of this disorder?

a. Surgical removal of selective regions of the cerebral cortex
b. Administration of serotonergic agonists that act specifically on cerebral cortical neurons
c. Administration of cholinergic antagonists directed against nicotinic receptors in the cerebral cortex
d. Administration of noradrenergic agonists directed against α_2 receptors in the cerebral cortex
e. Administration of compounds that slow aggregation of amyloid-β peptide into its fibrillar form

113. In their attempts to develop drugs that specifically act upon a given neurotransmitter system, pharmaceutical companies are beset with the problem that the neurotransmitter in question may have widespread presence throughout the CNS. Consequently, drugs aimed at blocking the biosynthesis or release of the neurotransmitter may generate unwarranted side effects by acting on neural systems unrelated to the neural systems the drug is designed to modulate. Of the following neurotransmitters, which one would appear to be the most difficult to work with because of its ubiquity within the CNS?

a. ACh
b. Glutamate
c. Norepinephrine
d. Dopamine
e. Substance P

Item 114–115

The following case relates to the next two questions. An individual was admitted to the emergency room and was diagnosed as having cortical damage and resultant neuronal degeneration due to an ischemic insult. The neurologist concluded that the brain damage involved neurotoxicity of those cells.

114. Which of the following neurotransmitter changes associated with neurotoxicity in this case was believed to have occurred?

a. Extracellular accumulation of norepinephrine
b. Extracellular accumulation of ACh
c. Extracellular accumulation of glutamate
d. Extracellular loss of serotonin
e. Extracellular loss of GABA

115. What is the likely mechanism underlying neurotoxicity as a result of ischemia?

a. Entry of Ca^{2+} into the cell
b. Reduction of extracellular chloride
c. Delayed removal of norepinephrine from the synapse
d. Hypersensitivity of the postsynaptic membrane to GABA
e. Failure of degradation of ACh

Item 116–117

The following case relates to the next two questions. A 50-year-old man suffered from anxiety attacks. A general medical, neurological, and psychiatric evaluation indicated that the patient was in good physical health, and, likewise, no neurological signs could be detected. Further analysis suggested that the anxiety attacks were brought on because of recent events at his place of employment, which led him to believe that his position might be terminated.

116. To treat this disorder, which of the following would most likely be administered to the patient?

a. Picrotoxin
b. Naloxone
c. Chlordiazepoxide
d. Bicuculline
e. Dopamine

117. Which of the following would be the most likely mechanism underlying the action of this drug of choice?

a. Blockade of chloride channel permeability
b. Opioid receptor blockade
c. Binding of the drug to the GABA benzodiazepine site
d. Activation of muscarinic cholinergic receptor
e. Competitive binding of the $GABA_A$-receptor site

Item 118–119

The following case relates to the next two questions. A 55-year-old female patient was admitted to the hospital for treatment of hypertension. Prior to her admission to the hospital, her blood pressure was slightly above normal, but in recent weeks, her blood pressure appeared to rise significantly. A general medical and neurological examination indicated that she was otherwise in acceptable health and that no medical or neurological signs could be detected.

118. To treat this disorder, which of the following drugs would be administered to the patient?

a. Yohimbine
b. Clonidine
c. Sodium lactate
d. Cholecystokinin
e. Carbon dioxide

119. The treatment of her hypertension by the appropriate drug (listed in question 118) was mediated by its actions on which of the following receptors?

a. Muscarinic ACh receptors
b. Dopaminergic receptors
c. α_2-adrenergic receptors
d. Serotonergic receptors
e. GABA receptors

Item 120–121

The following case relates to the next two questions. As a result of a leg injury, a 30-year-old male developed chronic pain and was subsequently treated with morphine. Consequently, he developed an addiction to morphine.

120. On which of the predominant receptor sites would this effect be mediated?

a. Opioid nociceptin receptor
b. Opioid μ receptor
c. Opioid δ receptor
d. Opioid κ receptor
e. Dopamine D$_2$-receptor

121. Based upon extensive research, which of the following regions of the brain would contain heavy concentrations of this receptor?

a. Mammillary bodies
b. Precentral gyrus
c. Midbrain periaqueductal gray
d. Inferior olivary nucleus
e. Deep pontine nuclei

Item 122–123

The following relates to the next two questions. Experimental studies aimed at providing neuroprotection against the hypoxic and ischemic effects of stroke discovered that its deleterious effects were due in part to excitotoxicity of neurons situated in the region of the stroke.

122. Based on this experimental evidence, which of the following drugs might be given to the patient in order to reduce the deleterious effects of the stroke?

a. GABA antagonist
b. Dopamine antagonist
c. Norepinephrine antagonist
d. NMDA antagonist
e. Serotonin antagonist

123. What would be the mechanism by which drug treatment (suggested from the answer to the previous question) could be effective?

a. Raising the blood pressure
b. Attempting to decrease disruption of the blood-brain barrier
c. Reducing seizure activity in the cerebral cortex and limbic system
d. Stabilizing body temperature
e. Reducing brain serotonin levels in the brainstem and cerebral cortex

Item 124–125

The following case relates to the next two questions. A patient was admitted to the hospital after experiencing increasing episodes of temporal lobe seizure activity.

124. To treat this disorder, which of the following drugs should be administered?

a. Physostigmine
b. Bicuculline
c. Pilocarpine
d. Kainate
e. Vigabatrin

125. What is the reason that the drug selected from among the choices in question 124 can be effective?

a. It blocks NMDA receptors
b. It activates noradrenergic receptors
c. It activates GABA receptors
d. It activates cholinergic receptors
e. It blocks dopamine receptors

126. Recent studies have revealed that nitric oxide may be a factor in brain injury, in particular, because nitric oxide is a source of reactive oxygen species to produce toxic compounds. If an investigator wished to reduce or eliminate the deleterious effects of nitric oxide, which of the following compounds would be used to try to block its conversion?

a. Glutamate
b. Choline
c. L-arginine
d. Tyrosine
e. Tryptophan

127. Which of the following best explains how nitric oxide differs from other "classical" neurotransmitters?

a. Nitric oxide is a gaseous transmitter
b. Nitric oxide has both excitatory and inhibitory functions
c. Nitric oxide occurs only in response to injury
d. The distribution of nitric oxide is limited to the peripheral nervous system
e. Nitric oxide is packaged in vesicles

128. A 60-year-old male has high blood pressure, and the diagnosis indicates that it is due in part to retention of water. Which of the following compounds would most likely relate to this process?

a. Oxytocin
b. Serotonin
c. Histamine
d. Vasopressin
e. Somatostatin

129. A 65-year-old man was experiencing considerable pain due to a chronic back problem and was administered morphine to alleviate the problem. Which of the following would constitute a possible mechanism by which morphine would provide effective action?

a. Release of somatostatin
b. Release of histamine
c. Release of vasopressin
d. Release of ACh
e. Release of substance P

130. Which of the following receptors requires the simultaneous binding of two different agonists for activation?

a. L-AP$_4$ receptor
b. Kainate receptor
c. NMDA receptor
d. AMPA receptor
e. GABA$_A$ receptor

131. A 16-year-old boy took the recreational drug of abuse phencyclidine (PCP or "angel dust"), resulting in an initial feeling of euphoria but followed by ataxia, sweating, seizures, and respiratory depression. To which of the following mechanisms would the deleterious effects of the drug in part be due?

a. Blockade of NMDA receptors
b. Blockade of AMPA receptors
c. Blockade of cholinergic receptors
d. Blockade of $GABA_A$ receptors
e. Blockade of $GABA_B$ receptors

132. A patient was diagnosed with a form of epilepsy. One approach in treating this disorder is to give the patient a drug that would have a selective blocking action upon neurotransmitter receptors. Which of the following receptors would such a drug block in order to serve as an effective treatment procedure?

a. GABA receptors
b. Glutamate receptors
c. Nicotinic receptors
d. Serotonin receptors
e. Glycine receptors

133. Monoamines differ from neuroactive peptides in which of the following ways?

a. Monoamines are synthesized only in the cell body of neurons
b. Synthesis of monoamines is governed by messenger RNA (mRNA) on ribosomes, which is not true for neuroactive peptides
c. Monoamines are generally synthesized as part of a larger precursor molecule, called a *prohormone*
d. Monoamine neurons are generally regarded as having only excitatory properties, while peptides are inhibitory
e. Monoamine neurons are principally found within brainstem nuclei, while peptide-containing neurons are found throughout the brain

134. Which of the following enzymes is directly responsible for the degradation of norepinephrine?

a. Tryptophan hydroxylase
b. Tyrosine hydroxylase
c. Dopamine β-hydroxylase
d. Catechol-O-methyltransferase
e. Choline acetyltransferase

135. A 50-year-old woman has been treated over the past six months with lithium for an ongoing emotional disorder. From which of the following disorders is this patient suffering?

a. Panic attacks
b. Schizophrenia
c. Obsessive-compulsive disorder
d. Bipolar disorder
e. Anxiety

136. Administration of which of the following could produce a long-lasting depletion of norepinephrine?

a. Amphetamine
b. Apomorphine
c. Clonidine
d. Reserpine
e. Yohimbine

137. In a recent study, catecholamine release was markedly attenuated when an agonist was administered to the experimental preparation. Which of the following could best account for this result?

a. The presence of a GABAergic neuron at the synapse
b. Postsynaptic inhibition
c. The presence of presynaptic autoreceptors
d. Destruction of the catecholamine cell body
e. Collateral inhibition

138. Removal of norepinephrine from the region of the synaptic cleft may be achieved by which of the following mechanisms?

a. Reuptake
b. Enzymatic degradation
c. Diffusion
d. A combination of enzymatic degradation and diffusion
e. A combination of enzymatic degradation, diffusion, and reuptake

Neurochemistry/ Neurotransmitters

Answers

94. The answer is d. *(Siegel et al., pp 244–246. Kandel, pp 282–284.)* The biosynthesis of catecholamines includes the following steps: Tyrosine is converted into L-dihydroxyphenylalanine (L-dopa) by tyrosine hydroxylase. L-dopa is then decarboxylated by a decarboxylase to form dopamine (and CO_2). The conversion of dopamine to norepinephrine comes about by the action of the enzyme dopamine β-hydroxylase. The rate-limiting enzyme in the biosynthesis of serotonin is tryptophan hydroxylase. In this process, tryptophan is converted to 5-hydroxytryptophan by tryptophan hydroxylase and by 5-hydroxytryptophan decarboxylase into serotonin.

95. The answer is b. *(Kandel, pp 282–284. Siegel et al., pp 284–285.)* As indicated in the answer to question 90, the rate-limiting step in the biosynthesis of dopamine is tyrosine hydroxylase, which converts tyrosine into L-dopa. The rate-limiting step in the biosynthesis of serotonin is tryptophan hydroxylase. The enzyme dopamine β-hydroxylase converts dopamine to norepinephrine. Phenylethanolamine-N-methyltransferase is involved in the conversion of norepinephrine to epinephrine. Choline acetyltransferase is involved in the biosynthesis of ACh.

96. The answer is e. *(Kandel, pp 36–37. Siegel et al., pp 244–245. Gilroy, pp 370–371.)* Phenylketonuria results in severe mental retardation and is caused by a defect in the gene that provides the code for Phe hydroxylase, the enzyme that converts Phe to tyrosine. As a result of this defective gene, there is an abundance of Phe in the brain, which produces a toxic metabolite, thus interfering in brain development and maturation.

97. The answer is b. *(Kandel, pp 187–197.)* The amplitude of the end plate potential differs from that of postsynaptic potentials observed in the CNS in that end plate potentials can be as great as 70 times larger than CNS postsynaptic potentials. The end plate potential is dependent upon the release of ACh from the nerve endings. Dopamine is not released at the neuromuscular junction. The end plate potential is a graded potential and is not an all-or-none response. Another important feature of this potential is that it is directly related to the quantity of neurotransmitter (ACh) released from the presynaptic terminals. The release of ACh onto the muscle membrane is associated with the opening of sodium and potassium channels, and not chloride channels.

98. The answer is d. *(Kandel, pp 196–198.)* The transmitter at the neuromuscular junction is ACh, and its actions are mediated by the nicotinic ACh-gated channel. As noted, it produces the end plate potential by permitting the passage of both sodium and potassium ions. Noradrenergic, muscarinic, and excitatory amino acid receptors are not known to function at the neuromuscular junction.

99–100. The answers are 99-c, 100-b. *(Kandel, pp 298–304. Gilroy, pp 623–639, 640–642. Siegel et al., pp 871–883.)* Myasthenia gravis is an autoimmune disease that causes cranial nerve and limb muscle weakness by producing antibodies that act against the nicotinic receptor at the neuromuscular junction. The result is that the action of nerve fibers that innervate skeletal muscle is affected, producing loss of the effects of ACh at the neuromuscular junction. The net result is a reduction of the size of the action potential in the muscle, producing a weakness in the affected muscle. This disorder is reversed by administration of drugs that inhibit the enzyme, acetylcholinesterase, that degrades ACh. MS, ALS, and combined system disease (see the chapter entitled "The Spinal Cord") involve damage to axons and/or nerve cells within the CNS, producing much more profound damage to motor functions and, in the case of combined system disease, damage to both motor and sensory systems. MD is typically characterized, in part, by progressive weakness of muscles and degeneration of the muscle fibers. The other disorders listed all affect the CNS, and thus the symptoms associated with these disorders differ significantly from those described in this case. Excessive release of ACh is not a realistic event that is likely to occur (except from the bite of a black widow spider). In theory, if it were to occur, there is no reason to believe that muscular weakness would be a symptom. Instead, there would be some rigidity and muscle spasms.

101. The answer is c. *(Siegel et al., pp 874–877.)* The α-toxins, including α-bungarotoxin, can produce postsynaptic effects similar to those observed with curare, by binding specifically to the α-subunits of the nicotinic ACh receptor. In the case of the neuromuscular junction, the binding is to the α-subunit of the nicotinic ACh receptor. Because of the selective actions of α-bungarotoxin upon the ACh receptor, it has been used effectively as an experimental tool to study the properties and actions of ACh and its associated receptors.

102–103. The answers are 102-a, 103-d. *(Kandel, pp 107–112, 294–295. Siegel et al., pp 342–343, 877–879.)* There are three basic mechanisms by which the transmitter is removed from the synaptic cleft: (1) enzymatic degradation, (2) reuptake, and (3) diffusion. In the case of the neuromuscular junction, ACh (and not glutamate) is the neurotransmitter and the primary mechanism involves enzymatic degradation. The enzyme involved is acetylcholinesterase, which helps break down ACh into acetate and choline. Choline is then taken up by the presynaptic terminal. Concerning the other choices, choline acetyltransferase is the enzyme involved in the synthesis of ACh; glutaminase and glutamine synthetase are involved in the formation of glutamate from glutamine and glutamine from glutamate, respectively. Serine hydroxymethyltransferase is the enzyme that converts serine into glycine.

104–106. The answers are 104-e, 105-d, 106-a. *(Siegel et al., pp 264–287. Kandel, pp 280–295.)* There is an increasing body of evidence that reductions in serotonin levels play an important role in depressive disorders. The raphe neurons, located along the midline of the brainstem, provide the basic sites of serotonergic neurons that project to all parts of the brain and spinal cord. The other choices refer to structures that concern motor and/or sensory functions mainly associated with cranial nerves. Since the raphe neurons were damaged, the neurotransmitter most likely responsible for the onset of depression in this instance is serotonin. It is possible that other transmitter systems, such as the catecholamines, may also play a role in this disorder; however, they would not be chiefly responsible for the disorder in this instance because of the restricted locus of the lesion. Recent practice has been to treat depression with serotonin reuptake inhibitors such as fluoxetine (Prozac), which has been found to be effective after several weeks of treatment. The other choices for question 106 would be inappropriate because they would likely have a depressant effect on CNS functions.

107. The answer is c. *(Kandel, pp 282–284. Siegel et al., pp 244–246, 268–270.)* Tyrosine is the amino acid substrate from which dopamine, norepinephrine, and epinephrine are formed. Tyrosine is converted into

L-dopa by tyrosine hydroxylase. L-dopa is decarboxylated by a decarboxylase into dopamine (and CO_2). Dopamine is converted into norepinephrine by dopamine β-hydroxylase. Norepinephrine is converted into epinephrine by phenylethanolamine-N-methyltransferase. Melatonin is formed from serotonin. 5-hydroxy-indole-O-methyltransferase is part of the final step in the conversion of serotonin into melatonin. Trytophan hydroxylase is the rate-limiting step in the biosynthesis of serotonin.

108. The answer is b. (*Kandel, pp 281–287.*) The rate-limiting step or controlling reaction in the biosynthesis of serotonin is tryptophan hydroxylase, which converts tryptophan into 5-hydroxytryptophan. Three of the other enzymes listed as choices—tyrosine hydroxylase, phenylethanolamine-N-methyltransferase, and dopamine β-hydroxylase—are, as noted in the explanation to question 107, involved in the biosynthetic pathways for norepinephrine and epinephrine. Glutamic acid decarboxylase is utilized in the synthesis of GABA.

109–112. The answers are 109-d, 110-c, 111-c, 112-e. (*Kandel, pp 1151–1157. Siegel et al., pp 950–965.*) The primary regions shown to be affected by Alzheimer's disease include the basal nucleus of Meynert (which contains cholinergic neurons that project widely to the forebrain, including the cerebral cortex), the hippocampal formation, and the cerebral cortex. The other choices included structures that have not been significantly implicated in this disorder. The neurotransmitter that has been most implicated in this disorder is ACh. Alzheimer's brains have been shown to have reduced levels of ACh and cholinergic markers, especially after damage to cholinergic neurons of the basal nucleus of Meynert. While reductions in other neurotransmitter levels may also occur, the other choices of neurotransmitters presented have not been clearly implicated in this disorder. One of the clearest neuropathological characteristics of Alzheimer's disease is the presence of amyloid deposits and neurofibrillary tangles in the cerebral cortex. In fact, there has been a new and promising strategy that has been applied for the treatment of Alzheimer's disease. It involves the attempt to administer small molecules that retard the aggregation of amyloid-β peptides that form fibrillar amyloid plaques, which affect the normal functions of neurons.

113. The answer is b. (*Purves, pp 153–155. Siegel et al., pp 328–332.*) The largest numbers of excitatory synapses in the CNS are mediated by glutamate, as it is believed that approximately half of the synapses in the brain release glutamate. For example, functions mediated by fibers that originate from the cerebral cortex and descend to such regions as the neostriatum, thalamus, brainstem, and spinal cord are generally believed to be mediated by glutamate. Many other neuronal systems throughout the brain and spinal cord utilize glutamate as well. Dopaminergic and noradrenergic neurons, while mostly excitatory, can also be inhibitory at some synapses and are less numerous than glutamate. Cholinergic and substance P synapses are also excitatory, but are likewise less numerous than glutamate.

114–115. The answers are 114-c, 115-a. *(Purves, p 130. Siegel et al., pp 328–332.)* It has been discovered that one mechanism of neurodegeneration involves prolonged activation of neurons by glutamate. It is believed that if glutamate accumulates in the extracellular space and is not removed, the presence of glutamate will effectively stimulate the neuron to death. It has been shown that neurotoxicity is linked to cell death after a stroke, which causes brain ischemia and oxygen deprivation. Glutamate receptors are involved in ischemic cell damage in the following way: glutamate released from the presynaptic terminal would normally activate NMDA and AMPA receptors in the postsynaptic membrane. This results in an increase in the intracellular concentration of Ca^{2+}, which remains long after the initial stimulus is removed, and thus prevents the cell from reestablishing a resting membrane potential. The net effect here is to produce injury (or death) to the cell.

116–117. The answers are 116-c, 117-c. *(Siegel et al., pp 336–340.)* One of the strategies used effectively for the treatment of anxiety disorders is to use classes of drugs that suppress CNS activity. One such class includes benzodiazepine agonists, such as chlordiazepoxide. This drug enhances GABA transmission by binding to the benzodiazepine site on the $GABA_A$-receptor benzodiazepine chloride ionophore complex. In this manner, it acts as a GABA agonist, producing anxiolytic, sedative, and anticonvulsant effects. The other choices for both questions relate to drugs that have opposite effects, namely, ones with excitatory effects on CNS neurons.

118–119. The answers are 118-b, 119-c. *(Kandel, pp 1214–1222. Siegel et al., pp 1080–1086.)* Clonidine has long been used effectively for the treatment of hypertension. The other choices listed are compounds that can induce panic attacks and are, therefore, inappropriate for the treatment of this patient. Clonidine is an adrenergic agonist whose functions are mediated by its actions upon α_2 receptors. Administration of this drug results in an overall decrease in noradrenergic transmission. Although the precise mechanism by which the effects of clonidine become manifest is unknown, it may be that it reduces noradrenergic transmission by acting upon α_2 presynaptic receptors, which typically produce autoinhibition of the noradrenergic pathways.

120–121. The answers are 120-b, 121-c. *(Kandel, pp 480–484. Siegel et al., pp 1096–1098.)* Research conducted over the past two decades has shown that the actions of morphine are mediated through opioid μ receptors, while other opioid receptors appear not to play a significant role. Likewise, dopamine receptors are not involved in this process. The region of the brain where opioid receptors are very heavily concentrated is the midbrain periaqueductal gray. This region plays an important role in the modulation of pain and is particularly responsive to opioid activation by morphine. While other areas of the brain indicated in question 117 may also contain opioid receptors, concentrations of this receptor are not known to be high (including a structure such as the mammillary bodies, for which no known functions have been identified). Moreover, none of these regions are known to play any role in the regulation of pain.

122–123. The answers are 122-d, 123-b. *(Siegel et al., pp 715–721.)* As mentioned earlier in the explanations for questions 114 and 115, glutamate has been implicated in ischemia-induced brain damage following brain trauma such as a stroke. It has also been shown that administration of NMDA-receptor antagonists following a stroke is effective by reducing tissue infarction and neuronal cell death. The other choices listed in question 122 are not known to relate to the reversal of the deleterious effects of stroke. The NMDA-receptor antagonist is effective, in part, by decreasing disruption of the blood-brain barrier. It has been suggested that this becomes manifest by a blockade of the neuronal production of reactive oxygen species that occurs as a result of activation of NMDA receptors. Again, the other choices listed for question 123 have no known relationship to the process in question.

124–125. The answers are 124-e, 125-c. *(Siegel et al., pp 755–763.)* One of the drugs that has been used effectively for the treatment of epilepsy, especially complex partial seizures involving the temporal lobe, has been vigabatrin. The other choices of drugs are ones that enhance convulsive activity either by facilitating excitatory transmitter function or by inhibiting inhibitory transmitter functions. Vigabatrin functions by enhancing GABA-mediated inhibition of neurons, perhaps by the inhibition of GABA-transaminase.

126. The answer is c. *(Kandel, p 295. Purves, pp 173–175, 460, 465. Siegel et al., pp 442–443.)* Nitric oxide is synthesized from L-arginine when stimulated by nitric oxide synthase. Choline is a precursor of ACh, tyrosine of dopamine and norepinephrine, and tryptophan of serotonin. Glutamate, a neurotransmitter, is synthesized from glutamine and can be converted into GABA by glutamic acid decarboxylase.

127. The answer is a. *(Purves, pp 173–175. Kandel, p 295. Siegel et al., pp 442–444, 725–727.)* Nitric oxide differs from more classical, or traditional, neurotransmitters in that, in addition to acting as a neurotransmitter, it is a gas and also acts as a second messenger. After nitric oxide is formed, it diffuses locally and interacts with specific molecules such as the enzyme catalyzing cyclic guanosine 5′-monophosphate (cGMP) synthesis, guanylyl. A number of different neurotransmitters can have either excitatory or inhibitory effects, depending upon the receptors with which they interact. Since nitric oxide is coupled to a variety of neurotransmitter systems, it is likely that it is also involved in both excitatory and inhibitory processes. Recent studies have shown that nitric oxide is likely involved in a wide variety of processes and is not limited to a single function. Moreover, it is widely distributed throughout both the CNS as well as in the peripheral nervous system. While many transmitters are packaged in synaptic vesicles, nitric oxide differs by diffusing widely without being packaged in synaptic vesicles.

128. The answer is d. *(Kandel, pp 978–980.)* Vasopressin is produced mainly from the magnocellular neurons of the hypothalamus. The hormone is released into the capillaries of the posterior pituitary. When it is released into the vascular system, it stimulates the kidneys to conserve water. The action of oxytocin is related to functions of the uterus and breasts. This hormone plays a role in the expulsion of the fetus at birth and in the milk ejection reflex following suckling. Substance P, histamine, and somatostatin are not known to relate specifically to this process.

129. The answer is b. *(Siegel et al., pp 294–310.)* When an opioid compound, especially a μ-receptor agonist (such as morphine), is administered in response to chronic pain, this causes the release of histamine in neurons. This leads to the activation of histamine H_2 receptors, which play a role in the relief of pain. In fact, there are ongoing attempts now to develop drugs, such as histamine H_3-receptor compounds, which have been shown to mediate antinociception and have anti-inflammatory properties as well. The other choices listed in this question are not known to relate to the alleviation of pain, in particular, with respect to morphine administration. In fact, substance P is associated with the elicitation of pain impulses.

130. The answer is c. (*Siegel et al., pp 315–325.*) NMDA receptors are unique among receptors in that they require the simultaneous binding of two different agonists for their activation. NMDA ion channels are opened after such compounds as glutamate and glycine are applied to the membranes that include NMDA receptors. Recent evidence has shown that a metabotropic glutamate receptor, L-AP$_4$, is present in the retina. Activation of this receptor may serve to hyperpolarize bipolar neurons within the retina. Glutamate activation (of this receptor) constitutes an unusual action because most neurons in the CNS are depolarized by glutamate. AMPA is one of several classes of ionotropic glutamate receptors and functions as a synaptic receptor for fast excitatory synaptic transmission mediated through glutamate. The other choices, kainate and GABA receptors, do not have this property.

131. The answer is a. (*Siegel et al., pp 319–321.*) NMDA ion channels are opened by both glutamate and glycine. On the other hand, Mg^{2+} generates a voltage-dependent block of this ion channel. The drug of abuse, phencyclidine (PCP), also utilizes a similar mechanism to block NMDA-receptor channels. The other choices do not relate to this mechanism with respect to PCP.

132. The answer is b. (*Siegel et al., pp 326–333.*) Excitatory amino acids and, in particular, the glutamate family of compounds have long been thought to play an important role in epileptiform activity. Epileptiform activity typically includes AMPA-receptor activation. However, as the seizure becomes more intense, there is increased involvement of NMDA receptors. This is evidenced by the facts that NMDA antagonists can reduce the intensity and length of the seizure activity and that, following removal of human epileptic hippocampal tissue, there is an up-regulation of both AMPA and NMDA receptors. Metabotropic glutamate receptors have been shown to be present in the retina but have not yet been demonstrated to be present in regions of the brain that are typically epileptogenic. GABA and glycine are inhibitory transmitters; therefore, seizures would logically block such receptor activation. There has been no substantive evidence concerning the role of cortical nicotinic receptors in epilepsy.

133. The answer is e. *(Purves, pp 117–137.)* Peptides differ from other neurotransmitters in several ways. Monoamines can be formed in all parts of the neuron with the completion of synthesis in the nerve terminal. In contrast, peptides are formed as a result of mRNA that is directed upon ribosomes, thus limiting the site of synthesis to the cell body, where the processing is accomplished by the endoplasmic reticulum and Golgi apparatus. Typically, different neuroactive peptides are cleaved from a single, much larger molecule (a prohormone) that has no biologic activity. The active peptide is cleaved by specific peptidases and is ultimately transported down the axon to the nerve terminal. In addition, the overwhelming majority of monoamine neurons are situated in the brainstem, while neuroactive peptides can be found over widespread regions of both the brainstem and the forebrain, and, in particular, the limbic structures. Both monoamines and peptides may display inhibitory as well as excitatory properties. For example, enkephalins are generally inhibitory, while substance P neurons are excitatory. Monoamine neurons may have excitatory effects in one region of the brain and inhibitory effects in another region.

134. The answer is d. *(Kandel, pp 280–286. Purves, pp 127–137.)* Tryptophan hydroxylase, tyrosine hydroxylase, and choline acetyltransferase are enzymes that are critical for the biosynthesis of serotonin, catecholamines, and ACh, respectively. Dopamine β-hydroxylase converts dopamine to norepinephrine. Catechol-O-methyltransferase and monoamine oxidase are critical for the metabolic degradation of catecholamines.

135. The answer is d. *(Siegel et al., pp 1080–1082. Kandel, pp 1213–1216.)* Lithium has been used for a number of years as an effective drug for the treatment of bipolar disorders. It has been shown to decrease the length, severity, and recurrence of manic states as well as the depressive components of this disorder. The mechanism of action of lithium in effectively combating bipolar disorder is not absolutely clear, since it has a wide variety of biological effects. In part, these include changes in the expression of some G-proteins and subtypes of adenyl cyclase, alteration of the coupling of G-proteins to neurotransmitter receptors, alterations of monoamine levels and receptors, and effects upon ion channels. Monoaminergic drugs are generally used for the treatment of panic disorders and, to some extent, to treat anxiety. Anxiety attacks are also treated with benzodiazepine drugs.

Drugs for the treatment of epilepsy generally include those that increase or maintain GABA levels or decrease glutamate levels. For schizophrenia, a wide range of drugs have been used; these include those that affect monoaminergic, cholinergic, and GABAergic systems. See question 453 and its answer for further discussion.

136. The answer is d. (*Kandel, pp 280–286. Purves, pp 127–137.*) Reserpine interferes with the uptake-storage mechanism associated with amine granules, which results in destruction of these granules. Administration of this drug will produce long-lasting depletion of norepinephrine. Amphetamine blocks the reuptake mechanism and, thus, produces a net increase in the release of norepinephrine. Apomorphine is a nonspecific dopamine agonist; clonidine is an α_2-receptor agonist, and yohimbine is an α_2-receptor antagonist.

137. The answer is c. (*Kandel, pp 280–286. Siegel et al., pp 247, 1078. Purves, pp 127–137.*) These findings can best be explained in terms of a mechanism that involves presynaptic autoreceptors. These receptors modulate the release of a catecholamine by responding to the concentration of this transmitter within the synapse. It thus represents a specific negative feedback mechanism. For example, if the concentration of transmitter in the synapse is high, then release will likely be inhibited. Less inhibition (i.e., more transmitter release) will occur if concentrations are low. Other choices are incorrect. The presence of a GABAergic neuron at the synapse, postsynaptic inhibition, and collateral inhibition are unrelated, since they refer to events that are associated with the postsynaptic neuron, not the catecholamine (presynaptic) neuron. As a result of the phasic nature of this phenomenon, destruction of the catecholamine cell body would produce events that were not phasic; indeed, there would be permanent loss of the neuron's capacity to release transmitter.

138. The answer is e. (*Kandel, pp 281–286. Purves, pp 120–135.*) There are three mechanisms by which a transmitter is removed from the region of the synaptic cleft. The most common one is reuptake, in which transporter molecules mediate high-affinity reuptake that is specific for the transmitter in question. Other mechanisms include diffusion, which removes some components of the transmitter substance, and enzymatic degradation of the amine achieved by the enzymes monoamine oxidase and catechol-O-methyltransferase.

The Spinal Cord

Questions

DIRECTIONS: Each item below contains a question or incomplete statement followed by suggested responses. Select the **one best** response to each question.

139. A college student received an injury as a result of being tackled in a football game. After the game, the student was treated at a local hospital and was found to be unable to abduct and rotate the left arm at the shoulder, flex the elbow, and extend the wrist of the left side. Further examination revealed depression of the biceps reflex of this limb, but the reflex activity involving the other limbs was normal. Which of the following is the most likely site of the injury?

a. Precentral gyrus
b. Basilar pons
c. Ventral horn cells at C1
d. Nerve roots of C5–C6
e. Triceps muscle

140. A neurological examination of a 75-year-old male revealed that when the abdominal wall was stroked, the muscles of the abdominal wall of the side of the body stimulated failed to contract. Other neurological tests appeared normal. Which of the following is the most likely region of the injury?

a. C1–C5 spinal segments
b. C6–T1 spinal segments
c. T2–T7 spinal segments
d. T8–T12 spinal segments
e. L1–L5 spinal segments

141. A 65-year-old female found that she had weakness when attempting to flex her left knee and extend the hip. Neurophysiological analysis of the affected regions revealed a reduced number of motor units firing with fasciculations and slowed conduction velocity. There was no depression of tendon reflexes or muscle wasting. Likewise, plantar and abdominal reflexes were normal, and there was little sensory loss, nor were there any signs of sphincter disturbances. Which of the following is the best explanation for this disturbance?

a. Peripheral neuropathy of nerves on the left side of the body that exit the spinal cord at L4–S1
b. Damage of the neuromuscular junctions associated with nerves that exit the left side of the spinal cord between T8 and L3
c. Degeneration of nerve cells in the ventral horn of the left side of the spinal cord between T8 and T12
d. Degeneration of fibers contained in the lateral funiculus of the left side of the thoracic spinal cord
e. Damage to the dorsal horn of the spinal cord of the left side between L1 and L4

142. A 55-year-old man discovered that he had pain in the neck and right arm and weakness in extending the fingers of his right hand, with loss of sensation in the right thumb and middle fingers. A neurological examination further revealed a weakness of the right biceps reflex, but other neurological signs could not be detected. What is the most likely diagnosis of this individual?

a. Syringomyelia involving the cervical cord
b. A knife wound of the right arm completely severing nerves innervating the biceps muscle
c. Prolapse of a cervical disk
d. Poliomyelitis involving the cervical cord
e. AIDS

143. A 60-year-old woman was hospitalized with a severe respiratory infection for several weeks. Afterward, she displayed symptoms of myalgia and weakness of the lower limbs. In addition, she also showed loss of muscle tone and some flaccidity, with loss of tendon reflexes. Examination also revealed a weakness of facial muscles. This constellation of symptoms progressed for approximately two weeks and persisted for more than a year, at which time recovery took place at a slow rate. There was also some demyelination coupled with lymphatic inflammation at the site of the demyelination. What is the most likely cause of this patient's condition?

a. Myasthenia gravis
b. Muscular dystrophy (MD)
c. Multiple sclerosis (MS)
d. Guillain-Barré syndrome
e. Lumbar disk prolapse

Item 144–145

The following case relates to the next two questions. A 46-year-old man found that, over a period of time, he developed progressive bilateral weakness of both upper and lower limbs beginning with the muscles of the hands. However, testing revealed that sensory functions appeared normal. Eventually, this individual was found to have wasting of muscles, fasciculations, and evidence of UMN dysfunction, together with an increase in tendon reflexes. After a few additional months, the patient developed facial weakness and an inability to swallow (dysphagia). Further analysis revealed abnormalities in the electromyegram (EMG) of the upper and lower extremities, denervation atrophy. However, the CSF remained normal.

144. From what was this patient most likely suffering?

a. Multiple sclerosis (MS)
b. Amyotrophic lateral sclerosis (ALS)
c. Poliomyelitis
d. Myasthenia gravis
e. A cerebral cortical stroke

145. What are the regions affected by this disorder?

a. Dorsal horns of the spinal cord
b. Lateral columns of the spinal cord
c. Ventral horns of the spinal cord
d. Dorsal columns and ventral horns of the spinal cord
e. Ventral horns and lateral columns of the spinal cord

146. A 38-year-old woman was referred to a neurologist because she complained of visual loss and muscle weakness. Subsequent examination revealed additional signs: impairment of other sensations, which included tingling and burning sensations, weakness of the lower limbs, paralysis of the upper limbs, progressive impairment of gait, signs of UMN involvement (i.e., spasticity and increased tendon reflexes), and bladder disturbances. No signs of infection were detected as measured by blood analysis, cultures, and chest x-ray. However, elevations in CSF protein were noted as well as an abnormal IgG synthesis. Which of the following is the most appropriate diagnosis of this patient?

a. Diffuse cerebellar degeneration
b. Amyotrophic lateral sclerosis (ALS)
c. Multiple sclerosis (MS)
d. A peripheral neuropathy
e. A prefrontal cortical brain tumor

DIRECTIONS: Each group of questions below consists of lettered options followed by a set of numbered items. For each numbered item, select the **one** lettered option with which it is most closely associated. Each lettered option may be used once, more than once, or not at all.

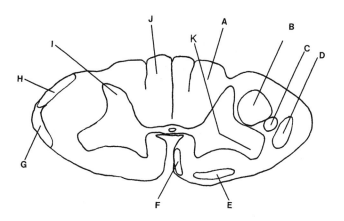

Item 147–155

Use the figure to answer these questions.

147. An 18-year-old male received a knife wound in his right arm, partially severing the peripheral nerve. Afterward, he complained about loss of some sensation. A neurological examination indicated a loss of ability to experience vibration sensation, two-point discrimination, and some pain. Which of the structures shown in the figure mediate two-point discrimination and vibration sensation that would normally be transmitted to the brain but which was affected by the injury?

148. A 44-year-old woman experienced excruciating pain emanating from her left leg. It was concluded that she was suffering from a disorder of unknown etiology for which drug treatment proved ineffective. A decision was made to surgically cut the pathway mediating pain from the left leg to the brain. Which of the structures shown in the figure was cut by the neurosurgeon?

149. A middle-aged woman was admitted to the hospital after suffering a stroke limited to the motor cortex. The patient presented with a classic UMN paralysis. Which pathway degenerated as a result of the stroke?

150. An elderly man was brought to the emergency room after fainting in his home. A subsequent MRI suggested the presence of a small stroke limited to the medial aspect of the rostral part of the midbrain tegmentum. Which pathway would most likely be affected by the stroke?

151. A 30-year-old man was brought to the emergency room after sustaining a work-related injury that damaged part of his spinal cord. A neurological examination revealed that the patient presented with a considerable loss of extensor muscle function. Which of the structures shown in the figure was damaged that could account for this defect?

152. A vascular lesion of the spinal cord resulted in loss of muscle spindle information to the cerebellum from the left leg. Which structure shown in the figure was most likely affected by this lesion?

153. A clinical procedure was formulated that enabled a neurosurgeon to microinject a neurotransmitter-receptor blocking agent into the region occupied by terminal endings of first-order neurons in the spinal cord in order to prevent transmission of pain impulses to the brain. Which of the sites shown in the figure would be most appropriate for administration of the drug?

154. A massive stroke of the motor regions of the cerebral cortex caused voluntary loss of movement. Among the fiber pathways that were affected by the stroke was a component that passes through the ipsilateral spinal cord. Which of the pathways shown in the figure would most likely be affected by the stroke?

155. A compression of the spinal cord could affect a variety of fiber tracts. Following such a compression, one such pathway would include fibers that convey information concerning whole limb movement from the lower limb and that reach the cerebellum via the superior cerebellar peduncle. Which of the pathways shown in the figure would sustain damage that is associated with this function?

Item 156–158

Each of the following effects may be caused by a lesion at a particular site. **Using the previous diagram,** where are the loci of each of the causative lesions listed below?

156. LMN paralysis

157. UMN deficit

158. Ataxia of movement

DIRECTIONS: Each item below contains a question or incomplete statement followed by suggested responses. Select the **one best** response to each question.

159. The level of the section of the spinal cord depicted on the previous diagram represents the location at which an individual received a knife wound that destroyed the right half of the spinal cord. Which of the following deficits would result from the knife wound?

a. Impaired bladder functions only
b. Impaired movements of the lower limb only
c. Impaired movements of the upper limb only
d. Loss of sensory functions of the lower limb only
e. Loss of both sensory and motor functions of the upper and lower limbs

160. Which of the following would excite the polar regions of the muscle spindle?

a. Unmyelinated C fibers
b. 1A fibers
c. Gamma motor neurons
d. Alpha motor neurons
e. General visceral efferent fibers

Item 161–164

An individual suffered a severe injury that resulted in the crushing of the peripheral nerves that normally enter the spinal cord at levels C7–T1, causing both motor and sensory loss.

161. Which region of the body would be affected by the injury?

a. Back of the head
b. Neck
c. Shoulder
d. Hand
e. Back

162. Concerning sensory loss in the affected region, which of the following sensations in first-order sensory neurons were affected and which normally terminate in laminae I and II of the spinal cord?

a. Tactile sensation
b. Pain and temperature sensation
c. Unconscious proprioception limited to inputs from muscle spindles
d. Unconscious proprioception limited to inputs from Golgi tendon organs
e. Inputs associated with pressure receptors

163. Which of the following is the principal transmitter that would have been released by the axon terminals of the affected first-order pain and temperature fibers?

a. Enkephalins
b. Acetylcholine (ACh)
c. Substance P
d. γ-aminobutyric acid (GABA)
e. Serotonin

164. Of the overall affected sensory fibers that enter the spinal cord, one group passes through Lissauer's marginal zone. Which of the following statements correctly characterizes the fibers in this region?

a. They mediate unconscious proprioception
b. This zone is composed of coarse, heavily myelinated fibers
c. Fibers within Lissauer's marginal zone may ascend or descend several segments
d. These fibers synapse with alpha motor neurons of extensor muscles
e. Cells in this zone typically project to thalamic nuclei

165. A small peripheral nerve injury involving some of the axons that enter the spinal cord at L1 affected principally fibers that innervate the nucleus dorsalis of Clarke. Which of the following is (are) the primary dysfunctions resulting from this injury?

a. Loss of autonomic functions
b. Loss of unconscious proprioceptive information
c. Loss of pain and temperature sensation
d. UMN paralysis
e. LMN paralysis

166. A patient was diagnosed with a form of motor neuron disease that initially affects neurons situated in the dorsolateral aspect of the ventral horn at L1–L4. Which of the following arrangements best describes the deficit likely to be present?

a. LMN paralysis involving the hand
b. UMN paralysis of the upper limb
c. LMN paralysis of the back muscles
d. LMN paralysis of the leg
e. UMN paralysis of the leg

167. A small vascular lesion that affected the region of the ventromedial white matter of the cervical cord was discovered in a middle-aged man during a neurological examination. The neurologist came to the conclusion that the lesion affected the descending fibers of the medial longitudinal fasciculus (MLF). What deficit did the neurologist observe that led him to this conclusion?

a. The patient presented with a UMN paralysis
b. The patient displayed difficulties in regulating his head position in response to postural changes
c. The patient displayed an LMN paralysis
d. The patient displayed ataxia of movement
e. The patient experienced significant difficulties in regulating blood pressure and bladder functions

Item 168–169

A 26-year-old woman complained about loss of some sensation on both sides of her body that seemed to be localized around the region of her waist. A neurological examination revealed that the primary sensations lost were pain and temperature, although some bilateral loss of light touch was also noted.

168. Which of the following was the most likely locus of the lesion?

a. Dorsal funiculus on both sides
b. Dorsal root ganglion, bilaterally
c. Region surrounding the central canal
d. Midline region of the lower medulla
e. Region of the ventral horn, bilaterally

169. Which of the following pathways were most likely affected by the lesion?

a. Lateral spinothalamic tract, anterior spinothalamic tract, posterior spinocerebellar tract
b. Anterior spinothalamic tract, lateral spinothalamic tract, anterior corticospinal tract
c. Anterior spinocerebellar tract, posterior spinocerebellar tract, lateral vestibulospinal tract
d. Anterior corticospinal tract, lateral spinothalamic tract, dorsal columns
e. Medial vestibulospinal tract, lateral spinothalamic tract, anterior spinothalamic tract

170. Which of the following statements concerning muscle spindles is true?

a. They detect the rate of change of muscle length
b. They are high-threshold receptors
c. They are arranged in series with the extrafusal muscle fibers
d. They contain a single type of intrafusal fiber
e. They are primarily tension detectors

171. An 18-year-old male was involved in a fight, which resulted in his being shot in the back. He was taken to the emergency room and a neurological examination revealed that there was a hemisection of the right half of the spinal cord that extended from T8 to T12. Which of the following deficits would result from this injury?

a. Loss of pain and temperature sensation from the right leg; loss of conscious proprioception from the left leg; UMN paralysis of the left leg
b. Loss of pain and temperature sensation from the left leg; loss of conscious proprioception from the right leg; UMN paralysis of the left leg
c. Loss of pain and temperature sensation from the left arm and leg; loss of conscious proprioception from the right leg and arm; flaccid paralysis of the right leg
d. Loss of pain and temperature sensation from the left leg; loss of conscious proprioception from the right leg; UMN paralysis of the right leg
e. Bilateral loss of pain and temperature sensation and conscious proprioception, both from the lower half of the body; UMN paralysis of the left leg and flaccid paralysis of the right leg

Item 172–176

The next five questions relate to this case history. Audrey was a 45-year-old woman who was brought to her local hospital's emergency room by her husband because of several days of progressive weakness and numbness in her arms and legs. Her symptoms had begun with tingling in her toes, which she assumed to be her feet "falling asleep." However, this feeling did not disappear, and she began to feel numb, first in her toes on both feet, then ascending to her calves and knees. Two days later, Audrey began to feel numb in her fingertips and had difficulty lifting her legs. When she finally was unable to climb the stairs of her house because of her leg weakness, had difficulty gripping the banister, and experienced shortness of breath, her husband urged her to go to the emergency room. The neurologist who examined Audrey in the emergency room noticed that she was short of breath while sitting in bed. He asked the respiratory therapist to measure her vital capacity (the greatest volume of air that can be exhaled from the lungs after a maximal inspiration), and the value for this was far lower than would be expected for her age and weight. Her neurologic examination showed that her arms and legs were very weak, so that she had difficulty lifting them against gravity. She was unable to feel a pin or a vibrating tuning fork at all on her legs and below her elbows, but was able to feel the pin on her upper chest. The neurologist could not elicit any reflexes from her ankles or knees. He subsequently advised the emergency room staff that Audrey needed to have a spinal tap and be admitted to the intensive care unit immediately.

172. Where in the nervous system was the damage?

a. Frontal lobe
b. Temporal lobe
c. Peripheral nerves and nerve roots
d. Spinal cord
e. Muscle

173. Audrey couldn't feel a pinprick in certain locations. Which receptor carries this information?

a. Merkel's tactile disk
b. Ruffini's corpuscle
c. Pacinian corpuscle
d. $C\delta$ and $A\delta$ fibers
e. Meissner's corpuscle

174. Which receptor should be activated by the tuning fork?

a. $C\delta$ and $A\delta$ fibers
b. Merkel's tactile corpuscle
c. Pacinian corpuscle
d. Ruffini's corpuscle
e. Meissner's corpuscle

175. The absent reflexes are a sign of a lesion of which portion of the nervous system?

a. The frontal lobe
b. The dorsal horn of the spinal cord or any point distal to this structure
c. The brainstem
d. The cervical corticospinal tract
e. Any point that is proximal to the upper cervical spinal cord

176. Damage to which nervous system structure caused the difficulty breathing?

a. Medullary respiratory center
b. Diencephalon
c. Pons
d. Phrenic nerve innervating the diaphragm
e. Trigeminal nerve

Item 177–181

Gary is a 35-year-old man who was previously healthy until one day he noticed that his right leg was weak. As the day progressed, he found that he was dragging the leg behind him when he walked, and he finally asked a friend to drive him home from work because he was unable to lift his right foot up enough to place it on the gas pedal. He also noticed that his left leg felt a little bit numb. Finally, his wife convinced him to go to the emergency room of his local hospital.

When Gary arrived at the emergency room, he was having a great deal of difficulty walking. The physician who examined him asked him when this had begun, and when Gary thought about it in more depth, he realized that perhaps this had started slowly several days before and he had ignored the symptoms. Gary's language function, cranial nerves, and motor and sensory examinations of his arms were within normal limits. When the physician examined Gary's right leg, it was markedly weak, with very brisk reflexes in the knee and ankle. Vibration and position sense in the right leg were absent. Pain and temperature testing were normal in the right leg, but these sensations were absent on the left leg and abdomen to the level of his umbilicus. Reflexes in the left leg were normal, but when the physician scratched the lateral portion of the plantar surface on the bottom side of Gary's right foot, the great toe moved up. The remainder of Gary's examination was normal.

177. What area of Gary's nervous system was damaged?

a. Brainstem
b. Cervical spinal cord
c. Thoracic spinal cord
d. Frontal lobe
e. Peripheral nerves

178. Damage to which tract could give Gary the loss of vibration and position sense on the right side?

a. Right fasciculus cuneatus
b. Right fasciculus gracilis
c. Left fasciculus cuneatus
d. Left fasciculus gracilis
e. Right Lissauer's tract

179. Gary's loss of left-sided pain and temperature sensation could be due to damage to which tract?

a. Right fasciculus cuneatus
b. Right fasciculus gracilis
c. Right spinothalamic tract
d. Left spinothalamic tract
e. Left corticospinal tract

180. Why was Gary's right leg weak?

a. There was muscle damage in the right leg
b. There was damage in his left frontal lobe
c. There was damage to the right corticospinal tract
d. The dorsal root was damaged
e. There was damage to the right femoral nerve

181. The upward movement of Gary's toe when the plantar surface of his foot was scratched was indicative of a lesion in which portion of the nervous system?

a. UMN
b. LMN
c. Peripheral nerves
d. Muscles
e. Sural nerve

The Spinal Cord

Answers

139. The answer is d. (*Simon et al., pp 164–168. Gilroy, pp 592–594.*) In this case, disruption of the root fibers of C5–C6 involve components of the brachial plexus and affect muscle groups such as the deltoid, supraspinatus, intraspinatus, biceps, and flexor carpi radialis. These muscles govern abduction of the arm, rotation of the arm at the shoulder, and flexion of the elbow and wrist. Reflex activity would also be affected due to disturbance of both alpha and gamma motor neurons serving the biceps muscle. Lesions involving the cerebral cortex or pons, especially the region of the pyramidal tracts, would produce a UMN paralysis, which would include hyperreflexia and hypertonia. An LMN paralysis involving the ventral horn cells at C1 would not affect the brachial plexus and the muscle groups indicated in this question. The triceps muscle is not involved in producing the movements affected by the injury.

140. The answer is d. (*Simon et al., pp 163–164.*) In this case, there is a loss of superficial abdominal reflexes, which require that spinal segments T8–T12 be intact. The test for these reflexes is to stroke a quadrant of the abdominal wall with an object such as a wooden stick. The normal response is for the muscle of the quadrant stimulated to contract and for movement of the umbilicus in the direction of the stimulus.

141. The answer is a. (*Simon, pp 168–187.*) The nerves innervating the knee and hip exit the spinal cord between L4 and S1. Typical characteristics of a peripheral neuropathy include muscle weakness directed in a more pronounced manner upon the proximal muscles. Depression of tendon reflexes is generally not seen, and muscle wasting might occur only at a very late stage of the disease. Damage to the neuromuscular junction, such as myasthenia gravis, produces a different constellation of deficits. These include muscle fatigue and weakness that is fluctuating. This disorder also typically affects cranial nerves. In addition, the spinal segments indicated (T8–L3) are not associated with the muscle groups in question. Damage to the ventral horn would produce an LMN (flaccid) paralysis, which is not characteristic of the muscle weakness of this patient. Likewise, damage to the lateral funiculus would produce a UMN (spastic) paralysis, and dorsal horn damage would produce sensory deficits as well as affect muscle tone. In addition, the spinal segments indicated in this last choice (e) do not relate to the muscle groups affected in the patient.

142. The answer is c. (*Simon, pp 173–183.*) The most likely cause of the condition in this patient is a cervical disk prolapse. This disorder would produce pain in the neck and arm, which increases with movement of the head. It would also cause loss of some sensation in the thumb and other fingers, as well as weakness in both finger extension and of the biceps reflex. Syringomyelia would produce bilateral segmental loss of pain and temperature. A knife wound completely severing the nerve would result in a functional loss similar to that experienced with an LMN paralysis. Polio results in loss of LMNs, thus also producing an LMN paralysis. One of the effects of AIDS is that it produces damage to the lateral and dorsal columns, resulting in the appearance of a UMN disorder.

143. The answer is d. (*Gilroy, pp 612–628. Simon et al., pp 182–184.*) Guillain-Barré syndrome is an acute polyneuropathy whose occurrence frequently follows a respiratory infection. It results in myalgia of the lower limbs, loss of muscle tone and tendon reflexes, and some flaccidity. The disorder can also affect the seventh cranial nerve. The disorder can produce diffuse demyelination of the peripheral nerves with an increase in lymphocytes present at the sites of demyelination. The other disorders listed are generally progressive where eventual recovery without intervention is not known to occur. Myasthenia gravis and lumbar disk prolapse would not show demyelination and lymphocyte increases near the sites of demyelination. MS involves CNS structures; therefore, the constellation of symptoms would be different. As indicated earlier, MD is progressive, with effects upon both proximal muscles and later in distal muscles.

144–145. The answers are 144-b, 145-e. (*Gilroy, pp 201–215, 357–362. Simon, pp 170–171, 179.*) ALS is characterized by a progressive loss of motor functions, first seen as weakness in limb muscles, especially those of the fingers, and later of the other limbs. Sensory functions are not significantly affected. Over time, there is wasting, atrophy, and fasciculations of limb muscles, followed by UMN signs. Electromyogram abnormalities can also be observed of the upper and lower extremities. In MS, there is also sensory loss, such as loss or blurring of vision, as well as bladder problems.

Poliomyelitis and myasthenia gravis involve LMN symptoms, while a cerebral cortical stroke would result in a UMN disorder without LMN signs. In ALS, there is damage initially to ventral horn cells of the spinal cord, producing LMN signs. As the disease progresses, there is involvement of UMNs located in the lateral columns of the spinal cord (i.e., corticospinal dysfunction), thereby producing UMN signs such as an increase in tendon reflexes and the presence of an extensor plantar response. Sensory neurons are not involved in this disorder.

146. The answer is c. (*Gilroy, pp 199–211.*) MS is a demyelinating autoimmune disease that affects CNS function. This disorder produces a wide variety of symptoms, including sudden sensory dysfunction and loss, which affect vision and the somatosensory system, causing tingling, pain, and hypesthesia. Broad functional motor disturbances also occur, including weakness of the upper or lower limbs, UMN signs, and gait impairment. There is also bladder dysfunction as well as an increase in CSF protein and IgG synthesis. Diffuse cerebellar degeneration would produce gait ataxia and deficits in the accuracy of intentional movements. As noted earlier, ALS would produce both a UMN and an LMN paralysis, which typically does not extend to sensory functions. Likewise, a peripheral neuropathy would not produce UMN signs, visual deficits, and extensive motor disturbances as described in this case. A tumor of the prefrontal cortex would affect some cognitive and emotional functions, but it would not affect sensory processes such as vision and somatosensation, nor would it produce signs of a UMN disorder or muscle weakness.

147–155. The answers are 147-A, 148-D, 149-B, 150-C, 151-E, 152-H, 153-I, 154-F, 155-G. (*Afifi, pp 59–83. Nolte, pp 220–235.*) Sensory fibers that terminate in the medulla are located in the dorsal columns. Fibers mediating conscious proprioception from the upper limb are contained in the fasciculus cuneatus (A). The lateral spinothalamic tract (D) transmits pain and temperature information directly to the thalamus. The lateral corticospinal tract (B) originates in the contralateral cortex and crosses over at the level of the lower medulla. This important pathway mediates control over volitional movements. When these fibers are cut, there is a clear loss of ability to produce volitional movements. The rubrospinal tract (C), situated adjacent to the lateral corticospinal tract, originates from the red nucleus of the midbrain and facilitates the actions of flexor motor neurons. The lateral vestibulospinal tract (E) powerfully facilitates alpha motor neurons of extensor muscles. This tract is located in the ventral funiculus adjacent to the gray matter. The axons of the cells situated in this part of the gray matter (i.e., ventral horn) innervate extensor motor neurons. The posterior (or dorsal) spinocerebellar tract (H) transmits information from muscle spindles to the cerebellum via the inferior cerebellar peduncle. This tract is located on the lateral aspect of the lateral funiculus of the cord, just above the anterior (or ventral) spinocerebellar tract. Pain and temperature fibers from the periphery terminate directly in the region of the dorsal horn, called the *substantia gelatinosa* (I). A smaller component of the corticospinal tract, the anterior corticospinal tract (F), originates from the cerebral cortex and passes ipsilaterally to the spinal cord. In its ventromedial position, the fibers are ipsilateral to their cortical origin. Just prior to their termination, many of the fibers are distributed to the contralateral side of the cord. The anterior (or ventral) spinocerebellar tract (G) arises from wide regions of the gray matter of the cord. These fibers pass contralaterally to the lateral aspect of the lateral funiculus to reach a position just below the dorsal spinocerebellar tract. These fibers then ascend to the cerebellum via the superior cerebellar peduncle, conveying information from Golgi tendon organs located in the lower limbs.

156–158. The answers are 156-K, 157-B, 158-J. *(Afifi, pp 59–83, 91–104. Nolte, pp 255–259.)* Ventral horn cells (K) constitute the final common path for descending motor pathways controlling movement, since they directly innervate skeletal muscle. Therefore, they are referred to as *lower motor neurons* (LMNs), and lesions involving any component of these neurons result in an LMN deficit. The deficit is characterized by a flaccid paralysis of the muscle groups innervated by these neurons. In contrast, neurons from the cerebral cortex (and elsewhere in the brain) that pass in the lateral funiculus of the cord (B) and innervate ventral horn cells rather than skeletal muscle are referred to as *upper motor neurons* (UMNs). Lesions of these fibers produce a UMN syndrome, which is characterized by a spastic paralysis. The fasciculus gracilis (J) conveys, in part, information from joint capsules of the lower limbs to the brain. Disruption of these fibers will block the transmission to the cerebral cortex of these signals that indicate the position of the lower limb following or preceding movement of that limb. Such loss will prevent the necessary feedback signals concerning one's position in space to reach the cortex. As a result, there will be a compensatory motor response characterized by a wide ataxic gait. In contrast, the fasciculus cuneatus mediates similar sensory modalities to the brain, but from the upper limb, and therefore damage to this pathway could not account for ataxia of movement.

159. The answer is e. *(Afifi, pp 64–66. Nolte, pp 221–224.)* The section depicted in the diagram is taken from the lower cervical cord. The cervical level of the spinal cord can be distinguished from other levels of the cord by the following characteristics: the presence of a well-defined fasciculus cuneatus medullae spinalis, situated immediately lateral to the fasciculus gracilis medullae spinalis; the presence of well-defined motor nuclei that are clumped into six different groups, three of which can be distinguished; an absence of an intermediolateral cell column; and relatively extensive quantities of both white and gray matter. Thus, a knife wound that destroyed the right half of the spinal cord results in a Brown-Séquard syndrome. The knife wound would cause loss of sensory and motor functions of both upper and lower limbs. The sensory loss of lower limbs would occur because of the damage to ascending fibers from spinothalamic and the fasciculus gracilis (causing loss of pain and temperature of the contralateral side of the body and conscious proprioception of the ipsilateral side), which would also include some loss of these sensations from the upper limb. At the lesion, there is additional loss of these sensations from the upper limb, which enter the cord at this level of spinal cord. Here, there would also be some bilateral pain and temperature loss at the level of the lesion because of the presence of crossing fibers. Because the lesion occurred at the cervical level, it would result in an LMN paralysis of the upper limb and a UMN paralysis involving the lower limb.

160. The answer is c. *(Kandel, pp 715–724.)* Gamma motor neurons innervate the polar regions of the muscle spindle and, when excited, cause resetting of the spindle by stretching it, resulting in a lowering of the threshold for activation of that receptor by an external force. Unmyelinated C fibers mediate nociceptive sensations from the periphery to the spinal cord and thus do not relate to this question. 1A fibers arise from the nuclear region of the spindle and mediate spindle activity to the spinal cord, and thus form the afferent limb of the monosynaptic stretch reflex. Alpha motor neurons arise in the ventral horn of the spinal cord and innervate extrafusal muscle fibers, causing movement of the limb when excited. It does not innervate the polar regions of the spindle. General visceral afferent fibers exit from the intermediolateral cell columns (at T1–L3 for sympathetics and S2–S4 for parasympathetics) of the spinal cord and innervate postganglionic neurons for these respective autonomic systems. Such fibers, therefore, do not relate to muscle spindles, including their polar regions.

161. The answer is d. (*Nolte, pp 225–232. Afifi, pp 59–89.*) First-order neurons that convey pain and temperature sensations to the spinal cord from C7–T1 are associated with innervation of the region of the hand. The back of the head is innervated from fibers that enter the spinal cord at C2, the neck at C3, the shoulder at C3–C6, and the back at T2–T12.

162. The answer is b. (*Nolte, pp 225–232. Afifi, pp 59–89.*) First-order neurons that convey pain and temperature sensations to the spinal cord terminate principally in laminae I and II upon dendrites of cells located in other laminae. For the most part, tactile and pressure sensations are carried by dorsal column–medial lemniscal systems, which terminate in the lower medulla. Fibers that mediate unconscious proprioception terminate in the nucleus dorsalis of Clarke.

163. The answer is c. (*Afifi, pp 59–89, 126–130.*) Immunocytochemical studies have demonstrated that the sensory neurons that terminate in laminae I and II of the dorsal horn of the spinal cord stain intensely for substance P. These neurons are believed to mediate pain impulses. Other transmitter substances, while present within the spinal cord, have not been associated directly with first-order sensory afferent fibers.

164. The answer is c. (*Nolte, pp 234–237. Afifi, pp 59–89.*) Lissauer's marginal zone, located on the dorsolateral margin of the dorsal horn of the spinal cord, receives many incoming fibers that are either unmyelinated or finely myelinated. These fibers principally mediate pain and temperature sensations. The fibers contained in this bundle may ascend or descend several segments, serving to integrate different levels of the substantia gelatinosa, which receives these inputs. These fibers are not known to make synaptic contact with motor neurons. Neurons in the substantia gelatinosa do not generally ascend beyond the spinal cord.

165. The answer is b. (*Afifi, pp 59–89.*) Clarke's nucleus dorsalis is situated in the medial aspect of lamina VII of the cord at thoracic and lumbar levels, but does extend up to C8. It receives first-order inputs from fibers that convey muscle spindle and Golgi tendon organ information (i.e., unconscious proprioception). Fibers from Clarke's nucleus dorsalis run laterally to form the dorsal spinocerebellar tract on the ipsilateral side, which terminates mainly in the anterior lobe of the cerebellum.

166. The answer is d. (*Afifi, pp 59–89. Nolte, p 227.*) The fact that the disorder affected the neuronal cell bodies of the ventral horn indicates that the patient will present with an LMN paralysis. The affected neurons from L1–L4 innervate the muscles of the lower limb; therefore, the LMN paralysis would affect the leg normally innervated by these neurons.

The neurons situated in the ventral horn of the gray matter of the cord are somatotopically organized. This relationship is most clearly seen at cervical levels of the cord. The neurons innervating flexors lie dorsal to those innervating extensors, and the neurons innervating the muscles of the trunk are situated medial to those innervating the hand. These relationships take on added significance when one considers the nature of the descending motor pathways that synapse with these cells. For example, fibers associated mainly with the control of the flexor musculature, such as the corticospinal and rubrospinal tracts, are situated at relatively dorsal levels of the lateral funiculus of the cord. Similarly, fibers associated with the regulation of antigravity muscles (i.e., generally the extensor musculature) are situated in a more ventral position. Thus, the somatotopic organization is maintained throughout the brainstem as well as the spinal cord.

167. The answer is b. (*Nolte, p 227.*) A principal descending component of the MLF arises from the medial vestibular nucleus, and, accordingly, this bundle is sometimes referred to as the *medial vestibulospinal tract.* The overall function of the MLF is to help coordinate changes in position or balance with the position of the head and eyes. The descending fibers of the MLF provide the anatomic substrate by which the inputs from the vestibular apparatus can influence the manner in which the head will be positioned. It accomplishes this by modulating upper cervical neurons that innervate muscles of the neck that control the position of the head. Since the projection is to the cervical cord, it would not likely have any direct effect upon extensor reflex activity of the lower limbs. Likewise, these descending fibers do not affect any structures that would cause alterations in blood pressure. This pathway does not innervate neurons of the spinal cord that supply the upper or lower limbs. Therefore, a UMN paralysis would not be expected. In addition, these fibers do not innervate the cerebellum or mediate conscious proprioception. Only if there were damage to the cerebellum or fibers mediating this form of sensation would one expect ataxia to occur.

168–169. The answers are 168-c and 169-b. (*Afifi, pp 59–89.*) Both the lateral and the anterior spinothalamic tracts cross over to the contralateral white matter of the cord relatively close to the central canal. Therefore, a lesion of this region would result in segmental loss of pain and temperature (plus some tactile sensation) because these fibers would be damaged. The dorsal funiculus mediates conscious proprioception; the dorsal root ganglion mediates all sensory processes, which are not limited to pain and temperature sensation; the midline region of the lower medulla contains second-order neurons that mediate conscious proprioception from the body; and the ventral horn contains motor but not sensory neurons. Concerning other pathways in the spinal cord, the anterior corticospinal tract represents approximately 10% of the fibers descending from the cortex as corticospinal fibers. These fibers pass ipsilaterally through the brainstem to the spinal cord, reaching the anterior funiculus of the cord. Near the level at which these fibers terminate, most anterior corticospinal fibers cross over in the commissure of the spinal cord to supply the intermediate gray of the ventral horn. The anterior spinocerebellar tract crosses over to the contralateral side and ascends as a distinct fiber pathway in the far lateral aspect of the white matter immediately below the position occupied by the dorsal spinocerebellar tract. Posterior spinocerebellar fibers, which arise from Clarke's nucleus dorsalis, do not cross in the spinal cord. Instead, they pass laterally from their cell of origin and ascend within the dorsal half of the far lateral aspect of the white matter to the cerebellum. Lateral vestibulospinal fibers arise from the lateral vestibular nucleus and descend ipsilaterally within the ventral funiculus to all levels of the spinal cord, where they terminate upon neurons in the ventral horn. Dorsal column fibers are first-order neurons that arise from the periphery and enter the spinal cord at all levels. They ascend ipsilaterally in the fasciculus gracilis and cuneatus to the level of the dorsal column nuclei of the medulla, where they terminate.

170. The answer is a. *(Kandel, pp 715–724.)* In contrast to Golgi tendon organs, which detect tension, muscle spindles respond to the rate of change in the length of the muscle and are referred to as *velocity detectors.* They are low-threshold detectors and are connected in parallel with the extrafusal muscle fibers. Stretching the muscle results in an elongation of intrafusal fibers, which stretches the sensory nerve endings in the spindle, producing an increase in the discharge rate. The muscle spindle actually contains three different types of intrafusal fibers—dynamic nuclear bag, static nuclear bag, and nuclear chain fibers—all of which are innervated by a single 1A afferent fiber. Static nuclear bag fibers and nuclear chain fibers are innervated by group II afferent fibers. The various properties of these intrafusal fibers combine in generating the firing patterns of the spindle.

171. The answer is d. *(Afifi, pp 94–97.)* Hemisection of the right side of the spinal cord that involves segments T8 to T12 will result in contralateral loss of pain and temperature sensation below the level of the lesion and ipsilateral loss of conscious proprioception below the level of the lesion. Thus, this patient will experience loss of pain and temperature in the left leg and loss of conscious proprioception in the right leg. In addition, there will be damage to the descending corticospinal fibers that normally are essential for activation of the LMNs that control muscles of the right leg (i.e., UMN paralysis of the right leg). However, since the lesion is situated below the entry of sensory fibers as well as the origin of anterior horn cells that innervate the upper limbs, no loss of sensation to the upper limbs will ensue, nor will there be an LMN or UMN paralysis of the upper limbs. The pain and temperature fibers ipsilateral to the site of the lesion are unaffected because the second-order neurons decussate at the approximate level of their cell bodies of origin and ascend on the side contralateral to the lesion, leaving this system intact.

172. The answer is c. *(Adams, pp 43–48, 1312–1318.)* This patient does not have a UMN lesion (spinal cord or above) because of the absent reflexes and ascending paralysis bilaterally involving all of the extremities. Lesions in the brain almost always give unilateral findings, and spinal cord lesions give a distinct level. The damage cannot be in the muscle, because the patient has sensory involvement as well. This case is an example of Guillain-Barré syndrome, or an inflammatory disease of the peripheral nerve resulting from demyelination. Inflammatory cells are found within the nerves, as well as segmental demyelination and some degree of wallerian degeneration. This damage can cause an ascending paralysis and sensory loss, affecting the arms, face, and legs. The CSF often has a high protein level, making a spinal tap a useful test for the diagnosis of Guillain-Barré syndrome. Nerve conduction studies are also helpful in making the diagnosis. Most neurologists believe Guillain-Barré syndrome to be an immunologic reaction directed against the peripheral nerve, and some patients have a history of having had some type of infection prior to developing Guillain-Barré syndrome. However, a clear-cut cause is rarely found. Despite a known cause, most patients recover from Guillain-Barré syndrome, although the speed of recovery varies. Treatment is currently available (administration of gamma globulin), and, if instituted early in the course of the disease, decrease in the length of the illness is possible.

173. The answer is d. (*Kandel, pp 430–440.*) Pain is mediated by Cδ and Aδ fibers in the skin.

174. The answer is c. (*Kandel, pp 430–440.*) Pacinian corpuscles best mediate vibration.

175. The answer is b. (*Adams, pp 43–48.*) The reflexes are lost because the LMNs, which are affected by this process, are unable to participate in the reflex arc necessary for a knee or ankle jerk to take place. These LMNs originate with stretch receptors in the tendons. Answers a, c, d, and e are all examples of UMN lesions, usually characterized by hyperactive reflexes.

176. The answer is d. (*Adams, pp 43–48.*) This is an example of an LMN problem. Answers a, b, and c are UMN structures. The trigeminal nerve is a cranial nerve that mediates sensation on the face and the muscles of mastication. Loss of diaphragmatic function causes respiratory distress.

177. The answer is c. (*Afifi, pp 91–103.*) Gary has a spinal cord syndrome called *Brown-Séquard's syndrome,* or hemisection of the spinal cord. The lesion is not at the cervical level because motor functions of the upper limbs were considered normal. The examiner can pinpoint the location of the lesion by using the "sensory level," or level at which the loss of pain and temperature begin, by remembering that the lesion affects fibers that have entered the spinal cord one or two levels below it, and then cross to the contralateral side. Therefore, a loss of sensory function at the T10 level indicates a lesion at the T8 or T9 level. A level at which motor deficits begin can be helpful as well, but in lesions of the thoracic spinal cord, muscles innervated by thoracic nerves are difficult to test. The examiner still expects weakness in the lower extremities, and this helps to make the diagnosis. Brown-Séquard's syndrome may occur as a result of different types of tumors or infections of the spinal cord.

178. The answer is b. *(Afifi, pp 91–103.)* Because one-half of the spinal cord is damaged, the dorsal columns are damaged, and the patient will have loss of proprioception and vibration ipsilateral to and below the level of the lesion. The loss must be ipsilateral because fibers mediating this type of sensation cross above the level of the lesion. The fasciculus gracilis carries fibers originating from the sacral, lumbar, and lower thoracic levels, and the fasciculus carries those from the upper thoracic and cervical levels. Lissauer's tract carries pain and temperature fibers via the dorsal root entry zone. Brown-Séquard's syndrome may occur as a result of different types of tumors or infections of the spinal cord.

179. The answer is c. *(Afifi, pp 91–103.)* The spinothalamic tract carries fibers mediating pain and temperature. The primary pain fibers enter the spinal cord and pass one or two segments in Lissauer's marginal zone before making a synapse with neurons that form the lateral spinothalamic tract. Fibers of the lateral spinothalamic tract then cross to the contralateral side one or two segments above or before where the primary afferent fibers have entered the cord. Accordingly, pain and temperature are lost below the lesion on the contralateral side. The cuneate and gracile fasciculi mediate proprioception and vibration, and the corticospinal tract mediates voluntary motor function.

180. The answer is c. *(Afifi, pp 91–103.)* The corticospinal tract mediates voluntary motor function. The fibers cross in the medullary pyramids, thus lesions below this structure cause ipsilateral weakness. The reflexes are brisk, since in a UMN lesion there is a loss of inhibition to spinal reflexes. Muscle, dorsal root, and femoral nerve damage are all examples of lesions distal to the spinal cord. A frontal lobe lesion would not cause sensory or motor level damage, and would probably cause problems more proximally, such as slurred speech.

181. The answer is a. *(Afifi, pp 91–103.)* A positive Babinski's sign, or dorsiflexion of the great toe when the lateral portion of the plantar surface of the foot is scratched, is a sign of corticospinal tract dysfunction, a tract consisting of UMNs. Peripheral nerve (including the sural nerve) lesions are LMN lesions.

The Autonomic Nervous System

Questions

DIRECTIONS: Each item below contains a question or incomplete statement followed by suggested responses. Select the **one best** response to each question.

182. A new discovery was made that allowed for the administration of a drug that selectively blocked synaptic transmission in autonomic ganglia in order to control blood pressure. Which of the following best characterizes this drug?

a. Cholinergic antagonist
b. Noradrenergic antagonist
c. Serotonergic antagonist
d. GABAergic antagonist
e. Peptidergic antagonist

183. In designing the drug described in question 182, the researchers also have to consider that peptides play a role. Which of the following statements accurately depicts the locus and function of peptides in autonomic function?

a. They are present only at preganglionic axon terminals of the parasympathetic nervous system
b. They are present only at postganglionic axon terminals of the parasympathetic nervous system
c. They are present in sympathetic ganglia, where they function primarily as neurotransmitters
d. They are present in sympathetic ganglia, where they function primarily as neuromodulators
e. They have not been localized in any of the autonomic ganglia

184. A patient with elevated heart rate and blood pressure is examined by a battery of physicians and they conclude that his condition is due to a deficiency or loss of the carotid sinus reflex. What is a component of this reflex?

a. Baroreceptor afferent fibers from cranial nerve XI
b. Glossopharyngeal efferent fibers
c. Interneurons within the nucleus ambiguus of the medulla
d. Efferent fibers contained in the intermediate component of the facial nerve
e. Vagal efferent fibers

185. A patient has a tendency to have elevated blood pressure and heart rate, which can be controlled in part by a calcium channel blocker. Which of the following statements most accurately characterizes the effects of neurotransmitters upon calcium currents in heart muscle cells?

a. They are reduced by norepinephrine acting through β receptors
b. They are increased by norepinephrine acting through β receptors
c. They are increased by acetylcholine acting on muscarinic receptors
d. They are increased by acetylcholine acting on nicotinic receptors
e. They are increased by serotonin acting on serotonin 1_A receptors

186. A 78-year-old male presents with loss of voluntary control of bladder functions. Which of the following possible conditions could account for the loss of bladder functions?

a. Loss of vagal and sacral efferent fibers only
b. Loss of vagal, sacral, and descending fibers from the cerebral cortex
c. Loss of lumbar and sacral efferent fibers only
d. Loss of lumbar, sacral, and descending fibers from the cerebral cortex
e. Loss of lumbar, thoracic, and cervical fibers only

187. After receiving a diagnosis of having elevated blood pressure, an attempt is made to control blood pressure by preventing the synthesis and storage of norepinephrine. Which of the following would be applied to achieve this result?

a. Guanethidine sulfate
b. Reserpine
c. Phenoxybenzamine hydrochloride
d. Hexamethonium chloride
e. Metoprolol

188. A patient is diagnosed with a hypothalamic tumor that results in significant alteration of autonomic functions, including loss of regulation of blood pressure and heart rate. Such effects upon autonomic functions can be understood in terms of the functional connections of the hypothalamus with a brainstem or spinal cord structure. Which structure would normally receive such inputs?

a. Ventrolateral nucleus of the thalamus
b. Nucleus accumbens
c. Solitary nucleus
d. Red nucleus
e. Ventral horn cells at the level of C8–T12 of the spinal cord

The Autonomic Nervous System

Answers

182. The answer is a. (*Kandel, pp 970–974.*) The transmitter released from preganglionic endings of both sympathetic and parasympathetic fibers is acetylcholine (ACh). The other transmitters listed are not involved at this synapse. Evidence in support of this view is derived, in part, from studies that demonstrated that drugs that block nicotinic receptors (e.g., hexamethonium chloride, curare) also block the output of these systems.

183. The answer is d. (*Kandel, pp 970–972.*) Recent studies demonstrate that a wide variety of peptides are found within most sympathetic ganglia. Evidence further suggests that these peptides do not act as transmitters, but instead serve as neuromodulators. In this manner, the action of peptides in autonomic ganglia is to alter the efficiency of neuronal excitability and the effectiveness of cholinergic transmission at autonomic synapses.

184. The answer is e. (*Kandel, pp 879–880.*) The carotid sinus reflex involves several neuronal elements. The afferent side of the reflex begins with stretch receptors in the walls of the carotid sinus. These receptors signal pressure as a result of stretch of the low-capacitance vessel. This causes an afferent volley of action potentials to pass along the glossopharyngeal nerve into the medulla, where the fibers synapse with neurons in the solitary nucleus. These neurons, in turn, synapse upon neurons in the dorsal motor nucleus (and nucleus ambiguus) of the vagus nerve whose axons innervate the heart. Activation of this reflex results in a decrease in heart rate and force of contraction. As a consequence of the decrease in cardiac output, there is an ensuing decrease in blood pressure as well.

185. The answer is b. (*Kandel, pp 964–973.*) The calcium current of heart muscle cells is enhanced by the release of norepinephrine, which acts on β-adrenergic receptors. This effect is additionally mediated by modulation of the potassium current, which serves to keep the action potential of the muscle cells constant. The pacemaker current is also affected by this process since its threshold is decreased as a result of activation of the β receptors (which further involves the second messenger system–cAMP-dependent protein kinase). Lowering the threshold of the pacemaker current serves to increase heart rate. Serotonin is not involved in postsynaptic regulation of the heart. Acetylcholine has an inhibitory effect upon the heart muscle by acting through different mechanisms.

186. The answer is d. *(Kandel, pp 963–972.)* The smooth muscle of the bladder is innervated by postganglionic fibers of the sympathetic nervous system that arise from the inferior mesenteric ganglion. This ganglion, in turn, receives its inputs from T12–L2 of the intermediolateral cell column of the spinal cord. The smooth muscle of the bladder also receives inputs from postganglionic parasympathetic fibers that are innervated by preganglionic fibers arising from S2–S4. The external sphincter of the bladder (striated muscle) is innervated by ventral horn cells from the spinal cord. These ventral horn cells, in turn, receive inputs from supraspinal neurons that arise, in part, from the cerebral cortex. It is these neurons that form a part of the substrate for voluntary control over bladder functions (in combination with the parasympathetic and sympathetic fibers from sacral and lumbar levels, respectively).

187. The answer is b. *(Cooper et al., pp 197–222, 227–290. Siegel et al., pp 221–240, 243–259.)* Noradrenergic activity can be blocked by a number of mechanisms. Reserpine, for example, prevents the synthesis and storage of norepinephrine in sympathetic nerve terminals. Guanethidine sulfate affects noradrenergic transmission by blocking the release of norepinephrine at the sympathetic endings. Competitive α-receptor blockers include phenoxybenzamine hydrochloride and phentolamine, whereas metoprolol blocks β_1 receptors. Since ACh is the transmitter at preganglionic synapses of both the parasympathetic and the sympathetic nervous systems, hexamethonium chloride is an effective ganglionic blocker at these synapses.

188. The answer is c. *(Kandel, pp 965–967.)* The solitary nucleus of the medulla plays a significant role in the neural control of autonomic functions because it receives input from several different regions of the brain that regulate such functions. These inputs include fibers that arise from the hypothalamus, central nucleus of the amygdala, midbrain periaqueductal gray, and sensory processes (i.e., visceral afferents) of the glossopharyngeal and vagus nerves. The last signal changes in blood pressure and levels of oxygen and carbon dioxide in the blood. The ventrolateral nucleus of the thalamus, red nucleus of the midbrain, and ventral horn cells of the spinal cord are associated with somatomotor rather than autonomic function. The nucleus accumbens is believed to be associated with motivational processes.

The Brainstem and Cranial Nerves

Questions

DIRECTIONS: Each item below contains a question or incomplete statement followed by suggested responses. Select the **one best** response to each question.

Item 189–190

The following test was administered to a patient: A cotton applicator was gently applied to the cornea of the eye as the patient was asked to look upward. The patient did not blink in response to stimulation of the cornea.

189. Which cranial nerves are normally involved in this reflex?

a. Nerves II and III
b. Nerves III and IV
c. Nerves III and V
d. Nerves V and VII
e. Nerves VII and IX

190. Which of the following best characterizes the nerves involved in this reflex?

a. Special sensory afferent and general somatic efferent
b. General somatic efferent alone
c. General somatic afferent and special visceral efferent
d. General somatic afferent and general somatic efferent
e. Special visceral afferent and special visceral efferent

Item 191–193

As a result of an infection, a 56-year-old woman experienced a loss of taste affecting the front of her tongue and the ability to smile.

191. If the sensory loss involved damage of cell bodies, which specific group of neurons would be so affected?

a. Otic ganglion
b. Nodose (inferior) ganglion
c. Pterygopalatine ganglion
d. Geniculate ganglion
e. Trigeminal ganglion

192. Which cranial nerve was most immediately affected?

a. Nerve V
b. Nerve VI
c. Nerve VII
d. Nerve IX
e. Nerve X

193. Which are the components of the nerve that would be affected?

a. General somatic afferent and general somatic efferent
b. Special visceral afferent and special visceral efferent
c. General visceral afferent and general somatic efferent
d. General somatic afferent and general visceral efferent
e. Special visceral afferent and general visceral efferent

Item 194–197

A 55-year-old man, who had been suffering from hypertension for the past eight years, experienced attacks of pain in the regions of the pharynx and ear, which were usually preceded by swallowing and coughing spells. These attacks, each of which lasted for an average of one minute, occurred a number of times; ultimately, this condition showed remission. Although the neurological examination was basically normal, a subsequent MRI was taken and revealed an abnormality at the base of the skull.

194. Which cranial nerve was most likely involved in this disorder?

a. Nerve V
b. Nerve VII
c. Nerve IX
d. Nerve XI
e. Nerve XII

195. From which structure did the motor component of this cranial nerve arise?

a. Otic ganglion
b. Nodose ganglion
c. Nucleus ambiguus
d. Inferior salivatory nucleus
e. Lateral reticular nucleus

196. Where are the cell bodies of the sensory component of the affected nerve located?

a. Solitary nucleus
b. Superior ganglion
c. Geniculate ganglion
d. Vestibular nuclei
e. Trigeminal ganglion

197. Which of the following best characterize the motor and sensory components of the affected nerve?

a. General visceral efferent and general visceral afferent
b. Special visceral efferent and general somatic afferent
c. General somatic efferent and special visceral afferent
d. Special visceral efferent and special visceral afferent
e. General somatic efferent and general somatic afferent

Item 198–199

In a classic experiment performed by Sherrington in the cat, marked rigidity was demonstrated in a decerebrate preparation. Similarly, an 80-year-old woman displayed rigidity, which resembled that shown in the cat after having a stroke.

198. Where was the most likely location of the stroke?
a. Thalamus
b. Hypothalamus
c. Upper midbrain
d. Pons
e. Spinal cord

199. Which of the following pathways could best account for the rigidity when its actions were unopposed?
a. Rubrospinal tract
b. Lateral vestibulospinal tract
c. Corticospinal tract
d. Medial vestibulospinal tract
e. Lateral reticulospinal tract

Item 200–202

A 43-year-old male was recovering from an infectious disease and experienced a marked instability in his blood pressure, with episodes of spiking of blood pressure. After a series of extensive examinations, it was concluded that this disorder was due to the effects of the infectious agent upon a component of the peripheral nervous system.

200. Which of the following constitute logical sites where an infectious agent could produce such an effect?
a. Superior ganglia of cranial nerves IX and X
b. Geniculate and trigeminal ganglia
c. Otic and superior salivatory ganglia
d. Carotid sinus and aortic arch
e. Carotid and aortic bodies

201. To which stimuli do (the appropriate) receptors situated in the sites listed in question 200 respond best?
a. Stretch
b. Change in chloride ion concentration
c. Contractions of the gut
d. Decrease in oxygen concentration
e. Increase in carbon dioxide concentration

202. To which of the following sites do neurons indicated in question 200 project in order to mediate their effects?

a. Trigeminal spinal nucleus
b. Fastigial nucleus
c. Midbrain reticular formation
d. Solitary nucleus
e. Autonomic nuclei of the facial nucleus (cranial nerve VII)

203. An individual has difficulty in adjusting his head, especially after he changes his posture. Which of the following is the most likely pathway affected that might cause this deficit?

a. Lateral vestibulospinal tract
b. Medial vestibulospinal tract
c. Medial reticulospinal tract
d. Lateral reticulospinal tract
e. Rubrospinal tract

Item 204–206

An individual experiences an ipsilateral paralysis of the soft palate and pharynx, producing hoarseness and dysphagia (inability to swallow) and, in addition, displays a loss of the carotid sinus reflex.

204. Which nerve group is most likely affected?

a. Cranial nerve XII
b. Cranial nerve XI
c. Cranial nerve X
d. Cranial nerve VII
e. Ventral horn cells of the cervical cord

205. Which of the following are the most probable nuclei damaged in this case?

a. Solitary and lateral reticular nuclei
b. Deep pontine and facial nuclei
c. Dorsal motor nucleus and nucleus ambiguus
d. Ventral horn of the cervical segment of the spinal cord
e. Inferior salivatory and medial vestibular nuclei

206. Which of the following best characterizes the neurons associated with the loss of functions described in this case?

a. General somatic efferent and special visceral efferent
b. General visceral efferent and special visceral efferent
c. General somatic efferent and general visceral efferent
d. General visceral efferent and general visceral afferent
e. Special visceral efferent and special visceral afferent

207. A patient complains that he cannot move his right eye to the right and that the right side of his face is expressionless. Where is the likely locus of the lesion?

a. Dorsal aspect of the medulla
b. Ventromedial medulla
c. Dorsal pons
d. Ventromedial pons
e. Medial midbrain

208. Upon examination, the patient is unable to move his right eye medially. Where is the likely locus of the lesion?

a. Dorsal medulla
b. Ventromedial medulla
c. Dorsal pons
d. Ventromedial pons
e. Medial midbrain

Item 209–211

The patient experiences difficulty in walking down stairs and reports some double vision as well.

209. In this instance, where is the most likely locus of the lesion?

a. Medulla
b. Dorsal pons
c. Ventromedial pons
d. Midbrain
e. Spinal cord

210. Which structure is included in the lesion?

a. Cervical spinal cord ventral horn cells
b. Cranial nerve VII
c. Cranial nerve VI
d. Cranial nerve IV
e. Cranial nerve III

211. How is this nerve classified?

a. General somatic efferent
b. Special visceral efferent
c. General visceral efferent
d. Combined general visceral and somatic efferent
e. Combined general visceral and special visceral efferent

212. Which of the following are the principal afferent fiber systems that supply the inferior olivary nucleus?

a. Hypothalamus and amygdala
b. Caudate nucleus and subthalamic nucleus
c. Solitary nucleus and nucleus of the ventrolateral medulla
d. Red nucleus and spinal cord
e. Deep pontine nuclei and vestibular nuclei

213. Which of the following is a principal projection target of the inferior olivary nucleus?

a. Cerebral cortex
b. Midbrain periaqueductal gray
c. Vestibular nuclei
d. Dorsal column nuclei
e. Cerebellar cortex

Item 214–215

An elderly female patient complains that she cannot taste the food that she eats. A careful neurological examination reveals no evidence of peripheral damage of the taste receptors. The evidence suggests, instead, that there was selective damage of certain regions of the brainstem.

214. Which of the following sites would include damage that could result in the selective loss of taste?

a. Superior olivary nucleus
b. Inferior salivatory nucleus
c. Solitary nucleus
d. Spinal nucleus of the trigeminal nerve
e. Reticular tegmental nucleus of the pons

215. Which of the following is a principal target of this brainstem structure (used as your answer to question 214)?

a. Anterior thalamic nucleus
b. Reticular thalamic nucleus
c. Ventral posteromedial thalamic nucleus
d. Ventrolateral thalamic nucleus
e. Dorsomedial thalamic nucleus

Item 216–219

A 68-year-old woman suffered from an infectious disorder for several weeks. Following recovery from this disorder, she experienced some loss of taste and an increase in salivation, together with pain spasms in the region of the pharynx, which extended into the ear. She also experienced some bradycardia and cardiac arrhythmia, as well as deviation of the uvula to the unaffected side.

216. Which of the following cranial nerves was most directly involved in this deficit?

a. Cranial nerve VII
b. Cranial nerve IX
c. Cranial nerve X
d. Cranial nerve XI
e. Cranial nerve XII

217. What is the name of the cell bodies of origin of the nerve fibers that directly innervate the organ responsible for an increase in salivation?

a. Inferior salivatory nuclei
b. Superior salivatory nuclei
c. Otic ganglion
d. Geniculate ganglion
e. Nucleus ambiguus

218. What is the origin of the fibers that were affected, causing deviation of the uvula?

a. Solitary nucleus
b. Inferior salivatory nucleus
c. Facial nucleus
d. Nucleus ambiguus
e. Dorsal motor nucleus of the vagus

219. Which of the following is the likely site of the lesion affecting this nerve?

a. Upper medulla
b. Lower medulla
c. Lower pons
d. Upper pons
e. Base of the skull

Item 220–222

A 40-year-old male who suffered from a disorder of unknown origin complained to his physician that he had difficulty in producing a smile from the left side of his face and that he couldn't salivate or produce tears from the left eye. Further analysis showed some loss of taste and that the affected muscles were flaccid and the eyelids were open.

220. Where do the cell bodies of origin within the CNS lie whose peripheral innervation of skeletal muscles were affected by this disorder?

a. Upper medulla
b. Lower pons
c. Upper pons
d. Lower midbrain
e. Upper midbrain

221. From which of the following structures do the preganglionic parasympathetic fibers of this nerve arise?

a. Dorsal motor nucleus of the vagus
b. Nucleus ambiguus
c. Inferior salivatory nucleus
d. Superior salivatory nucleus
e. Edinger-Westphal nucleus of cranial nerve III

222. Where was the most likely locus of this lesion?

a. Nucleus of the facial nerve
b. Inferior and superior ganglia of cranial nerve IX
c. Geniculate ganglion
d. Cerebral cortex
e. Reticular formation

DIRECTIONS: Each group of questions below consists of lettered options followed by a set of numbered items. For each numbered item, select the **one** lettered option with which it is most closely associated. Each lettered option may be used once, more than once, or not at all.

Item 223–227

Match each description with the appropriate site shown in the figure.

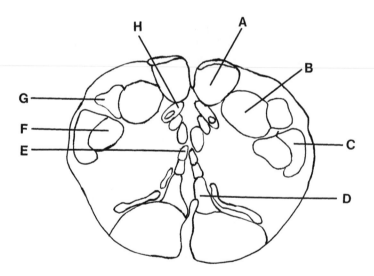

223. A middle-aged woman suffers a vascular occlusion involving part of the brainstem, resulting in selective loss of sensation in the leg and concomitant ataxia. Which structure is most likely affected?

224. If the vascular lesion described in the previous question were expanded to cause loss of sensation in the hand, which structure is associated with such a loss of sensation?

225. A 47-year-old male is brought into the emergency room and is diagnosed with a small brainstem stroke. The patient presents with an inability to display reflex movements of the head in response to vestibular stimulation. Which structure is most likely affected by this lesion?

226. In order to alleviate excruciating pain to the face, a surgical lesion of the fiber bundle mediating pain sensation from the face is made. Which structure is associated with the surgical lesion?

227. A vascular lesion of the lower brainstem in a patient results in the loss of conscious proprioception in the limbs contralateral to the lesion. Which structure is affected by this lesion?

Item 228–236

Match each description with the appropriate site shown in the figure.

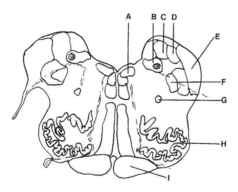

228. A young adult male suffers an injury to the region of the face that affects in part the peripheral nerve innervating the tongue, which results in some loss of ability to identify the taste of foods. Which structure in the brainstem would normally receive these peripheral taste inputs?

229. A stroke involving a part of the lower brainstem resulted in loss of the ability to coordinate movements of the head in response to changes in posture. Which structure is associated with this loss of function?

230. A midbrain stroke results in significant damage to the red nucleus, causing major degeneration of the descending fibers from this nucleus. Which structure present in the lower brainstem is now devoid of this input?

231. A localized vascular lesion results in a sudden increase in blood pressure. Which structure is affected, resulting in this change in blood pressure?

232. Which neurons contribute the largest number of fibers that are contained in the inferior cerebellar peduncle?

233. As a result of a stroke involving the lower brainstem, a 64-year-old man presents with a loss of swallowing and the gag reflex. Which structure is so affected?

234. A stroke involving part of the lower brainstem results in a contralateral UMN paralysis. Which structure is so affected?

235. Following a vascular lesion of the lower brainstem, a patient is tested for cranial nerve functions. When asked to stick out his tongue, it deviates to the side. Which structure is so affected?

236. Which bundle of fibers arises from the spinal cord and the brainstem and projects directly to the cerebellum?

Item 237–242

Match each description with the appropriate site shown in the figure.

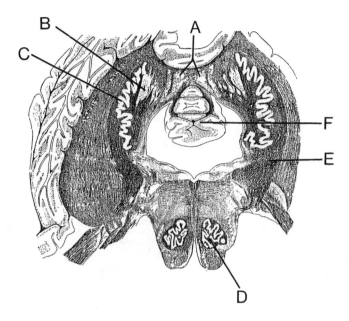

237. A vascular lesion results in loss of balance, ataxia, and some loss of regulation of blood pressure. Which structure, if damaged, would likely result in this group of deficits?

238. Which are the neurons that project to the vestibular nuclei and reticular formation?

239. A middle-aged male was admitted to the hospital having suffered a stroke. The patient presented with loss of ability to produce coordinated movements of the upper limbs with little loss of balance. Which is the most likely site of this lesion?

240. Which is the site that comprises part of a feedback pathway to the red nucleus from the cerebellum?

241. Which structure receives inputs from the vermal region of the cerebellar cortex?

242. Which neurons receive inputs from the lateral aspects of the cerebellar hemispheres?

Item 243–249

Match each description with the appropriate site shown in the figure.

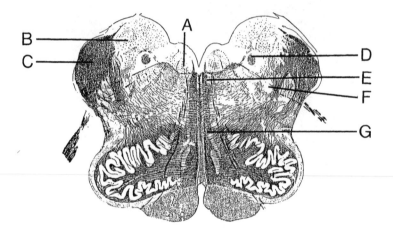

243. A person suffered a facial injury that resulted in dizziness and some loss of balance. Which structure would lose inputs as a result of the injury?

244. An individual suffered from a discrete brainstem lesion affecting ascending and descending axons. The patient presented with loss of postural adjustment of the head in response to changes in position of the body and some nystagmus. Which structure was affected by the lesion?

245. A patient complained that she lost her sense of taste. A subsequent MRI suggested the presence of a small vascular lesion of the brainstem. Which structure was likely affected by this lesion?

246. When a patient attempted to protrude his tongue, it deviated to the side. Damage to which structure would account for this loss?

247. Where is the lesion that would result in contralateral loss of conscious proprioception and some tactile sensation of the limbs?

248. A patient presented with loss of pain sensation from one side of the face. It was discovered that it was probably due to a small brainstem lesion. Where was the likely locus of this lesion?

249. Which fibers convey muscle spindle afferents to the cerebellum?

Item 250–254

Match each description with the appropriate site shown in the figure.

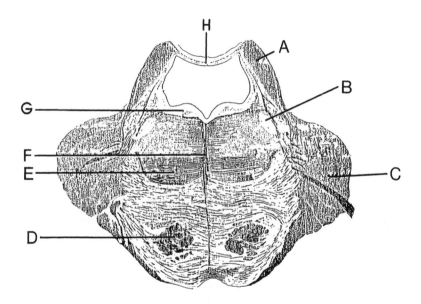

250. An individual suffered from a rare autoimmune disorder that destroyed neuronal cell bodies situated in the basilar aspect of the pons. The patient presented with loss of coordination of movements of the forelimbs when attempting to make a purposeful response. Which fibers degenerated as a result of the autoimmune disorder?

251. A discrete brainstem lesion resulted in significant reduction in reflexes involving mastication. Which was the likely structure affected by the lesion?

252. An individual was admitted to a hospital after falling unconscious. Later, he presented with a UMN paralysis and was told that he had had a stroke involving part of his brainstem. Damage to what structure would account for his deficit?

253. If the stroke described in question 252 had been more expansive and caused loss of conscious proprioception and tactile sensation on the same side of the body where the UMN paralysis was present, damage to what structure would account for this sensory loss?

254. A person suffered from a degenerating disease that selectively destroyed his deep cerebellar nuclei. The axons of which structure would likely show significant degeneration as a result of this disorder?

Item 255–259

Match each description with the appropriate site shown in the figure.

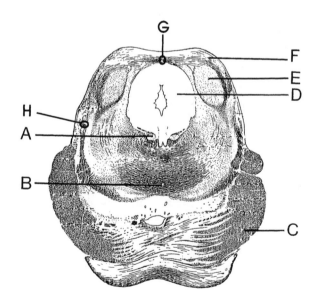

255. An individual suffered a stroke involving part of his midbrain and, when tested by an audiologist, it was revealed that he had lost some ability in auditory discrimination, acuity, and ability to localize sound in space. The loss of which structure could possibly account for these deficits?

256. A person was admitted to a hospital after inhaling a toxic agent, which was later found to produce significant cerebellar damage. The patient subsequently died, an autopsy was performed, and brainstem sections were taken. The pathologist noted significant damage of a structure within the midbrain. Which structure would most likely show such a deficit?

257. A 79-year-old woman was admitted to the emergency room after suffering a stroke. The stroke involved parts of the cerebral cortex, resulting in a contralateral UMN paralysis. Which fibers would be degenerated?

258. A middle-aged man was admitted to the emergency room after falling down stairs. Later, he complained about having double vision and, during a neurological examination, was found to have difficulty moving his eye downward, especially when attempting to look medially. The neurologist concluded that the patient had a small vascular lesion of the brainstem. Which structure was most likely affected by the lesion?

259. An individual was diagnosed with a brainstem tumor and presented with increased sensitivity to pain, a reduction in blood pressure, and a general change and irregularity in emotionality. Which structure was most likely affected by the tumor?

Item 260–264

Match each description with the appropriate site in the figure.

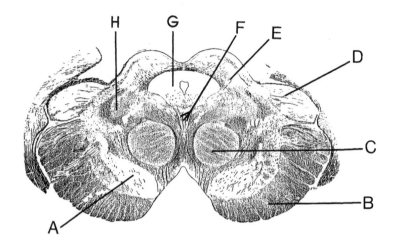

260. A patient was observed to have difficulty moving his eyes up or down as well as following moving objects. Subsequent diagnosis suggested that there was compression of part of the brainstem. Which was the principal structure most likely affected by this compression?

261. Concerning the patient described in question 260, if the compression of the brainstem also resulted in reduced auditory acuity, discrimination of sounds, and localization, damage to which structure could account for this sensory loss?

262. A patient presented with motor dysfunctions characterized by rigidity, tremor, and akinesia. At which site could a lesion produce such a constellation of motor deficits?

263. A person presented with a contralateral limb ataxia, together with a weakness of the medial rectus muscle and a fixed dilated pupil. The neurologist concluded that the patient sustained an infarction of the brainstem. Which structure constituted the principal focus of the infarction?

264. A rare autoimmune disorder that specifically destroys neuronal cell bodies affected a 72-year-old female. As a result, she was unable to direct her eyes medially or vertically, and her pupils did not constrict in response to light. Which structure was damaged by this disorder?

DIRECTIONS: Each item below contains a question or incomplete statement followed by suggested responses. Select the **one best** response to each question.

265. A 60-year-old male suffered from excruciating pain on the left side of his face. Since drug therapy was found to be ineffective in alleviating the pain, it was decided that surgery was indicated. Which of the following structures would be surgically cut or destroyed in order to alleviate the pain?

a. First-order descending sensory fibers contained in the ipsilateral spinal tract of cranial nerve V
b. Neurons in the ventral posterolateral nucleus of the thalamus
c. Cells contained in the main sensory nucleus of the trigeminal nerve
d. Substantia gelatinosa
e. Midbrain periaqueductal gray

266. After eating a meal that contained food that was spoiled, a 15-year-old boy experienced a rather extensive bout of emesis. Which of the following structures would most closely relate to this function?

a. Ventromedial hypothalamus
b. Posterior thalamus
c. Primary motor cortex
d. Dorsolateral pontine tegmentum
e. Area postrema

267. An individual experienced the following constellation of symptoms following a brainstem lesion associated with a stroke of that region: hoarseness, difficulty in swallowing, diminished gastric secretions, and loss of some cardiovascular reflex functions. To which of the following structures can these symptoms be attributed?

a. Cranial nerve VII
b. Cranial nerve IX
c. Cranial nerve X
d. Cranial nerve XI
e. Pontine reticular formation

268. After examining a patient, a neurologist concluded that he suffered a stroke involving the dorsolateral medulla. What deficit did the neurologist see that allowed him to reach this conclusion?

a. Loss of pain and thermal sensation on the ipsilateral half of the face
b. Loss of pain and temperature sensation on the ipsilateral side of the body
c. Dysphonia
d. Hemiparesis
e. Intention tremor

269. Which of the following statements concerning the olivocochlear bundle is correct?

a. It arises from the inferior olivary nucleus and projects to the cochlea
b. Stimulation of it inhibits acoustic fiber responses to auditory stimuli
c. It communicates directly with the medial lemniscus
d. It can be seen easily in brainstem sections taken from the upper pons
e. It is part of the ascending auditory pathway to the dorsal cochlea nucleus

270. An elderly woman was brought to see an audiologist after complaining about some hearing difficulties. The audiologist noted that she was suffering from unilateral deafness and referred her to a neurologist for further examination. On the basis of his examination, damage to which of the following structures could account for her present condition?

a. The auditory cortex of one side
b. The lateral lemniscus of one side
c. Cranial nerve VIII on one side
d. The medial geniculate
e. The medial lemniscus

271. Which of the following contains first-order sensory neurons with their cell bodies located within the CNS?

a. Geniculate ganglion
b. Spiral ganglion
c. Mesencephalic nucleus of cranial nerve V
d. Solitary nucleus
e. Scarpa's ganglia

272. A middle-aged person was referred to a neurologist after experiencing certain visual deficits. Through the use of an MRI and other diagnostic procedures, it was concluded that there was some damage to a part of his nervous system. The patient presented with a lateral gaze paralysis, in which both eyes were conjugatively directed to the side opposite the lesion. In this condition, where was the locus of the lesion?

a. Root fibers of cranial nerve III
b. Nucleus of cranial nerve III
c. Root fibers of cranial nerve VI
d. Nucleus of cranial nerve VI
e. Nucleus and root fibers of cranial nerve IV

273. An individual was sent to a neurologist because he was having difficulty moving his eyes horizontally to one side. The neurologist concluded that the individual had a vascular lesion. Which of the following structures was affected by this lesion?

a. Paramedian pontine reticular formation
b. Ventrolateral medulla
c. Cranial nerve IV
d. Primary motor cortex
e. Ventral posterolateral nucleus of thalamus

274. A patient displayed an ipsilateral paralysis of lateral gaze coupled with a contralateral hemiplegia. Which of the following was the most likely site of the lesion?

a. Ventromedial medulla
b. Dorsomedial medulla
c. Ventrocaudal pons
d. Dorsorostral pons
e. Ventromedial midbrain

275. Which of the following sets of cranial nerves carry special visceral afferent fibers?

a. V, VII, and IX
b. III, VI, and XII
c. IX, X, and XI
d. II, VII, and VIII
e. I, VII, and IX

276. A patient displayed the following constellation of symptoms: UMN paralysis of the left leg, paralysis of the lower half of the left side of the face, and a left homonymous hemianopsia. Which of the following regions would most likely contain the lesion?

a. Medulla
b. Basilar pons
c. Pontine tegmentum
d. Midbrain
e. Forebrain

277. When a patient was asked to follow an object placed in the right side of his visual field, he was unable to move his right eye either up or down. Which of the following regions would most likely contain the lesion?

a. Medulla
b. Basilar aspect of the pons
c. Pontine tegmentum
d. Midbrain
e. Cerebellum

278. A patient was capable of displaying pupillary constriction during an accommodation reaction but not in response to a direct-light stimulus. Which of the following was the most likely site of the lesion?

a. Optic nerve
b. Ventral cell column of cranial nerve III
c. Pretectal area
d. Visual cortex
e. Edinger-Westphal nucleus of cranial nerve III

279. A person complained that he had a hard time sensing the taste of foods. A subsequent neurological examination revealed that he had a significantly diminished sense of taste. Which of the following groups of structures could be logical sites where a lesion would lead to impaired sensation of taste?

a. Geniculate ganglion, chorda tympani, and medial lemniscus
b. Solitary nucleus, parabrachial nucleus, and ventral posteromedial nucleus
c. Solitary nucleus, ventral posterolateral nucleus, and postcentral gyrus
d. Solitary nucleus, ventral posteromedial nucleus, and superior parietal lobule
e. Geniculate ganglion and ventral posterolateral nucleus

Item 280–283

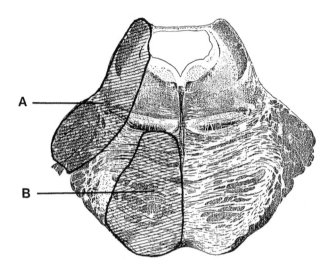

280. An occlusion of which of the following arteries would result in the lesion at A?

a. Basilar artery
b. Superior cerebellar artery
c. Anterior spinal artery
d. Vertebral artery
e. Posterior inferior cerebellar artery

281. An occlusion of which of the following arteries would result in the lesion at B?

a. Paramedian branch of the basilar artery
b. Circumferential branch of the basilar artery
c. Superior cerebellar artery
d. Anterior inferior cerebellar artery
e. Anterior spinal artery

282. Which structure was affected by the lesion at B?

a. Medial lemniscus
b. Lateral lemniscus
c. Corticospinal tract
d. Medial longitudinal fasciculus
e. Tectospinal tract

283. The lesion at B would most likely result in which of the following deficits?

a. Paralysis of the contralateral limbs
b. Loss of conscious proprioception of the contralateral side of the body
c. Nystagmus
d. Lateral gaze paralysis
e. Facial paralysis

Item 284–286

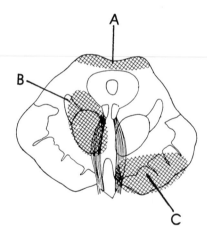

284. A patient with the lesion at A will generally show which of the following deficits?

a. Partial blindness
b. Loss of ability to gaze medially
c. Loss of ability to show tracking movements
d. Loss of accommodation reflex
e. Nystagmus

285. Which of the following deficits is likely to occur as a result of the lesion at B?

a. Contralateral loss of conscious proprioception
b. Transient tremor of the ipsilateral limb
c. Ipsilateral fourth-nerve palsy
d. Hearing loss
e. Contralateral loss of taste sensation

286. The deficits associated with the lesion at C are the result of damage to which of the following structures?

a. Substantia nigra and crus cerebri
b. Red nucleus and crus cerebri
c. Crus cerebri and cranial nerve III
d. Red nucleus and substantia nigra
e. Substantia nigra and cranial nerve III

287. Which of the following statements best describes the regions of the ventral tegmental area and pars compacta of the substantia nigra?

a. Both regions contain dopaminergic neurons but project to different populations of forebrain structures
b. Both regions provide converging dopaminergic inputs to the hypothalamus
c. Both regions provide converging dopaminergic inputs to the neostriatum
d. Both regions are innervated by GABAergic fibers and project to the cerebral cortex
e. Lesions of either region result in the development of a parkinsonian-like syndrome

288. Which of the following is the principal ascending auditory pathway of the brainstem?

a. Medial lemniscus
b. Lateral lemniscus
c. Trapezoid body
d. Trigeminal lemniscus
e. Brachium of the superior colliculus

Item 289–293

Emma was a 64-year-old woman who had heart disease for many years. While carrying chemicals down the stairs of the dry-cleaning shop where she worked, she suddenly lost control of her right leg and arm. She fell down the stairs and was able to stand up with some assistance from a coworker. When attempting to walk on her own, she had a very unsteady gait, with a tendency to fall to the right side. Her supervisor asked her if she was all right, and noticed that her speech was very slurred when she tried to answer. He called an ambulance to take her to the nearest hospital. The physician who was called to see Emma in the emergency room noted that her speech was slurred as if she were intoxicated, but the grammar and meaning were intact. Her face appeared symmetric, but when asked to protrude her tongue, it deviated toward the left. She was unable to tell if her right toe was moved up or down by the physician when she closed her eyes, and she couldn't feel the buzz of a tuning fork on her right arm and leg. In addition, her right arm and leg were markedly weak. The physician could find no other abnormalities in the remainder of Emma's general medical examination.

289. Where in the nervous system did the damage occur?

a. Right lateral medulla
b. Occipital lobe
c. Left lateral medulla
d. Right cervical spinal cord
e. Left medial medulla

290. Where in the nervous system could a lesion occur that would cause arm and leg weakness but spare the face?

a. Right corticospinal tract in the cervical spinal cord
b. Left inferior frontal lobe
c. Right medullary pyramids
d. Occipital lobe
e. Right side of basilar pons

291. Other than the weakness on her right side, what type of deficit could cause Emma's gait problem, and where could a lesion causing this deficit occur?

a. Proprioceptive, left medial lemniscus
b. Sight, left eye
c. Descending component of the medial longitudinal fasciculus
d. Pain, left spinothalamic tract
e. Proprioceptive, right medial lemniscus

292. Deviation of the tongue to the left, away from the right hemiparesis, implies a lesion in which area of the nervous system?

a. Right hypoglossal nucleus
b. Left hypoglossal nucleus
c. Right inferior frontal lobe
d. Left inferior frontal lobe
e. Right cerebral peduncle

293. What type of speech problem does Emma have?

a. Broca's aphasia
b. Wernicke's aphasia
c. Mixed aphasia
d. Dysarthria
e. Agnosia

Item 294–298

Julie was a 29-year-old office worker with diabetes, who awoke one morning with the inability to close her left eye and a left facial droop. Her left eye felt a bit dry as well. She had run out of sick days and, hoping that the problem would go away, went to work. After several coworkers noticed that her face was drooping and that she was especially sensitive to loud noises on her left side, they convinced her to go to the nearest emergency room to make sure that she had not had a stroke. She was examined immediately because of her age. The doctor noted right away that her mouth drooped on the left side. Her left eye was slightly closed. He tested her speech and mental status, which were normal, other than some slight slurring of her speech. Her vision and eye movements were also normal. Sensation and jaw movement were also normal, but when she was asked to wiggle her eyebrows, only the right side of her forehead moved. When asked to close her eyes tightly and not allow him to open her eyes, her right eye would not open, but her left eye could not oppose the force. She was not able to hold air in her cheeks when asked to hold her breath, and when asked to smile, only the right side of her mouth elevated. She was very sensitive to noise on her left side. When asked to protrude her tongue, it did not deviate to either side, but if she closed her eyes and sugar water was placed on the left side of the anterior portion of her tongue, she could not identify it. The remainder of her examination was normal. A nurse asked if a head CT should be ordered in order to look for a stroke or tumor, but the doctor said that it wasn't necessary. He told Julie that he would draw some blood and give her a medication to take for a while.

294. Assuming that the doctor was correct and this wasn't a stroke, where in the nervous system did the damage occur?

a. Buccinator muscle
b. Trigeminal nerve
c. Facial nerve
d. Glossopharyngeal nerve
e. Hypoglossal nerve

295. Julie's facial weakness is characteristic of which of the following?
a. A muscle lesion
b. A lesion of the internal capsule
c. A superior brainstem lesion
d. A UMN seventh-nerve lesion
e. An LMN seventh-nerve lesion

296. Damage to which area may have produced the defect in taste in the anterior two-thirds of her tongue?
a. Intermediate nerve
b. Glossopharyngeal nerve
c. Lingual nerve
d. Facial nerve, distal to the chorda tympani nerve
e. Facial nerve, proximal to the chorda tympani nerve

297. Assuming that Julie had no prior problems with her ears or cochlear nerve, damage to the nerve supply of which muscle could cause the sensitivity to or distortion of noises?
a. Digastric
b. Platysma
c. Buccinator
d. Geniohyoid
e. Stapedius

298. If Julie did not have the loss of taste and noise sensitivity, but did have the inability to move her left eye to the left, which area would now be damaged?
a. The trigeminal and abducens nerves
b. The facial and trigeminal nerves, distal to their exit from the brainstem
c. The facial and abducens nerve nuclei within the pons
d. The facial nerve, distal to the chorda tympani nerve
e. The facial nerve, distal to the geniculate ganglion

Item 299–303

A second-year medical student was asked to see a nursing home patient as a requirement for a physical diagnosis course. The patient was a 79-year-old man who was apparently in a coma. The student wasn't certain of how to approach this case, so he asked the patient's wife, who was sitting at the bedside, why this patient was in a coma. The wife replied, "Oh, Paul isn't in a coma. But he did have a stroke." Slightly confused, the student leaned over and asked Paul to open his eyes. He opened his eyes immediately. However, when asked to lift his arm or speak, Paul did nothing. The student then asked Paul's wife whether she was certain that his eye opening was not simply a coincidence and whether he really was in a coma, since he was unable to follow any commands. Paul's wife explained that he was unable to move or speak as a result of his stroke. However, she knew that he was awake because he could communicate with her by blinking his eyes. The student appeared rather skeptical, so Paul's wife asked her husband to blink once for "yes" and twice for "no." She then asked him if he was at home, and he blinked twice. When asked if he was in a nursing home, he blinked once. The student then asked him to move his eyes, and he was able to look in his direction. However, when the student asked him if he could move his arms or legs, he blinked twice. He also blinked twice when asked if he could smile. He did the same when asked if he could feel someone moving his arm. The student thanked Paul and his wife for their time, made notes of his findings, and returned to class.

299. Where in the nervous system could a lesion occur that can cause paralysis of the extremities bilaterally, as well as in the face, but not of the eyes?

a. High cervical spinal cord bilaterally
b. Bilateral thalamus
c. Bilateral basal ganglia
d. Bilateral basilar pons
e. Bilateral frontal lobe

300. An infarct in what vascular distribution could cause this lesion?

a. Anterior spinal artery
b. Vertebral artery
c. Basilar artery
d. Middle cerebral artery
e. Posterior cerebral artery

301. Damage to which tracts caused Paul's inability to move his arms and legs?

a. Corticospinal and corticobulbar tracts
b. Spinothalamic tract
c. Solitary tract
d. Superior cerebellar peduncle
e. Inferior cerebellar peduncle

302. Damage to which tract caused Paul's lack of perception of someone moving his arm?

a. Corticospinal and corticobulbar
b. Middle cerebellar peduncle
c. Spinothalamic tract
d. Rubrospinal tract
e. Medial lemniscus

303. What area is spared to preserve consciousness?

a. Deep frontal white matter
b. Pontine reticular formation
c. Temporal lobes
d. Prefrontal cortex
e. Occipital lobe

Item 304–308

Herb, a 62-year-old man who smoked two packs of cigarettes per day for 35 years, was suffering from a chronic cough that was attributed to his smoking habit by his physician. One day Herb noticed that his right eyelid drooped slightly and that his right pupil was smaller than the left. He also noticed that the inner side of his right hand was numb and that he had begun to drop things from his right hand. He had no other symptoms. Herb consulted his physician, who directed him to a neurologist. The neurologist noted that although the right pupil was smaller than the left, it was still reactive to light. Although Herb's right eyelid drooped slightly, he could close his eyes tightly when asked to do so. The neurologist noted that Herb did not sweat on the right side of his face. He was unable to feel a pinprick on the inner surface of his right hand, and his right triceps and hand muscles were weak.

304. Where in the nervous system did damage occur?

a. Left oculomotor nerve
b. Right oculomotor nerve
c. Edinger-Westphal nucleus
d. Sympathetic fibers coursing from the hypothalamus to the intermediolateral cell column
e. Parasympathetic fibers coursing from the Edinger-Westphal nucleus

305. Herb's small pupil was due to which of the following?

a. Unopposed action of the muscles with parasympathetic innervation
b. Unopposed action of the muscles with sympathetic innervation
c. Both sympathetic and parasympathetic damage
d. A lesion in the nucleus of the third nerve
e. A lesion in distal branches of the trochlear nerve

306. Why was Herb able to close his eye tightly, despite a drooping eyelid?

a. The facial nerve does not innervate muscles mediating eye closure
b. The facial nerve is only partially affected
c. The facial nerve is unaffected by this lesion
d. The trigeminal nerve compensates for eye closure
e. This lesion affects only involuntary eye closure

307. Which pair of neurotransmitters is involved in the pathway that has been damaged?

a. Substance P and acetylcholine (ACh)
b. Norepinephrine and epinephrine
c. 5-HT and GABA
d. GABA and ACh
e. ACh and norepinephrine

308. Damage to which fibers caused the numbness and weakness of his hand?

a. Damage to the ipsilateral cerebral peduncle
b. Damage to the corticospinal tract
c. Damage to the cervical spinal roots entering the brachial plexus
d. Infarction of the basilar artery
e. Damage to the median nerve

Item 309–313

Mike was a 35-year-old man who had had optic neuritis (an inflammation of the optic nerve causing blurred vision) several years before. He was told that he had a 50% chance of eventually developing multiple sclerosis (MS), a degenerative disease of the CNS white matter. One day he noticed that he had double vision and felt weak on his right side. Although he noted that the symptoms were becoming steadily worse throughout the day, he attributed this to stress from his job as a stockbroker, and in order to relax he decided to take a drive in his car. While he was driving, his vision became steadily worse. As he was about to pull over to the side of the road, he saw two trees on the right side of the road. Uncertain which was the actual image, he attempted to place his right foot on the brake pedal. Mike suddenly realized that he was unable to lift his right leg, and his car collided with the tree. A pedestrian on the side of the road called the EMS, and Mike was brought to a nearby emergency room.

A neurologist was called to see Mike because the emergency room physicians thought he might have had a stroke, despite his young age. The neurologist spoke to Mike, then examined him. He found that his left eye was deviated to the left and down. When he attempted to look to his right, his right eye moved normally, but his left eye was unable to move farther to the right than the midline. His left pupil was dilated and did not contract to light from a penlight. His left eyelid drooped, and he had difficulty raising it. In addition, the right side of his mouth remained motionless when he attempted to smile, but his forehead was symmetric when he raised his eyebrows. Mike's right arm and leg were markedly weak. The neurologist told Mike that he wasn't certain that this was necessarily a stroke, but admitted him to the hospital for observation and tests.

309. A lesion in which of the following nerves caused Mike's double vision?

a. Optic nerve
b. Oculomotor nerve
c. Cervical sympathetic fibers
d. Trochlear nerve
e. Abducens nerve

310. Which of the following muscles were affected by nerve damage, causing Mike's eye to be deviated toward the left side and down?

a. Superior rectus, superior oblique, inferior rectus, inferior oblique
b. Superior rectus, inferior rectus, inferior oblique, lateral rectus
c. Superior rectus, inferior rectus, inferior oblique, medial rectus
d. Lateral rectus, superior oblique, medial rectus, inferior rectus
e. Lateral rectus, superior oblique, inferior oblique, medial rectus

311. Where in the nervous system did the damage occur?

a. Left frontal lobe
b. Right frontal lobe
c. Left eye
d. Cervical spinal cord
e. Midbrain

312. Damage to which fibers caused the enlarged, unreactive pupil on the left?

a. Medial longitudinal fasciculus
b. Frontal or pontine eye fields
c. Edinger-Westphal nucleus or preganglionic parasympathetic fibers
d. Trochlear nerve
e. Cervical sympathetic fibers

313. Damage to which area caused Mike's weakness?

a. Left precentral gyrus
b. Right precentral gyrus
c. Left cervical spinal cord
d. Right cervical spinal cord
e. Left cerebral peduncle

Item 314–318

A 17-year-old high school football player presented to a neurology clinic because his mother thought that he may have acquired neck problems during a game. A month before, he had sustained a concussion from a blow to his head from another player. Shortly after, she noted that he intermittently tilted his head to the side. When asked what was the matter, he simply said that sometimes he had double vision and that the images were situated on top of each other vertically, making it difficult to go down stairs. When he was examined, there was no neck pain or limitation of motion. He tended to keep his head tilted to the right side. When asked to follow the doctor's finger with his head in a straight position, his left eye would not move downward when his eyes were turned to the right, and they tended to remain slightly deviated toward the left. At this point, he stated that he had double vision and felt better if his head was tilted to the right. The remainder of his eye movements, as well as the remainder of his exam, was normal.

314. Where did the damage occur?

a. The oculomotor nerve
b. The abducens nerve
c. The trochlear nerve
d. The trigeminal nerve
e. The facial nerve

315. Which muscle was weakened?

a. Superior rectus
b. Inferior rectus
c. Lateral rectus
d. Superior oblique
e. Inferior oblique

316. From which portion of the brainstem did the damaged nerve emerge?

a. Right ventral midbrain
b. Right dorsal midbrain
c. Left ventral midbrain
d. Left dorsal midbrain
e. Left ventral pons

317. What was the action of the weak muscle?

a. Outward and upward rotation of the orbit
b. Outward and downward rotation of the orbit
c. Inward and upward rotation of the orbit
d. Inward and downward rotation of the orbit
e. Deviation of the orbit laterally

318. How could the head trauma have caused the double vision?

a. Direct damage to the eye
b. Damage to the occipital lobes
c. Damage to the midbrain
d. Damage to the pons
e. Damage to the cranial nerve peripherally

The Brainstem and Cranial Nerves

Answers

189–190. The answers are 189-d and 190-c. (*Gilroy, p 33. Simon et al., p 347. Afifi, p 175.*) The reflex described in this question is the corneal reflex. It involves the reflex activation of the ophthalmic division of the sensory component of cranial nerve V in response to touching of the cornea and the motor division of the facial (cranial nerve VII), which produces the motor component (i.e., the blinking response). The sensory component of cranial nerve V is classified as a general somatic afferent fiber and the somatic motor component of cranial nerve VII is classified as a special visceral efferent fiber.

191–193. The answers are 191-d, 192-c, 193-b. (*Gilroy, pp 587–589. Afifi, pp 163–165.*) Taste associated with the anterior two-thirds of the tongue is mediated by the facial (cranial nerve VII) nerve. The geniculate ganglion contains the cell bodies associated with the sensory (gustatory) component of the seventh nerve. The somatic motor component of the seventh nerve mediates the muscles of facial expression. Thus, the sensory and motor components of the seventh nerve affected in this individual can be characterized as special visceral afferent (because this afferent contains chemoreceptors) and special visceral efferent (because the motor component innervates skeletal muscle and is derived from a branchial arch), respectively.

194–197. The answers are 194-c, 195-c, 196-b, 197-b. (*Gilroy, pp 590–591. Afifi, pp 131–132.*) Cranial nerve IX, the glossopharyngeal nerve, innervates the skeletal muscles of the pharynx. The motor component involved arises from the nucleus ambiguus of the medulla. This cranial nerve also contains afferents, a component of which arises from the superior ganglion. These sensory neurons convey somatosensory sensation, including pain afferents that ultimately synapse in the spinal trigeminal nucleus. The motor component of the glossopharyngeal nerve mediating swallowing and coughing constitutes a special visceral efferent (because it is derived from a visceral arch), and the sensory component conveying pain is referred to as a general somatic afferent fiber.

198–199. The answers are 198-d and 199-b. *(Afifi, p 232. Kandel, pp 668–669, 817.)* Rigidity can occur by experimentally producing a decerebrate preparation (i.e., severing the brainstem at the level of the pons), and it appears clinically as well. In both situations, there has to be extensive destruction of brain tissue below the midbrain in the region of the pons, but the medulla is spared. In this way, the lateral vestibulospinal tract remains intact. This pathway powerfully facilitates extensor motor neurons and extensor reflexes, thus contributing significantly to the expression of decerebrate rigidity, in particular when the descending inhibitory pathways, which arise from more rostral levels, are disrupted by the experimental procedure or stroke.

200–202. The answers are 200-d, 201-a, 202-d. *(Afifi, pp 133–135. Kandel, pp 972–975.)* Specialized peripheral receptors, which specifically respond to changes in blood pressure, include the carotid sinus (associated with cranial nerve IX) and the aortic arch (associated with cranial nerve X). If these receptors (or the cell bodies associated with these receptors) are damaged, then one of the fundamental regulatory mechanisms for the control of blood pressure would be disrupted. The results of such a disruption would likely lead to increases and instability in blood pressure, with evidence of spiking of blood pressure. Because these sensory receptors in these structures respond to increases in blood pressure, they are, in effect, stretch receptors and are consequently referred to as *baroreceptors*. The principal projection of the axons associated with these baroreceptors is the solitary nucleus of the medulla, which in turn projects to autonomic nuclei such as the dorsal motor nucleus of the vagus nerve, ventrolateral medulla, and higher regions associated with autonomic functions, which include the PAG, hypothalamus, and limbic system.

203. The answer is b. *(Afifi, pp 82–85.)* The medial vestibulospinal tract arises from the medial vestibular nucleus and descends in the medial longitudinal fasciculus to cervical levels, where it controls LMNs, which innervate (flexor) muscles controlling the position of the head. The lateral vestibulospinal tract facilitates extensor motor neurons of the limbs, the rubrospinal tract facilitates flexor motor neurons of the limbs, and the reticulospinal tracts modulate muscle tone of the limbs.

204–206. The answers are 204-c, 205-c, 206-b. *(Martin, pp 42–44. Afifi, pp 125–133.)* This individual who suffers a paralysis of the soft palate and pharynx, as well as loss of the carotid sinus reflex, sustains damage that includes cranial nerve X. It should be noted that several of these symptoms could have been incurred by damage to cranial nerve IX as well. However, in this question, cranial nerve IX was not listed as a choice. The axons of the nucleus ambiguus of cranial nerve X innervate the soft palate and pharynx. Damage to these neurons would frequently cause dysphagia, hoarseness, and paralysis of the soft palate. In addition, damage to the dorsal motor nucleus of the vagus constitutes an efferent limb for expression of the carotid sinus reflex. Thus, damage to these two nuclear groups would produce the constellation of deficits described for this case. The nucleus ambiguus is classified as a special visceral efferent fiber because it innervates skeletal muscle and it is derived from a visceral arch, while the dorsal motor nucleus innervates thoracic and abdominal viscera and is therefore classified as a general visceral efferent fiber.

207. The answer is c. (*Martin, pp 42–49. Afifi, pp 148–153.*) The combined deficit in which the patient loses ability to (use his lateral rectus muscle to) abduct his right eye and display facial expression on the right side of the face means that the lesion is located in the dorsal pons at the site where the facial nerve curves around (just above) the motor nucleus of cranial nerve VI. Thus, a lesion at this site will affect both cranial nerves, causing the combined deficits described previously.

208. The answer is e. (*Afifi, pp 209–213.*) The cranial nerve involved in adduction of the eye is cranial nerve III, in which the act of moving the eye medially is governed by the medial rectus muscle. Cranial nerve III is located near the midline of the rostral half of the midbrain just below the midbrain periaqueductal gray.

209–211. The answers are 209-d, 210-d, 211-a. (*Martin, pp 42–49. Afifi, pp 194–195.*) To walk down stairs, one has to have the ability to move the eyes down when they are in the medial position. This involves the use of cranial nerve IV (trochlear nerve), which innervates the superior oblique muscle (whose action is to pull the eye downward when in the medial position). If there is damage to this nerve on one side, the eyes will not be able to focus on the same visual field, thus producing double vision. Cranial nerve IV is classified as a general somatic efferent fiber because it innervates skeletal muscle and it is derived from somites.

212. The answer is d. *(Afifi, pp 118–120.)* Two of the principal afferent fiber systems that project to the inferior olivary nucleus include the red nucleus and the spinal cord. These inputs serve important functions of enabling the inferior olivary nucleus of transmitting information related to both sensory (spinal cord) and motor (red nucleus) processes to the cerebellar cortex. The other structures indicated in this question do not have known projections to the inferior olivary nucleus.

213. The answer is e. *(Afifi, pp 118–120.)* The primary projection pathway of the inferior olivary nucleus exits this nucleus, enters the inferior cerebellar peduncle of the contralateral side of the brain, and passes into the cerebellar cortex, terminating on apical dendrites of Purkinje cells throughout the cerebellar cortex in a somatotopic manner. As indicated previously in the explanation of the previous question, this pathway represents an important source of input to the cerebellum from significant regions mediating sensory and motor information (via the inferior olivary nucleus). Other suggested answers do not include known projection targets of the inferior olivary nucleus.

214–215. The answers are 214-c and 215-c. *(Afifi, pp 133–134.)* The central pathways mediating taste include the following: primary afferent taste fibers associated with taste receptors of cranial nerves VII, IX, and X synapse in the solitary nucleus. Many fibers from the solitary nucleus project to the ventral posteromedial nucleus of the thalamus, which in turn project to the ventrolateral aspect of the postcentral gyrus.

216–219. The answers are 216-b, 217-a, 218-d, 219-e. *(Afifi, pp 130–134. Gilroy, pp 590–591. Simon et al., pp 92–93.)* The cranial nerve that was directly affected was the glossopharyngeal nerve (cranial nerve IX). This is a mixed and complex nerve containing (1) special visceral efferents from the nucleus ambiguus that supply the stylopharyngeus muscle (for elevation of pharynx in speech); (2) special visceral afferent fibers that transmit taste impulses from the posterior third of the tongue and general visceral afferent fibers associated with the inferior ganglion whose receptors lie in the carotid sinus that regulates cardiovascular functions; (3) general somatic afferents whose cell bodies lie in the superior ganglion of cranial nerve IX and which mediate somatosensory information, including pain from the pharynx; and (4) general visceral efferent fibers that originate in the inferior salivatory nucleus, which are preganglionic and synapse in the otic ganglion. The postganglionic fiber from the otic ganglion innervates the parotid gland and mediates, in part, salivation. Thus, when this nerve is affected by an infectious agent, it results in the constellation of symptoms presented earlier in this case. Since the cell bodies of motor (or visceral motor) fibers (mediating motor and visceral effects) as well as the terminals of sensory afferents (mediating pain from the pharynx) lie in different regions of the medulla, it is very unlikely that such an effect could be the result of damage centrally. A much more likely occurrence is that the infectious agent produced disruption of the glossopharyngeal nerve peripherally, such as at the base of the skull or jugular foramen, where all the components run together and can be more easily affected.

220–222. The answers are 220-b, 221-d, 222-c. *(Afifi, pp 163–166. Gilroy, pp 588–589. Simon et al., pp 347–348.)* The nerve affected by this disorder is cranial nerve VII (facial nerve). The cell bodies of origin, which innervate the muscles of facial expression (special visceral efferents), arise from the facial nucleus, which are located in the ventrolateral aspect of the lower pons. The preganglionic parasympathetic neurons, which synapse with postganglionic neurons in the submandibular and pterygopalatine ganglia, arise from the superior salivatory nucleus of the lower pons. Based on the same reasoning as indicated in the answer to question 215, the most likely locus of the defect is the geniculate ganglion. The region of the geniculate ganglion and regions adjacent to it contain sensory, skeletal, and visceral motor components of this nerve. Therefore, disruption of this nerve in the region of the geniculate ganglion will produce the constellation of deficits described in this case. The other choices are not appropriate. Cranial nerve IX is not involved. Neither are the regions of the reticular formation and facial nucleus, because lesions at either of these locations could not account for the totality of deficits described in this case. The lesion could not have involved the cerebral cortex because the motor effects were described as a flaccid facial paralysis. A cortical lesion does not produce flaccidity of these muscles.

223–227. The answers are 223-A, 224-B, 225-E, 226-C, 227-D. *(Afifi, pp 104–117.)* The nucleus gracilis (A) contains cells that respond to movement of the lower limb as a result of joint capsule activation. Damage to this region will result in loss of conscious proprioception associated with the leg, and, additionally, the loss of conscious proprioception will result in ataxia because this input is essential for normal ambulation to occur. The nucleus cuneatus (B) contains cells that respond to a variety of stimuli applied to the upper limb, including vibratory stimuli. One component of the descending medial longitudinal fasciculus (E) contains fibers that arise from the medial vestibular nucleus that project to cervical levels and contribute to reflex activity associated with the position of the head. The descending track of the trigeminal nerve (C) contains first-order fibers mediating pain and temperature information from the head region. Because of its lateral position in the brainstem, a surgical procedure is sometimes carried out to cut these fibers as a means of alleviating excruciating pain. Fibers of the medial lemniscus (D) arise from the contralateral dorsal column nuclei and ascend to the ventral posterolateral nucleus of the thalamus. These fibers transmit the same information noted earlier for the dorsal column nuclei, which includes two-point discrimination and conscious proprioception from the opposite side of the body.

228–236. The answers are 228-B, 229-C, 230-H, 231-B, 232-H, 233-G, 234-I, 235-A, 236-E. (*Nolte, pp 254–276. Afifi, 117–135.*) Different groups of neurons of the solitary complex (B) respond to taste stimuli and to inputs that signal sudden changes in blood pressure. The medial vestibular nucleus (C) receives direct vestibular inputs from the otolith organ and semicircular canals. Axons of medial vestibular neurons descend to the spinal cord in the medial longitudinal fasciculus and serve to regulate reflexes associated with the head. The inferior vestibular nucleus (D) also receives vestibular inputs, but does not project its axons to the spinal cord. The inferior olivary nucleus (H) receives inputs from the red nucleus and spinal cord, and it projects its axons through the inferior cerebellar peduncle (where it constitutes its largest component) to the contralateral cerebellar cortex, where they synapse with the dendrites of Purkinje cells.

The nucleus ambiguus (G) is a special visceral efferent nucleus that is situated in a position ventrolateral to that of the hypoglossal nucleus. Its axons innervate the muscles of the larynx and pharynx and, therefore, are essential for the occurrence of such responses as the gag reflex. The pyramids (I), located on the ventromedial aspect of the brainstem, contain fibers that arise from the sensorimotor cortex. These neurons serve as essential upper motor neurons that mediate voluntary control of motor functions. The hypoglossal nucleus (A), a general somatic efferent nucleus, is located in the dorsomedial aspect of the medulla. Its axons innervate the muscles of the tongue and cause extrusion of the tongue toward the opposite side, but when this structure is damaged, the tongue protrudes to the side of the lesion when extended. Fibers contained in the inferior cerebellar peduncle (E) arise from cells located in both the spinal cord and the brainstem.

237–242. The answers are 237-A, 238-A, 239-C, 240-B, 241-A, 242-C. (*Afifi, pp 147–167, 303–320. Nolte, pp 470–484.*) The efferent projections of the cerebellum arise from three distinct groups of nuclei called *deep cerebellar nuclei.* The nucleus located in the most medial position is the fastigial nucleus (A). It gives rise to at least two important projections: one that is distributed to the reticular formation and another that is distributed to the vestibular nuclei. In this manner, the fastigial nucleus contributes to the regulation of balance and ambulation via its connections with the vestibular system and to the regulation of blood pressure (as well as muscle tone) via its connections with reticular formation. The nucleus situated most laterally is the dentate nucleus (C). It projects through the superior cerebellar peduncle and its axons innervate principally the ventrolateral nucleus of the thalamus, which in turn projects to the motor cortex. In this way, the dentate nucleus contributes to the regulation of coordinated movements of the distal musculature. Damage to any component of this circuit would seriously affect the capacity to produce coordinated movements of the arms and hands.

Neurons of the emboliform (B) and globose (not labeled) nuclei lie in an intermediate position between the fastigial and dentate nuclei and therefore are often referred to as the *interposed nuclei.* Their axons project through the superior cerebellar peduncle principally to the red nucleus. The projections from the cerebellar cortex to the deep cerebellar nuclei are topographically organized. Cells located in the far medial aspect of the cerebellar cortex, the vermal region, project (via Purkinje cell axons) to the fastigial nucleus (A). In contrast, the lateral aspects of the cerebellar hemispheres project to the dentate nucleus (C), which is the most lateral of the deep cerebellar nuclei.

243–249. The answers are 243-B, 244-E, 245-D, 246-A, 247-G, 248-F, 249-C. (*Afifi, 118–139. Nolte, pp 230–239, 255–274, 284–307.*) The inferior vestibular nucleus (B) lies immediately medial to the inferior cerebellar peduncle (shown at C) and receives direct inputs from first-order vestibular fibers that arise from the vestibular apparatus. The medial longitudinal fasciculus (E) contains second-order vestibular fibers, the majority of which ascend in the brainstem to innervate cranial nerve nuclei III, IV, and VI. A small component of this bundle also descends to cervical levels of the spinal cord from the medial vestibular nucleus. As noted previously, the descending component of the MLF integrates vestibular signals, which help to regulate the position of the head with changes in position of the body. Damage to this structure will also affect the ascending fibers, which innervate the neurons controlling the extraocular eye muscles. Such damage would result in nystagmus. The solitary nucleus (D) receives inputs from first-order taste fibers and is thus a special visceral afferent nucleus that transmits taste signals to the ventral posteromedial nucleus of the thalamus. The solitary nucleus also receives cardiovascular inputs from cranial nerve IX and, for this reason, has properties of a general visceral afferent nucleus as well. The hypoglossal nucleus (A) innervates the muscles of the tongue, causing it to protrude outward and to the opposite side. Thus, when this nerve is damaged, the opposite (normal) nerve causes the tongue to deviate to the side of the lesion when the patient attempts to stick out his tongue.

The medial lemniscus (G) ascends to the thalamus and transmits information associated with conscious proprioception from the contralateral side of the body as a result of the decussating fibers of the medial lemniscus. This bundle constitutes a second-order neuron that arises from the dorsal column nuclei of the lower medulla. The dorsal column nuclei receive first-order signals that mediate conscious proprioception from fibers contained within the dorsal columns of the spinal cord. Damage to the medial lemniscus would result in loss of conscious proprioception on the side of the body opposite the lesion. The spinal nucleus of cranial nerve V (F) receives pain and temperature fibers from first-order trigeminal neurons that arise from the head. Damage to this region would result in loss of pain sensation from the ipsilateral side of the face. The inferior cerebellar peduncle (C) is one of two principal cerebellar afferent pathways. One major fiber group contained within the inferior cerebellar peduncle arises from brainstem structures such as the contralateral inferior olivary nucleus and reticular formation. The other groups of fibers contained within this bundle arise from the spinal cord. Of the fibers that ascend in this bundle from the spinal cord, many constitute second-order muscle spindle afferents that arise from the nucleus dorsalis of Clarke.

250–254. The answers are 250-C, 251-B, 252-D, 253-E, 254-A.
(*Afifi, pp 147–167, 303–320. Nolte, pp 230–239, 256–259, 470–478.*) The middle cerebellar peduncle (C) serves as a relay nucleus for the transmission of information from the cerebral cortex to the cerebellum. Fibers in this peduncle arise from the contralateral deep pontine nucleus, which receives its principal afferents from the cerebral cortex. As noted previously, damage to this pathway would affect the cerebral cortex–cerebellar circuit, resulting in movements of the distal musculature that would lack coordination. The motor nucleus of cranial nerve V (B) is an LMN (special visceral efferent) because it innervates the muscles of mastication and controls, in particular, jaw-closing responses. Corticobulbar and corticospinal fibers (D) are situated in the ventral aspect of the basilar pons. Damage at any level of the corticospinal system would result in a contralateral UMN paralysis. The medial lemniscus (E) is a somatotopically organized pathway that arises from the dorsal column nuclei and projects to the ventral posterolateral nucleus of the thalamus. Fibers of this pathway that arise from the nucleus gracilis (associated with the leg) project to more dorsolateral aspects of the ventral posterolateral nucleus. Fibers arising from the nucleus cuneatus (associated with the arm) project to more ventromedial aspects of the ventral posterolateral nucleus. Thus, damage to this pathway would result in loss of conscious proprioception and some tactile sensation on the contralateral side of the body (i.e., the same side where the upper motor paralysis would be expressed). Fibers of the superior cerebellar peduncle (A) arise from the dentate and interposed nuclei of cerebellum and project to both the red nucleus and the ventrolateral nucleus of the thalamus. Therefore, if these cerebellar nuclei were destroyed, then the fibers contained in the superior cerebellar peduncle would show extensive degeneration.

255–259. The answers are 255-E, 256-B, 257-C, 258-A, 259-D.
(*Afifi, pp 187–213. Nolte, pp 266–277.*) The inferior colliculus (E) is situated in the caudal aspect of the tectum and is an important relay nucleus for the transmission of auditory information to the cortex from lower levels of the brainstem. Damage to the inferior colliculus would likely result in some loss of auditory discrimination, acuity, and ability to localize sound in space. The decussation of the superior cerebellar peduncle (B) is also present at caudal levels of the midbrain and is usually seen together with the inferior colliculus. These crossing fibers arise from the dentate and

interposed nuclei and terminate in the contralateral red nucleus and ven-trolateral nucleus of the thalamus. Damage to the cerebellum would likely result in degeneration of the fibers contained within the superior cerebellar peduncle. The crus cerebri (C) contains fibers that arise from all regions of the cortex and project to all the levels of the brainstem and the spinal cord. As noted previously, damage to the corticospinal tract at any level would result in a UMN paralysis. The trochlear nucleus (cranial nerve IV) (A), which is situated just below the periaqueductal gray at the level of the infe-rior colliculus, receives direct inputs from ascending fibers of the medial longitudinal fasciculus that arise from vestibular nuclei. The trochlear nucleus governs the downward movements of the eyes, in particular, when they are in a medial position. A fourth nerve paralysis is particularly seen when the patient is attempting to walk down a flight of stairs and cannot move his eyes downward. The midbrain periaqueductal gray (D) contains dense quantities of enkephalin-positive cells and nerve terminals. The transmitter (or neuromodulator) enkephalin plays an important role in the regulation of pain, cardiovascular functions, and emotional behavior.

260–264. The answers are 260-E, 261-D, 262-A, 263-C, 264-F. *(Afifi, pp 187–213. Nolte, pp 266–277. Waxman, p 94.)* The superior colliculus (E), situated at a more rostral level of the tectum, plays an important role in tracking or pursuit of moving stimuli as well as movements of the eyes up and down. Damage to this region would clearly affect the ability to produce these movements. The medial geniculate nucleus (D), which is part of the forebrain, actually sits over the lateral aspect of the midbrain and can be seen at rostral levels of the midbrain. It is part of an auditory relay system and receives its inputs from the inferior colliculus via fibers of the brachium of the inferior colliculus. Damage to this relay nucleus would affect auditory acuity and one's ability to localize and discriminate sound. The pars compacta is situated in the medial aspect of the substantia nigra (A) and contains dopamine neurons whose axons innervate the striatum. Damage to these dopamine neurons produces Parkinson's disease, which is characterized by rigidity, tremor, and akinesia. The red nucleus (C), a structure associated with motor functions, receives direct inputs from both the cerebral cortex and the cerebellum. The contralateral limb ataxia could be accounted for by the loss of inputs from the red nucleus to the cerebel-lum via the inferior olivary nucleus. The loss of pupillary constriction and ability to move the eye medially could be accounted for by the fact that the fibers of the oculomotor nerve pass ventrally in proximity to the red nucleus. Thus, damage to the red nucleus would also affect the oculomotor nerve. The oculomotor nerve (cranial nerve III) (F), located at the level of the superior colliculus, contains general somatic efferent components that innervate extraocular eye muscles and general visceral efferent components whose postganglionic fibers innervate smooth muscles associated with pupillary constriction and bulging of the lens. As just noted, damage to the oculomotor nerve would produce impairment of vertical and medial movements of the eyes as well as loss of the pupillary light reflex.

265. The answer is a. (*Afifi, pp 171–177. Nolte, pp 294–301.*) The spinal trigeminal nucleus receives its sensory inputs from first-order neurons contained in the ipsilateral descending tract of cranial nerve V. A central property of the spinal trigeminal nucleus is that it is uniquely associated with pain inputs (to the exclusion of the main sensory nucleus and mesencephalic nucleus). Fibers from this nucleus mainly project contralaterally to the ventral posteromedial nucleus of the thalamus. Surgical interuption of these descending first-order pain fibers is a practical approach and one that has been carried out by neurosurgeons. Destruction of the ventral posterolateral nucleus would not necessarily destroy the major pain inputs to the cerebral cortex and would additionally be a more difficult structure to destroy surgically. The main sensory nucleus of the trigeminal nerve is not known to convey pain inputs to thalamus and cortex. The substantia gelatinosa conveys pain and temperature sensation from the body and not the head. The midbrain periaqueductal gray constitutes part of a pain-inhibitory system, not one that transmits pain sensations to the cerebral cortex.

266. The answer is e. (*Kandel, pp 1292–1294. Nolte, pp 136, 138–139.*) The area postrema is of interest because it is a circumventricular organ associated with emetic functions. As a circumventricular organ, the area postrema constitutes a part of the ependymal lining of the brain's ventricular system (in this case, the fourth ventricle). The area postrema contains both fenestrated and nonfenestrated capillaries that allow for enhanced transport, which possibly accounts for the fact that it lies outside the blood-brain barrier. Axons and dendrites from neighboring structures (but not from the forebrain) innervate this structure, which is composed of astroblast-like cells, arterioles, sinusoids, and some neurons. Various peptides (but not monoamine-containing neurons) have also been shown to be present in this structure. Experimental evidence has strongly implicated the area postrema as a chemoreceptor trigger zone for emesis. It responds to digitalis glycosides and apomorphine.

267. The answer is c. (*Afifi, pp 129–131.*) Cranial nerve X is a highly complex nerve. Special visceral efferent fibers innervate the constrictor muscles of the pharynx and the intrinsic muscles of the larynx. Damage to this division results in hoarseness and difficulty in swallowing. General visceral efferent fibers constitute part of the cranial aspect of the parasympathetic nervous system; thus, they are preganglionic parasympathetic fibers that innervate the heart, lungs, esophagus, and stomach. Damage to the descending vagus would reduce gastric secretions and disrupt cardiovascular reflex activity. Special visceral afferents include fibers from chemoreceptors for taste associated with the epiglottis and chemoreceptors in the aortic bodies that sense changes in O_2-CO_2 levels in the blood. General visceral afferent fibers arise from the trachea, pharynx, larynx, and esophagus and signal changes in blood pressure to the brainstem. Cranial nerve IX shares a number of similarities with cranial nerve X. However, damage to cranial nerve IX would not affect gastric secretions. Cranial nerve VII does not relate to functions such as swallowing, speech, and gastric secretions. Cranial nerve XI is a purely motor nerve. The reticular formation of the pons does not regulate gastric secretions, swallowing, or speech.

268. The answer is a. (*Afifi, pp 142–144. Nolte, p 280.*) A primary characteristic of a lesion of the dorsolateral medulla is loss of pain and temperature sensation on the contralateral side of the body and ipsilateral half of the face. Damage to the descending tract of the trigeminal nerve and to the spinal nucleus of cranial nerve V will produce loss of sensation on the ipsilateral side of the face. There also will be damage to the lateral spinothalamic tract, which has already crossed at the level of the spinal cord and which conveys pain and temperature sensation from the contralateral side of the body. Hemiparesis would not result from this lesion since the pyramidal tract would remain intact. The cerebellum would also be spared, and intention tremor associated with cerebellar damage would not occur.

269. The answer is b. (*Martin, pp 212–213. Nolte, pp 326–342.*) The olivocochlear bundle is a most interesting pathway because it arises from the region immediately dorsal to the superior olivary nucleus and projects contralaterally back to the hair cells of the cochlea. Stimulation of this bundle results in inhibition or reduction of responses to auditory signals by auditory nerve fibers. There is no evidence that the olivocochlear bundle bears any anatomic or functional relationship to the medial lemniscus. Since the pathway arises from the superior olivary nucleus, which is present at the level of the lower pons, it would not be visible in a section taken from the upper pons.

270. The answer is c. (*Afifi, pp 481–484. Nolte, pp 326–342.*) Since the auditory relay system is a highly complex pathway in which auditory signals are bilaterally represented at all levels beyond the receptor level, lesions at these levels would not produce a solely unilateral deafness. Such a loss could only result when the lesion involves either the receptor or the first-order neurons of the nerve (i.e., cranial nerve VIII itself). The medial lemniscus is not related to the auditory system.

271. The answer is c. (*Afifi, pp 171–176. Nolte, pp 295–301.*) In general, first-order sensory neurons form ganglia outside the CNS. There is one exception: the mesencephalic nucleus of cranial nerve V, which transmits unconscious proprioception (i.e., muscle spindle activity) from jaw muscles. These inputs serve as the first-order neurons for a disynaptic pathway to the cerebellum, as well as for a monosynaptic pathway with the motor nucleus of cranial nerve V for the jaw-closing reflex.

272. The answer is d. (*Afifi, pp 168–171. Nolte, pp 290–294.*) Conjugate lateral gaze requires the simultaneous contractions of the lateral rectus muscle of one eye and the medial rectus of the other eye. Recent studies have indicated that there is a region that integrates and coordinates such movements and that the site is part of the nucleus of cranial nerve VI. It is likely that it accomplishes this phenomenon, in part because ascending axons from the abducens nucleus pass through the medial longitudinal fasciculus to the contralateral nuclei of cranial nerve III. Thus, the abducens nucleus serves not only to innervate the lateral rectus muscle but also to integrate signals necessary for conjugate deviation of the eyes. The abducens nucleus appears to be the only cranial nerve structure where lesions of the root fibers and nucleus fail to display identical effects.

273. The answer is a. (*Afifi, pp 169–171. Nolte, pp 288–294, 351–355, 359–373.*) The paramedian pontine reticular formation is an important integrating structure controlling the position of the eyes. It receives inputs from the cerebral cortex (presumably the region of the frontal eye fields) and fibers from the cerebellum, spinal cord, and vestibular complex. Its efferent fibers project to the cerebellum, vestibular complex, pretectal region, interstitial nucleus of Cajal, and nucleus of Darkschewitsch of the rostral midbrain. These are all nuclei concerned with the regulation of eye position and movements. It is not related to any other known motor or auditory functions, nor has it been shown to contain ascending noradrenergic neurons.

274. The answer is c. (*Afifi, pp 227–230. Nolte, pp 260–262, 290–294.*) For a lesion to produce both an ipsilateral gaze paralysis and contralateral hemiplegia, it must be situated in a location where fibers regulating both lateral gaze and movements of the contralateral limbs lie close to each other. The only such location is the ventrocaudal aspect of the pons, where fibers of cranial nerve VI descend toward the ventral surface of the brainstem and where corticospinal fibers are descending toward the spinal cord. The other regions listed in the question do not meet this condition.

275. The answer is e. (*Purves, pp 263–282.*) The group called special visceral afferent fibers is limited to those cranial nerves that convey impulses to the brain associated with olfaction (I) and taste (VII, IX, and X). Since olfaction and taste involve chemical senses, some authors also include cranial nerves IX and X in the group because these nerves contain components involved in signaling changes in O_2 and CO_2 levels in the blood.

276. The answer is e. (*Purves, pp 258–261. Nolte, pp 381–385.*) Because the deficit includes a homonymous hemianopsia, the lesion has to be located somewhere in the forebrain, such as in the region that includes the optic tract and internal capsule on the right side of the brain. The motor neurons of cranial nerve VII, as well as spinal cord motor neurons, receive cortical fibers that are crossed, which accounts for the fact that motor dysfunctions of the lower face and body involve lesions on the same side.

277. The answer is d. (*Afifi, pp 211, 227–231.*) Inability to move the eyes up or down when they are displaced laterally would result from a lesion of the midbrain involving cranial nerve III. Because the somatomotor neurons of cranial nerve III supply, in part, the superior and inferior recti muscles as well as the inferior oblique muscle, cranial nerve III is responsible for up-and-down movements of the eye when they are positioned laterally. Recall that when the eye is positioned medially, it is the superior oblique that is innervated by cranial nerve IV that pulls the eye downward.

278. The answer is c. *(Afifi, p 218. Nolte, pp 431–432.)* This disorder is referred to as the *Argyll Robertson pupil* and occurs with CNS syphilis (tertiary). Although the precise site of the lesion has never been fully established, it is believed to be in the pretectal area. The reasoning is that in the pupillary light reflex, many optic fibers terminate in the pretectal area and superior colliculus region and are then relayed to the autonomic nuclei of cranial nerve III. Impulses from this component of cranial nerve III then synapse with postganglionic parasympathetics that innervate the pupillary constrictor muscles, thus producing pupillary constriction. In the case of the accommodation reflex, retinal impulses first reach the cortex and are then relayed through corticofugal fibers to the brainstem. Some of these fibers are then relayed directly or indirectly to both motor and autonomic components of cranial nerve III, thus activating the muscles required for the accommodation reaction to occur, which includes pupillary constriction.

279. The answer is b. *(Kandel, pp 642–644. Nolte, pp 305–306, 313–316.)* The solitary nucleus receives first-order neurons from the taste system and thus serves as a critical relay nucleus for the taste pathway. Axons arising from the solitary nucleus project to the ventral posteromedial nucleus of the thalamus and may also synapse in the parabrachial nuclei of the upper pons. Structures such as the ventral posterolateral nucleus, medial lemniscus, and superior parietal lobule are not associated with the taste pathway.

280. The answer is b. *(Kandel, pp 1309–1313. Nolte, pp 259–267, 280.)* The superior cerebellar artery supplies the dorsolateral aspect of the upper pons. The basilar artery supplies the medial aspect of the pons. The other arteries (vertebral, anterior spinal, and posterior inferior cerebellar) supply different parts of the medulla. The lateral aspect of the upper pons contains spinothalamic fibers, the lateral lemniscus, and the locus ceruleus (situated just dorsal to the motor nucleus of cranial nerve V, which is also affected by the lesion). This lateral pontine lesion produces a syndrome that includes (1) loss of pain and temperature sensation from the contralateral side of the body (damage to the lateral spinothalamic tract), (2) ipsilateral loss of masticatory reflexes (damage to the motor nucleus of cranial nerve V), (3) diminution of hearing (disruption of secondary auditory pathways), and (4) Horner's syndrome (disruption of descending fibers from the hypothalamus and midbrain that mediate autonomic functions).

281. The answer is a. (*Kandel, pp 1309–1313.*) The paramedian branch of the basilar artery supplies the ventromedial pons (i.e., medial basilar pons). The circumferential branch supplies more lateral regions of the pons, as does the superior cerebellar artery. The anterior spinal and anterior inferior cerebellar arteries supply different parts of the medulla.

282. The answer is c. (*Afifi, pp 180–184. Kandel, pp 1309–1313.*) The lesion is restricted to the basilar pons. Thus, the only structure affected by this lesion among the choices given is the corticospinal tract. The other structures listed are situated in the tegmentum of the pons.

283. The answer is a. (*Afifi, pp 180–184. Kandel, pp 1309–1313.*) Since the lesion is restricted to the medial aspect of the basilar part of the pons, the corticospinal tract would be affected, producing paralysis of the contralateral limbs. Although other structures would also be affected and could produce additional deficits, such deficits are not listed in this question. The other dysfunctions listed would not occur because they are associated with structures situated in the pontine tegmentum, which is not included in this lesion.

284. The answer is c. (*Afifi, pp 227–229. Kandel, pp 1312–1314.*) The lesion involves the superior colliculus. This structure receives inputs from the cerebral cortex and optic tract, and its neurons respond to moving objects in the visual field. It is considered essential for the regulation of tracking movements. Lesions of the superior colliculus have not been shown to produce any of the other deficits listed in this question. Nystagmus is not likely to occur because the lesion does not involve the medial longitudinal fasciculus or the pontine gaze center.

285. The answer is a. (*Afifi, pp 227–229. Kandel, pp 1312–1314.*) The lesion will disrupt fibers of the medial lemniscus (lateral aspect of the lesion) and thus produce contralateral loss of conscious proprioception. It will also disrupt fibers passing from the cerebellum to the red nucleus and ventrolateral nucleus of the thalamus, which could account for a tremor of the contralateral limb. Note that there would be no ipsilateral motor loss because functions associated with the red nucleus are expressed on the contralateral side. Oculomotor palsy would also be present because the lesion disrupts root fibers of cranial nerve III. However, the lesion is too rostral to affect cranial nerve IV. There is no hearing loss because the auditory fibers are situated too far laterally. Since the taste pathway is essentially ipsilateral, if any fibers are damaged by the lesion, deficits in taste sensation would be ipsilateral.

286. The answer is c. (*Afifi, pp 227–229. Kandel, pp 1312–1314.*) The primary structures damaged by this lesion include the crus cerebri, which results in a UMN paralysis of the contralateral limbs, as well as a paresis of the lower facial and tongue muscles. The other outstanding syndrome present from this lesion is a paralysis that results from damage to cranial nerve III. Other structures may be marginally affected.

287. The answer is a. (*Siegel et al., pp 251–252. Afifi, pp 199–201.*) The pars compacta of the substantia nigra contains dopamine neurons whose axons project to the neostriatum. In contrast, the dopaminergic neurons of the ventral tegmental area project to other areas of the forebrain, such as the hypothalamus, limbic system, and cerebral cortex. There is no known overlap in the distribution of these dopaminergic projection systems. A parkinsonian-like syndrome results from damage to the pars compacta of the substantia nigra, but not from a lesion restricted to the ventral tegmental region.

288. The answer is b. (*Afifi, pp 154–156. Nolte, pp 340–342.*) The principal ascending pathway of the auditory system listed in this question is the lateral lemniscus. It transmits information from the cochlear nuclei to the inferior colliculus. The trapezoid body is a commissure that contains some of the fibers of the lateral lemniscus that cross from the cochlear nuclei of one side of the brainstem en route to the inferior colliculus of the other side. The trapezoid body is present at the level of the caudal pons. The brachium of the superior colliculus, trigeminal lemniscus, and medial lemniscus do not transmit auditory sensory information.

289–293. The answers are 289-e, 290-a, 291-a, 292-b, 293-d. (*Adams, pp 799, 1383. Afifi, pp 125–127, 141–143.*) Emma had a stroke resulting from occlusion of medial branches of the left vertebral artery, presumably secondary to atherosclerosis (i.e., cholesterol deposits within the artery, which eventually occlude it). The resulting syndrome is called the *medial medullary syndrome,* because the affected structures are located in the medial portion of the medulla. These structures include the pyramids, the medial lemniscus, the medial longitudinal fasciculus, and the nucleus of the hypoglossal nerve and its outflow tract. Emma's symptoms resulted from damage to the aforementioned structures and may have been caused by the same process (atherosclerosis) that resulted in her heart disease. The weakness of her right side was caused by damage to the medullary pyramid on the left side. Her face was spared because fibers supplying the face exited above the level of infarct. However, a lesion in the corticospinal tract of the cervical spinal cord above C5 could cause arm and leg weakness and spare the face, because facial fibers exit in the rostral medulla. A lesion in the inferior portion of the precentral gyrus of the left frontal lobe would cause right-sided weakness, but would include the face, because this area is represented more inferiorly than are the extremities. Her unsteady gait was a result of the weakness of her right side, but may also have been the result of the loss of position and vibration sense on that side from damage to the medial lemniscus (as demonstrated by the inability to identify the position of her toe with her eyes closed, and the inability to feel the vibrations of a tuning fork). Without position sense, walking becomes unsteady because it is necessary to feel the position of one's feet on the floor during normal gait. Damage to both the medial lemniscus and pyramids at this level causes problems on the contralateral side because this lesion is located rostral to the level where both of these fiber bundles cross to the opposite side of the brain. Damage to the descending component of the medial longitudinal fasciculus could only affect head and neck reflexes, but not gait. Gait is also unaffected by pain inputs. Deviation of the tongue occurs because fibers from the hypoglossal nucleus innervate the genioglossus muscle on the ipsilateral side of the tongue. This muscle normally protrudes the tongue toward the contralateral side. Therefore, if one side is weak, the tongue will deviate toward the side ipsilateral to the lesion when protruded. A lesion in the precentral gyrus causes protrusion of the tongue toward the side that is contralateral to the lesion because it is rostral to the crossing of fibers into the hypoglossal nucleus. Emma's speech was dysarthric (slurred) because her tongue was weak on the left side. The physician saw this during the exam when her tongue deviated to the left when protruded. Since the weakness of the tongue is purely a motor problem, rather than an effect that is manifested by a lesion to higher centers in the cortex (which mediate the structure and function of speech), the grammar, content, and meaning of Emma's speech remained intact, as would be expected with an aphasia or agnosia.

294–298. The answers are 294-c, 295-e, 296-e, 297-e, 298-c. *(Adams, pp 1376–1377. Afifi, pp 163–168, 179–181.)* This is an example of Bell's palsy, or damage to the facial nerve distal to its nucleus in the pons. The motor weakness is LMN because of the involvement of the upper one-third of the face (this has bilateral innervation within the CNS). The loss of taste on the anterior two-thirds of the tongue and the hyperacusis (sensitivity to noise) point to damage that is distal to the brainstem because these are functions whose nerves join the facial nerve distal to its exit from the pons. This type of palsy may be caused by a virus and is more common among people with diabetes. This type of facial paralysis, involving the upper one-third of the facial muscles, is characteristic of an LMN facial nerve lesion. Since there is bilateral innervation within the CNS, from the prefrontal gyrus bilaterally until their synapse at the facial nerve nucleus, all UMN facial weakness spares the forehead. Since there is motor weakness of the face and since the chorda tympani nerve (which subserves taste) joins the facial nerve, it is likely that the lesion exists proximal to where the chorda tympani joins the facial nerve. A lesion in the lingual nerve (a branch of the trigeminal) would result in a loss of taste as well, but would also result in a loss of sensation to the face, not motor weakness. If the lesion occurred distal to the chorda tympani nerve, taste would have been spared. The facial nerve sends a branch to the stapedius muscle distal to the geniculate ganglion, but proximal to the chorda tympani nerve. Lesions proximal to this branch will cause weakness of the stapedius muscle. Contraction of this muscle normally serves as a mechanism for dampening the motion of the ossicles, thus lowering the amount of stimulation reaching the organ of Corti. If this muscle is paralyzed, hyperacusis, or increased acuity, as well as hypersensitivity to low tones will occur. Since the genu of the facial nerve is in close proximity to the nucleus of the abducens nerve, the pons is a likely location for this particular type of combination of findings. Since the damage to the facial nerve has occurred distal to the facial nerve nucleus, an LMN facial palsy is present. The lack of hyperacusis and the presence of normal taste imply that the lesion is proximal to the geniculate ganglion. Therefore, the lesion must be between the facial nerve nucleus and the geniculate ganglion, and the location in the pons is the most likely choice. If this clinical picture is present, then an infarct or tumor in the pons must be suspected, and, in this case, an imaging study would be more appropriate.

299–303. The answers are 299-d, 300-c, 301-a, 302-e, 303-b. (*Adams, pp 802–805. Afifi, pp 163–168, 180–182.*) This is an example of the *locked-in syndrome,* or pseudocoma, caused by an infarction of the basilar pons. Because the tracts mediating movement of the limbs and face run through this region, the patient is unable to move the face, as well as both arms and legs. Consciousness and eye movements are preserved. The pontine basilar pons is supplied mainly by the basilar artery. Complete occlusion of this artery causes deficits on both sides, since this artery supplies both sides of the pons. Basilar artery occlusion causes damage to the basilar pons, where the corticospinal and corticobulbar tracts run. These tracts contain motor fibers mediating movement of the limb and face, respectively. This results in complete paralysis to both sides of the body and the face. None of the tracts in the other choices mediate conscious movement. Sensory loss, including loss of proprioception (feeling the movement of a limb), also occurs as a result of damage to the medial lemniscus bilaterally. This tract contains fibers from the dorsal columns and also runs through the pontine tegmentum. Patients with the locked-in syndrome are often mistaken for comatose patients due to their inability to move or speak. If the lesion spares the reticular formation, an area mediating consciousness in the pons, the patient will remain alert.

304–308. The answers are 304-d, 305-a, 306-c, 307-e, 308-c. (*Adams, p 280, 538. Afifi, pp 163–168, 179–184, 209–220, 227–229. Kandel, pp 962–974.*) Herb's drooping eyelid, small pupil, and lack of sweating on the right side are examples of Horner's syndrome. This is caused by the interruption of sympathetic fibers anywhere along their course from the hypothalamus and brainstem to the intermediolateral cell column in the upper thoracic levels of the spinal cord, where neurons, supplying sympathetic innervation to the pupil, the levator palpebrae superioris muscle of the eyelid, and sweat glands of the face, are located. Interruption of this sympathetic innervation will result in the drooping of the upper eyelid (ptosis), pupillary constriction (miosis; due to unopposed action of the parasympathetic innervation of the circular muscles of the iris), and lack of sweating on the face. Parasympathetic or oculomotor damage causes pupillary dilation, rather than constriction. Herb could close his eyes tightly because this function is mediated by the seventh nerve, which is not damaged by this lesion. Preganglionic sympathetic neurons are predominantly cholinergic, and postganglionic sympathetic neurons are predominantly noradrenergic. Horner's syndrome may be caused by either a preganglionic or a postganglionic lesion. The location may be determined by the use of eyedrops specifically targeted at a particular neurotransmitter. One cause of interruption of the sympathetic fibers is a tumor of the apex (top portion) of the lung, called a *Pancoast tumor.* Because the apex of the lung is in close proximity to the spine, a Pancoast tumor may compress the upper thoracic spinal cord where the sympathetic fibers exit from it. Compression of the adjacent spinal nerves between C8 and T2, entering the brachial plexus, also interrupts the nerve supply to the hand and triceps muscle, causing numbness and weakness in these areas. Pancoast tumors do not often cause respiratory symptoms early in their course because they are located far from the mainstem bronchi. Because these tumors have this unique location, the neurological abnormalities often predate the respiratory problems. The neurologist suspected that Herb may have a Pancoast tumor in the lung because of his long history of smoking.

309–313. The answers are 309-b, 310-c, 311-e, 312-c, 313-e. (*Afifi, pp 168–169, 194–196, 209–222, 227–232.*) The third cranial nerve (oculomotor) controls four of the six extraocular muscles that move the eye. When this nerve fails to function, the eye remains deviated laterally due to the unopposed action of the other two extraocular muscles. When the eyes no longer move together, patients have double vision because the visual cortex now receives two different images. In addition, fibers originating in the third nerve nucleus innervate the levator palpebrae superioris, a muscle that helps to lift the eyelid. Damage to the optic nerve causes loss of vision, blurred vision, and a central scotoma (blind spot in the center of the visual field). Damage to the cervical sympathetic fibers causes Horner's syndrome, consisting of ptosis (drooping of the eyelid), miosis (constriction of the pupil), and anhydrosis (loss of sweating), not eye movement abnormalities. The actions of the superior oblique, the muscle innervated by the trochlear nerve, include intorsion, depression, and abduction. The abducens nerve mediates the lateral rectus muscle, which abducts the eye. The eye is depressed and abducted due to the unopposed actions of the superior oblique and lateral rectus muscles, which together move the eye downward and abduct it (see earlier discussion for the actions of these muscles). The other four muscles are innervated by the oculomotor nerve, which presumably has been damaged. This is an example of Weber's syndrome, or a lesion involving the third cranial nerve outflow tract and the corticospinal and corticobulbar tracts in the cerebral peduncles of the midbrain. Weber's syndrome may occur as a result of an occlusion of the interpeduncular branches of the posterior cerebral artery (which supply this portion of the midbrain), a tumor pressing on this area, an aneurysm (circumscribed dilation of an artery) of the posterior communicating artery, or a plaque (lesion) related to multiple sclerosis. Fibers from the Edinger-Westphal nucleus are affected by lesions of the midbrain as well, and because they are instrumental in constricting the pupil, this lesion causes the patient to have a dilated pupil. If there is a mass that is external to the midbrain but pressing on the oculomotor nerve, then the preganglionic parasympathetic fibers traveling to the ciliary ganglion, which, in turn, innervate the pupillary constrictor muscles, can be damaged, also causing a dilated pupil. Cervical sympathetic fibers cause pupillary dilatation, so damage to these fibers causes pupillary constriction (see Horner's syndrome, earlier). Involvement of the cerebral peduncle causes damage to the corticospinal and corticobulbar tracts, resulting in weakness of the contralateral face, arm, and leg. The motor deficit is contralateral because the corticospinal tracts cross in the medullary pyramids, below the level of the lesion. The upper portion of Mike's face was spared in this case (as well as in any other UMN lesion) because the face is innervated bilaterally until the level of the caudal pons, so a unilateral lesion results in sparing of this portion of the face. The combination of a third-nerve palsy and contralateral hemiparesis can occur only in the midbrain. The observed effects relating to cranial nerve III could not be accounted for by cortical damage. Likewise, damage to the cervical cord would not affect the third nerve.

314–318. The answers are 314-c, 315-d, 316-b, 317-d, 318-e. (*Afifi, pp 194–203. Adams, p 270.*) Damage to the trochlear nerve causes weakness of the superior oblique muscle, resulting in the inability of the orbit to deviate downward when the eye is intorted. To compensate for the classically vertical double vision, the patient tends to tilt his head to the contralateral side, causing the contralateral eye to intort. The trochlear nerve supplies the superior oblique muscle. The trochlear nerve is the only nerve to decussate peripherally, and also to emerge from the dorsal aspect of the brainstem. In this case, the damaged nerve emerged from the right (contralateral) dorsal midbrain. The action of the superior oblique muscle is to rotate the orbit medially and downward. Because the trochlear nerve is not only the smallest cranial nerve but also has the longest course of any cranial nerve, it is especially vulnerable to trauma. One of the most common causes of trochlear nerve palsy is trauma.

Sensory Systems

Questions

DIRECTIONS: Each item below contains a question or incomplete statement followed by suggested responses. Select the **one best** response to each question.

319. The output of the retina is mediated by which of the following cells?
a. Bipolar cells
b. Horizontal cells
c. Rods
d. Cones
e. Ganglion cells

320. Which of the following constitutes a direct interneuron linking the receptor and ganglion cells?
a. Bipolar cell
b. Horizontal cell
c. Golgi cell
d. Amacrine cell
e. Optic nerve cell

321. Which of the following best characterizes how cones differ from rods?
a. A higher sensitivity to light than rods
b. More photopigment than rods
c. Pigments that are sensitive to different parts of the light spectrum
d. A lower temporal resolution with a long integration time and slow response relative to rods
e. Lower acuity and are present in fewer numbers in the fovea than rods

322. An individual is diagnosed with retinitis pigmentosa, which produces a defective opsin. Which of the following will most likely result from this deficit?
a. Degeneration of area 17 of the cerebral cortex
b. Degeneration of cone cells
c. Loss of central vision
d. Total loss of vision
e. Reduced response to light

323. Action potentials can be produced from which of the following cells?

a. Amacrine cells
b. Rods
c. Cones
d. Ganglion cells
e. Horizontal cells

Item 324–325

An individual is diagnosed by an optometrist as being nearsighted.

324. To correct this person's defect, which of the following lenses would the doctor recommend be put into his eyeglasses?

a. Cylindrical
b. Concave
c. Convex
d. Neutral
e. Rectangular

325. In this case, the corrective lens is applied because of which of the following conditions?

a. Retinal damage
b. The eyeball is too long
c. The eyeball is too short
d. The eyeball is oblong
e. The lens resists change

Item 326–327

Another individual is diagnosed by the same optometrist as being farsighted.

326. To correct this person's defect, which of the following lenses would the doctor recommend be put into his eyeglasses?

a. Cylindrical
b. Concave
c. Convex
d. Neutral
e. Spherical

327. In this case, the corrective lens is applied because of which of the following conditions?

a. Corneal damage
b. The eyeball is too long
c. The eyeball is too short
d. The eyeball is oblong
e. The lens resists change

328. A person is told that he has astigmatism. To correct this defect, the optometrist prescribes which of the following lenses and for which reason?

a. Cylindrical lens because the cornea or lens is oblong
b. Concave lens because the eyeball is too long
c. Convex lens because the lens is too short
d. Neutral lens because the eyeball is normal but the cornea is too thin
e. Concave lens because the cornea is opaque

329. A patient complains of having constant headaches involving the frontal region. Further examination reveals increased intraocular pressure. The pupil is dilated, but at the time of examination there is little evidence of visual deficits. Which is the likely diagnosis given to this person?

a. Cataracts
b. A tumor of the visual cortex or lateral geniculate nucleus
c. A tumor at the base of the brain impinging upon the optic chiasm
d. Glaucoma
e. Color blindness

330. A routine eye examination reveals the presence of inflammation limited to the left optic disk, probably due to neuritis of this region. Which is the likely visual deficit resulting from this disorder?

a. Total blindness of the left eye
b. Left homonymous hemianopsia
c. Left heteronymous hemianopsia
d. Left enlargement of the blind spot
e. Left upper quadrantanopia

331. As a result of calcification of the internal carotid artery, which impinged upon the lateral half of the right optic nerve prior to its entrance to the brain, a 68-year-old woman experienced certain visual deficits. Which is the most likely visual deficit?

a. Total blindness of the right eye
b. Right nasal hemianopsia
c. Right homonymous hemianopsia
d. Right bitemporal hemianopsia
e. Right upper homonymous quadrantanopia

332. It was discovered that a 29-year-old male had a tumor pressing on the base of the brain, where it impinged upon the optic chiasm. He discovered that his field of vision was seriously affected. Which defect was present in this individual?

a. Total blindness of both eyes
b. Bitemporal hemianopsia
c. Right homonymous hemianopsia
d. Binasal hemianopsia
e. Right lower homonymous quadrantanopia

333. A routine MRI revealed the presence of a tumor situated in the left optic tract proximal to the lateral geniculate nucleus. The patient complained of having a reduction in his field of vision. Which best characterizes the likely visual deficit?

a. Total blindness of the left eye
b. Bitemporal hemianopsia
c. Right homonymous hemianopsia
d. Left homonymous hemianopsia
e. Left homonymous quadrantanopia

334. A 70-year-old male was admitted to the emergency room and a subsequent MRI revealed the presence of a tumor involving parts of the left temporal lobe. In addition to certain short-term memory deficits, visual deficits were noted as well. Which of the following visual deficits would most likely result from this tumor?

a. Left homonymous hemianopsia
b. Right homonymous hemianopsia
c. Left upper quadrantanopia
d. Right upper quadrantanopia
e. Left lower quadrantanopia

335. A 55-year-old woman complained of headaches and was subsequently diagnosed as having a tumor localized to the left parietal lobe. In addition to a variety of sensory deficits, further examination also revealed a reduction in her visual fields. Which of the following visual deficits would most likely result from this tumor?

a. Left homonymous hemianopsia
b. Right homonymous hemianopsia
c. Left upper quadrantanopia
d. Right upper quadrantanopia
e. Right lower quadrantanopia

336. The conscious perception of movement is mediated by which of the following receptors?

a. Meissner's corpuscles
b. Free nerve endings
c. Merkel's receptors
d. Joint capsules
e. Pacinian corpuscles

337. Which of the following types of inhibition have been identified within the dorsal column nuclei?

a. Feed-forward inhibition utilizing local interneurons only
b. Feedback inhibition utilizing local interneurons only
c. Descending inhibition from fibers arising in the cerebral cortex only
d. Feed-forward, feedback, and descending inhibition
e. Feed-forward and descending inhibition only

338. A researcher is interested in studying the properties of neurons that are capable of responding to the direction or orientation of a given stimulus moved along a receptive field. Where would he place his microelectrodes to access these neurons?

a. Spinal cord
b. Medulla
c. Pons
d. Thalamus
e. Cerebral cortex

339. A patient had been seeing a physician for almost a year because she complained of pain in her shoulder. After extensive analysis, the physician determined that the pain in her shoulder reflected referred pain that arose from another source. In this case, which of the following best explains the basis for the referred pain?

a. Inhibitory fibers that block transmission of pain impulses along a given pathway and then transfer the impulses to a different pathway associated with a different part of the body
b. A massive discharge along a given pathway that results in the activation of a separate pathway because of the principle of divergence
c. A convergence of primary afferent fibers from a given region onto second-order neurons that normally receive primary afferents from a different body part
d. The disruption of lateral spinothalamic fibers
e. The blockade of substance P from primary afferent terminals

340. A car door was accidentally closed on the hand of a teenage boy. As a result, he experienced significant pain that persisted for a while. In terms of the neurochemical events that took place at the afferent terminals of the first-order pathway that conveyed the pain sensation to the spinal cord, which of the following transmitters would be released onto dorsal horn neurons of the spinal cord from these primary afferent fibers?

a. Enkephalins alone
b. Glutamate alone
c. Substance P alone
d. Glutamate and substance P
e. Enkephalins, substance P, and glutamate

341. A person is experiencing severe pain. If it were possible to place an electrode into the gray matter around the cerebral aqueduct of the midbrain and stimulate the cells in this region, it would induce an analgesic response. Which of the following would best explain such an effect?

a. Activation of a pathway that ascends directly to the cortex and mediates analgesia
b. A descending pathway that blocks nociceptive inputs at the level of the dorsal horn
c. Activation of local interneurons that block ascending nociceptive signals at the level of the midbrain
d. Activation of an ascending inhibitory pathway that projects to the ventral posterolateral nucleus of the thalamus
e. Activation of cholinergic neurons in the basal forebrain

342. Concerning the analgesic effects mediated by stimulation of the periaqueductal gray indicated in question 341, which of the following provides the best explanation of the neural substrate(s) underlying this phenomenon?

a. Fibers from the periaqueductal gray that synapse directly on dorsal horn cells
b. Fibers from the periaqueductal gray that synapse on neurons of the nucleus raphe magnus that then synapse on dorsal horn cells
c. Fibers from the periaqueductal gray that synapse on inferior olivary neurons that then synapse on dorsal horn cells
d. Hypothalamic fibers that synapse on neurons of the nucleus solitarius that then synapse on neurons of the dorsal horn
e. Hypothalamic fibers that synapse directly on dorsal horn neurons

343. A cell that responds with an *on-center* and *off-surround* to generate contrast within the receptive field can be identified in which of the following cells?

a. Retina (ganglion cell)
b. Lateral geniculate nucleus
c. Retina (ganglion cell) and lateral geniculate nucleus
d. Layer IV of the primary visual cortex (area 17)
e. Retina (ganglion cell), lateral geniculate nucleus, and area 18

344. Fibers in each optic tract synapse in which of the following structures?

a. The lateral geniculate nucleus only
b. The lateral geniculate nucleus and the pretectal area
c. The lateral geniculate nucleus, the pretectal area, and the superior colliculus
d. The lateral geniculate nucleus, the pretectal area, the superior colliculus, and the suprachiasmatic nucleus
e. The lateral geniculate nucleus, the pretectal area, the superior colliculus, the suprachiasmatic nucleus, and the nuclei of cranial nerves III and IV

345. At the level of the dorsal horn of the spinal cord, which of the following best explains how nociceptive transmission may be blocked by descending brainstem fibers?

a. Opioidergic, and only contact dendrites of postsynaptic neurons that contain opiate receptors
b. Opioidergic, and only contact opiate receptors located presynaptically on nociceptive terminals
c. Opioidergic, and contact both dendrites of postsynaptic neurons and presynaptic terminals, both of which contain opiate receptors
d. Serotonergic, and only contact dendrites of postsynaptic neurons that contain 5-HT receptors
e. Cholinergic, and contact dendrites of both postsynaptic neurons and presynaptic terminals, both of which contain muscarinic receptors

346. In the olfactory glomerulus, primary afferent fibers terminate principally upon which of the following structures?

a. Granule cell dendrites forming axodendritic synapses
b. Granule cell axon terminals forming axoaxonic synapses
c. Mitral cell dendrites forming axodendritic synapses
d. Mitral cell axon terminals forming axoaxonic synapses
e. Axon terminals of fibers arising from the olfactory tubercle, forming axoaxonic synapses

347. When a cone is hyperpolarized by light, which of the following occurs?

a. The on-center bipolar cell is excited and the off-center bipolar cell is inhibited
b. The on-center bipolar cell will inhibit the ganglion cell with which it makes synaptic contact
c. The ganglion cell that receives its input from an off-center bipolar cell will discharge because the bipolar cell is excited during the presence of the stimulus
d. An on-center bipolar cell excites a neighboring ganglion cell that receives its input from an off-center bipolar cell
e. A transmitter released from a cone cell has the same effect upon all processes with which it synapses

348. A middle-aged male is involved in an automobile accident that causes brain damage affecting a region of the cerebral cortex, resulting in loss of the conscious perception of smell. Which of the following regions of the cortex is most likely affected?

a. Temporal neocortex
b. Posterior parietal lobule
c. Cingulate gyrus
d. Prefrontal cortex
e. Precentral gyrus

349. Lateral inhibition within the retina is most effectively achieved through the action of which of the following cell types?

a. Rod cells
b. Cone cells
c. Bipolar cells
d. Ganglion cells
e. Horizontal cells

350. There are cells that respond to an image in a specific position, have discrete excitatory and inhibitory zones, and are associated with a specific axis of orientation. Which of the following cells would respond to such an image?

a. M cells of the lateral geniculate nucleus
b. P cells of the lateral geniculate nucleus
c. Simple cells of the visual cortex
d. Complex cells of the visual cortex
e. Hypercomplex cells of the visual cortex

351. Which part of the olfactory receptor mechanism initially responds to an olfactory stimulus?

a. Mitral cell
b. Granule cell
c. Sustentacular cell
d. Basal cell
e. Olfactory cilia

352. The neural basis of olfactory discrimination is believed to utilize which of the following properties?

a. Specific activation of different cell groups within the amygdala
b. Specific activation of different groups of olfactory glomeruli that are spatially organized and segregated within the olfactory bulb
c. Specific activation of different groups of cells within the olfactory tubercle
d. Temporal summation of olfactory signals in the anterior olfactory nucleus
e. Temporal summation of olfactory signals in the mediodorsal thalamic nucleus

353. The principal efferent pathway of the olfactory bulb arises from which of the following cells?

a. Granule cells
b. Golgi cells
c. Receptor cells
d. Mitral cells
e. Periglomerular cells

354. Direct efferent projections of the olfactory bulb supply which of the following structures?

a. Hypothalamus and prefrontal cortex
b. Amygdala and pyriform cortex
c. Hippocampus and amygdala
d. Prefrontal cortex and medial thalamus
e. Septal area and prefrontal cortex

355. A person was examined by a neurologist after complaining that he kept having a sensation of smell that he could not clearly define. A subsequent MRI revealed the presence of a brain tumor and that the patient was experiencing uncinate hallucinations. The tumor was most likely situated in which of the following regions?

a. Uncal region
b. Medial dorsal thalamic nucleus
c. Parietal cortex
d. Hypothalamus
e. Midbrain periaqueductal gray

356. Which of the following sensory systems is able to utilize a circuit that bypasses the thalamus for the transmission of sensory information from the periphery to the cerebral cortex?

a. Conscious proprioception
b. Taste
c. Olfaction
d. Vision
e. Audition

Sensory Systems

Answers

319. The answer is e. (*Kandel, pp 516–520.*) The output of the retina is mediated by the ganglion cells. Ganglion cells receive inputs from photoreceptor and bipolar cells. In turn, ganglion cells give rise to optic nerve fibers, which project through the optic chiasm and optic tracts to the lateral geniculate nucleus of the thalamus. Other cells mentioned in this question only produce local connections within the retina.

320. The answer is a. (*Kandel, pp 514–520.*) The bipolar cell receives inputs from the receptor cells (i.e., rods and cones). The response of the bipolar cell to the receptor cell input is then mediated to the ganglion cell. (See the discussion that follows for further consideration of the physiology of the retina.) Horizontal and amacrine cells connect neighboring receptor or bipolar cells, Golgi cells are not present in the retina, and optic nerve cells project out of the retina as indicated earlier.

321. The answer is c. (*Kandel, pp 508–515.*) Cones differ from rods in that cone cells contain pigments that are sensitive to different parts of the light spectrum, while rod cells are achromatic. The other choices are incorrect: rods have a greater sensitivity to light than cones and have more photopigment than cones. Cones also have a higher temporal resolution with a shorter integration time and more rapid response than cones. Cones also have greater acuity and are present in greater quantities in the fovea than rods.

322. The answer is e. (*Adams, pp 246–247.*) In one form of retinitis pigmentosa, there is a genetic defect with respect to rhodopsin. The result of this defect is the production of defective opsin. As a consequence, rod cells are affected, leading to a reduced response to light. However, central vision is spared, as are cone cells. CNS neurons, such as those located in area 17, are not directly affected and vision is not totally lost.

323. The answer is d. (*Kandel, pp 512–521.*) The only cell in the retina that is capable of producing an action potential is the ganglion cell. As indicated earlier, the ganglion cell gives rise to optic nerve fibers, which terminate as optic tract fibers in the lateral geniculate nucleus. As a result of action potentials generated in the ganglion cells, volleys of impulses are transmitted over these fibers, resulting in the appropriate responses in the neurons of the lateral geniculate nucleus.

324–325. The answers are 324-b, 325-b. *(Kingsley, pp 436–439. Purves, pp 225–227.)* To correct for myopia, a person is prescribed a concave (or flat) lens, because objects focus in front of the retina. The concave lens helps to refocus the object onto the retina. The reason that the focus of the object is in front of the retina is that the eyeball is too long.

326–327. The answers are 326-c, 327-c. *(Kingsley, pp 436–439. Purves, pp 225–227.)* To correct for farsightedness, a person is prescribed a convex lens, because objects focus in front of the retina. The convex lens helps to refocus the object onto the retina. The reason that the focus of the object is in front of the retina is because the eyeball is too short.

328. The answer is a. *(Kingsley, pp 436–439. Purves, pp 225–227.)* In astigmatism, the shapes of the cornea and possibly the lens become oblong, resulting in differences in the curvature of the lens along the long and short axes. Thus, astigmatism is corrected with a cylindrical lens.

329. The answer is d. *(Gilroy, pp 142–143.)* Glaucoma is a condition of elevated intraocular pressure caused (perhaps by infection) when debris accumulates in the spaces that lead to Schlemm's canal. If not treated, it can rapidly lead to blindness because the pressure can block conduction along the optic nerve. In addition, glaucoma can also be associated with frontal headaches; the diagnosis can be identified by determining the intraocular pressure.

330. The answer is d. *(Simon, pp 138–145.)* A neuritis involving the optic disk would affect the size of the visual field loss around the optic disk, which corresponds to the blind spot. In general, this kind of neuritis would expand somewhat the size of the blind spot but would cause no further visual loss.

331. The answer is b. *(Simon, pp 138–145.)* Calcification of the internal carotid artery could serve to disrupt nerve fibers proximal to it. One such group of fibers includes parts of the optic nerve. In this case, the component of the right optic nerve affected includes the lateral aspect, or those fibers that mediate vision associated with the nasal visual field of the right eye. If the damage were more extensive and if it involved the entire nerve, then total blindness of the right eye would have occurred.

332. The answer is b. (*Simon, pp 138–145.*) A tumor pressing on the optic chiasm will disrupt the optic nerve (and tract) fibers that cross to the opposite side. These fibers mediate vision associated with fibers arising from the nasal retina of each eye. Since the nasal retina of each eye is associated with the temporal visual field for each eye, the visual loss is referred to as a *bitemporal hemianopsia*.

333. The answer is c. (*Simon, pp 138–145.*) Disruption of optic tract fibers destined for the lateral geniculate nucleus will cause a homonymous hemianopsia because it affects fibers arising from the temporal retina of the ipsilateral side and from the nasal retina of the contralateral side. Since the damage occurred in the left optic tract, the loss of vision is reflected on the right visual field [i.e., the left temporal retina is associated with the nasal (or right) visual field of the left eye, and the right nasal retina is associated with the temporal (or right) visual field of the right eye]. Therefore, such a lesion would result in a right homonymous hemianopsia.

334. The answer is d. (*Simon, pp 138–145.*) From the lateral geniculate nucleus, there are two trajectories that the fiber pathways take en route to the visual cortex. One pathway passes dorsally through the parietal lobe and terminates in the upper bank of the calcarine fissure in the ipsilateral primary visual cortex. The second pathway takes a more circuitous (ventral) route—called the *Meyer-Archambault* loop—through the temporal lobe and terminates in the lower bank of the calcarine fissure in the ipsilateral primary visual cortex. The lower bank of the calcarine fissure is associated with the upper visual quadrants of the contralateral visual fields for both eyes, while the upper bank of the calcarine fissure is associated with the lower quadrants of the contralateral visual fields for both eyes. Thus, if there is a lesion of the left temporal lobe affecting the Meyer-Archambault loop, then the right upper quadrant for each eye will be affected. This deficit is referred to as a *right upper quadrantanopia*.

335. The answer is e. (*Simon, pp 138–145.*) The reasoning underlying the answer to this question is exactly as presented in the explanation of the answer to question 330. In brief, fibers from the left lateral geniculate destined for the upper bank of the calcarine fissure will mediate visual impulses associated with lower quadrants of the right visual fields for both eyes. This deficit is referred to as a *right lower quadrantanopia*.

336. The answer is d. *(Nolte, pp 192–212.)* Meissner's corpuscles, Merkel's receptors, and pacinian corpuscles respond to tactile, pressure, or possibly vibratory stimuli, while free nerve endings are associated with nociceptive stimuli. Joint capsules respond to movement of the limb, and the axons of these receptors contribute to the dorsal column–medial lemniscal system mediating the conscious perception of movement.

337. The answer is d. *(Kandel, pp 433–440, 451–457.)* To generate an excitatory focus with an inhibitory surround, three types of inhibition are present in the dorsal column nuclei. First-order neurons ascending in the dorsal columns make synaptic contact with different cells in the dorsal column nuclei and excite those cells. One such cell may be an inhibitory interneuron that makes synaptic contact with a neighboring dorsal column nuclear cell, thus inhibiting that cell (i.e., feed-forward inhibition). In addition, the dorsal column cell that is excited by the first-order neuron may make synaptic contact with another inhibitory interneuron (in addition to its classical ascending projection to the ventral posterolateral nucleus of the thalamus). This inhibitory interneuron makes synaptic contact with an adjacent dorsal column cell and inhibits that cell (i.e., feedback inhibition). Finally, a descending fiber from the postcentral gyrus can make synaptic contact with inhibitory interneurons that inhibit dorsal column cells (descending inhibition). The figure illustrates feedback, feed forward, and descending inhibition. Inhibitory neurons are depicted in black.

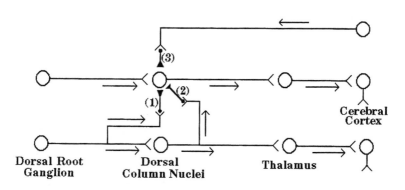

(1) **Feed-Forward Inhibition**
(2) **Feedback Inhibition**
(3) **Descending Inhibition**

338. The answer is e. (*Kandel, pp 456–468.*) As a general rule, neurons that are situated in the cortex in association with any of the sensory systems take on a much higher level of complexity than neurons that are situated at lower levels of the relay network. In the case of the somatosensory system, direction-sensitive cells in the somatosensory cortex will respond to one direction of movement of a stimulus along the receptive field and not to another direction. Orientation-sensitive neurons respond best to movement along one axis of the receptive field. This is not true of neurons that are situated in lower levels of the somatosensory pathway.

339. The answer is c. (*Kandel, pp 472–485.*) Referred pain is a phenomenon in which pain impulses, arising from primary afferent fibers from one part of the body (such as from deep visceral structures), terminate on dorsal horn projection neurons that normally receive cutaneous afferents from a different part of the body (such as the arm). In this situation, a person who is suffering a heart attack experiences pain that appears to be coming from the arm. It is the convergence of these distinctly different inputs onto the same projection neurons that provides the basis for this phenomenon. None of the other possible mechanisms listed in this question have an anatomic or physiologic basis.

340. The answer is d. (*Kandel, pp 472–485.*) Primary nociceptive afferent fibers would have to release an excitatory transmitter in order for normal transmission to take place. Two excitatory transmitters have been identified in association with different classes of primary nociceptive afferents: (1) substance P and (2) excitatory amino acids. The best candidate as an excitatory amino acid is glutamate. Since enkephalins have been shown to be inhibitory transmitters in the pain system, they are not likely to be released from the primary afferents. Instead, other CNS neurons impinge upon the primary afferents, and enkephalins are released from those neurons.

341. The answer is b. (*Kandel, pp 472–485.*) Perhaps one of the most important discoveries in pain research made over the past 15 years is that of a descending pathway that originates in the midbrain periaqueductal gray and makes synaptic contacts in the medulla. From the medulla, this pathway descends to the dorsal horn, where these fibers provide the anatomic substrate for suppression of pain inputs that enter the spinal cord from the periphery. There are no known inputs to the cortex that directly produce analgesia. The mechanism governing analgesia appears to operate at lower brainstem and spinal cord levels. The ascending fibers for transmission of pain impulses reach thalamic nuclei directly, and, thus, local interneurons within the midbrain would not be able to interfere with such transmission. The pathway to the ventral posterolateral nucleus of the thalamus is an excitatory one and is not known to have any inhibitory properties. Cholinergic neurons in the basal forebrain have been implicated in memory functions and are not known to have any role in the regulation of pain sensation.

342. The answer is b. (*Kandel, pp 485–487.*) The descending pathway for central inhibition of nociception involves the following: fibers that originate in the midbrain periaqueductal gray matter project caudally to the level of the nucleus raphe magnus, upon whose neurons they synapse. Fibers from the nucleus raphe magnus then project further caudally, where they synapse in the dorsal horn of the spinal cord.

343. The answer is c. (*Kandel, pp 512–533.*) Both retina ganglion cells and lateral geniculate neurons exhibit an on-center and off-surround with respect to objects in the receptive field. Cells in area 18 of the visual cortex are not known to possess these characteristics. Cells in layer IV of the primary visual cortex do not have circular receptive fields. Instead, these cells respond to such stimuli as lines and bars.

344. The answer is d. (*Afifi, pp 216–218, 404–406, 474–476.*) Fibers of the optic tract synapse in a number of regions associated with the processing of visual information or visual reflex activity. These include the lateral geniculate nuclei (part of the classical visual pathway for relaying visual information to the visual cortex), the pretectal area (for elicitation of the pupillary light reflex and reflex movements of the eyes), the superior colliculus (for bilateral control of rapid eye movements), and the suprachiasmatic nucleus (which relates to the control of circadian rhythms). There are no known monosynaptic projections from the retina to the nuclei of cranial nerves III and IV.

345. The answer is c. (*Kandel, pp 485–487.*) Evidence indicates that within the dorsal horn of the spinal cord, descending pain-inhibitory fibers from the lower brainstem (serotonergic and noradrenergic fibers) synapse upon interneurons that are enkephalinergic. These enkephalinergic neurons then synapse upon both presynaptic terminals of primary pain-afferent fibers and the dendrites of dorsal horn projection neurons (which also receive inputs from the primary nociceptive afferent fibers).

346. The answer is c. *(Kandel, pp 629–632. Nolte, pp 316–323.)* The olfactory receptor and its primary afferent fiber terminate upon dendrites of mitral cells. This relationship is of importance because it is the axon of the mitral cell that projects out of the olfactory bulb (forming the major component of the lateral olfactory stria). The granule cell processes make synaptic contact with dendrites of mitral cells, forming dendrodendritic synapses, but are not known to make synaptic contact with primary afferent terminals. Cells arising in the olfactory tubercle are not known to project to the olfactory bulb. Instead, projections of cells situated in the olfactory tubercle contribute fibers to the medial forebrain bundle and stria medullaris.

347. The answer is a. *(Kandel, pp 510–521.)* When a cone is hyperpolarized by light, there is a reduction in the release of transmitter substance (glutamate). This reduced amount of transmitter results in excitation of the on-center bipolar cell and inhibition of the off-center bipolar cell (presumably because the two types of bipolar cell contain different postsynaptic receptors). Since bipolar cells excite the ganglion cells, an off-center bipolar cell will be inhibited when light is present and, thus, will be unable to excite the ganglion cell to which it is connected. On-center bipolar cells are excited when light is present and so are the ganglion cells to which they are connected. In addition, on-center bipolar cells inhibit ganglion cells that receive their primary input from off-center bipolar cells. This serves to increase the likelihood that these ganglion cells will remain inhibited when the light stimulus is present. A cone cell may make synaptic contact with two types of bipolar cells (on-center or off-center). Because they possess different postsynaptic receptor mechanisms, the two types of bipolar cells will respond differently to input from cones.

348. The answer is d. *(Kandel, pp 63–635. Afifi, pp 461–462.)* Experimental evidence indicates the prefrontal cortex is a key region for the conscious perception of smell. This conclusion is based upon two observations. First, the prefrontal cortex receives major inputs from the olfactory bulb by the following routes: olfactory bulb to pyriform cortex to prefrontal cortex, or olfactory bulb to pyriform cortex (and olfactory tubercle) to mediodorsal thalamic nucleus to prefrontal cortex. Second, lesions of the prefrontal cortex result in a failure to discriminate odors. Olfactory functions are not known to be associated with any of the other choices. Instead, the primary auditory receiving area is located in the auditory cortex, the posterior parietal lobule is concerned with such processes as the programming mechanisms associated with complex motor tasks, the cingulate gyrus has been associated with such functions as spatial learning and the modulation of autonomic and emotional processes, and the prefrontal gyrus contains the primary motor area.

349. The answer is e. *(Kandel, pp 510–521.)* Lateral inhibition within the retina is generated most effectively by the horizontal cells. A horizontal cell receives inputs from a given receptor cell and, when activated, inhibits adjacent receptor cells. It is possible for a given cone cell to differentially affect two neighboring bipolar cells and for an on-center bipolar cell to hyperpolarize an adjacent off-center ganglion cell. However, the primary flow of information through these neuronal elements is in the plane of orientation that most directly connects the receptor cell to the ganglion cell through a bipolar cell. Therefore, the contribution of these elements to lateral inhibition is relatively minimal (if at all) in comparison to the effects generated by horizontal cells. The ganglion cell is not known to play any role in lateral inhibition.

350. The answer is c. *(Kandel, pp 523–543.)* Cells in the lateral geniculate nucleus respond very much like ganglion cells in the retina because of the point-to-point projection pathway from the retina to the lateral geniculate. Accordingly, lateral geniculate cells have small concentric receptive fields that are either on-center or off-center in which the cells respond best to small spots of light that are in the center of the receptive field. On the other hand, cells in the visual cortex display a much greater complexity in their responses to images in the visual field. Instead of responding to small spots of light, they respond to lines and borders in the different areas of the visual field. In particular, the simple cell responds as a function of the retinal position in which the line-stimulus is located, as well as its orientation (e.g., whether it is in a vertical or horizontal position). As a result, when a bar of light is positioned in the appropriate part of the visual field with the appropriate orientation, the cells in area 17 will respond maximally. When either of these parameters is altered, the firing pattern of the cell will be reduced or totally inhibited. Complex cells lack clear excitatory and inhibitory zones (i.e., these neurons respond to bars of light in a given orientation but they are not position-specific). Hypercomplex cells are stimulated by bars of light of specific lengths or by specific shapes.

351. The answer is e. *(Kandel, pp 625–634.)* The olfactory cilia are extensions of the receptor cell, and it is this part of the cell that initially responds to an olfactory stimulus. The cilia contain protein membranes that bind with different odorants, which constitutes a necessary condition for excitation of the olfactory cell. Mitral and granule cells are situated in the olfactory bulb and, consequently, are not part of the receptor mechanism. Sustentacular cells are supporting cells and are not part of the receptor mechanism. Basal cells are the precursors for receptor cells and, thus, are also not directly part of the receptor mechanism.

352. The answer is b. *(Kandel, pp 626–636.)* A number of recent studies have indicated that different olfactory glomeruli respond to different kinds of olfactory stimuli. In a sense, this represents a type of organization of the olfactory bulb that bears a functional similarity to the spatial organization that exists for other sensory systems. There is no evidence that such a spatial arrangement exists for other components of the olfactory system, nor is there any evidence that temporal summation plays any role in the process of olfactory discrimination.

353. The answer is d. *(Nolte, pp 316–323.)* The principal output pathways of the olfactory bulb arise from mitral cells and a related cell, called a *tufted cell*. The mitral cells project their axons out of the olfactory bulb to other regions of the forebrain associated with the transmission of olfactory information to the cerebral cortex. The major pathway subserving this is the lateral olfactory stria. Other cells that are mentioned in this question are either not present in the olfactory bulb (Golgi cells) or they have no known projections outside of the olfactory bulb. Receptor cells project only as far as the glomerulus. The granule cell has no axon. The periglomerular cell makes only local connections among neighboring glomeruli.

354. The answer is b. *(Kandel, p 633. Nolte, pp 316–323.)* Mitral cell axons enter the lateral olfactory stria and project caudally through this bundle to supply the medial amygdala and pyriform cortex. Olfactory projections to other nuclei, such as the hippocampal formation, prefrontal cortex, medial thalamus, and septal area, require at least one additional synaptic connection such as in the pyriform cortex, amygdala, or olfactory tubercle.

355. The answer is a. *(Afifi, p 489. Nolte, p 323.)* Uncinate fits (hallucinations) are characterized by seizure activity involving portions of the anterior aspect of the temporal lobe. The structures most often implicated include the uncus, parahippocampal gyrus, the region of the amygdala and adjoining tissue, and the pyriform cortex. During the occurrence of uncinate fits, a person experiences olfactory hallucinations of a highly unpleasant nature.

356. The answer is c. *(Nolte, pp 230–239, 295–304, 319–323, 547–560.)* The pathway for conscious proprioception from the body utilizes the ventral posterolateral nucleus as its thalamic relay. Conscious proprioception from the head utilizes the ventral posteromedial nucleus as its relay. The taste pathway utilizes the ventral posteromedial nucleus as well. The visual system utilizes the lateral geniculate nucleus, and the auditory system utilizes the medial geniculate nucleus. In contrast, the olfactory system can transmit olfactory information to the prefrontal cortex without engaging thalamic nuclei. Thus, olfactory information reaches the pyriform cortex and amygdala from the olfactory bulb and then is transmitted directly to the prefrontal cortex. However, it should be noted that olfactory information also can reach the prefrontal cortex by virtue of projections from the olfactory tubercle and pyriform cortex via the mediodorsal thalamic nucleus. Thus, the olfactory system may utilize a parallel processing mechanism in transmitting inputs to the prefrontal cortex.

Anatomy of the Forebrain

Questions

DIRECTIONS: Each group of questions below consists of lettered options followed by a set of numbered items. For each numbered item, select the **one** lettered option with which it is most closely associated. Each lettered option may be used once, more than once, or not at all.

Questions 357–361

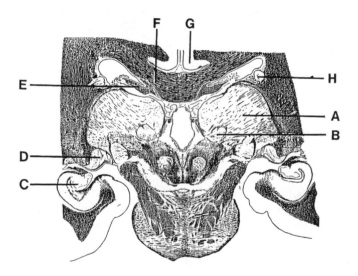

357. Which neurons in this figure project their axons to the inferior parietal lobule?

358. Which fiber bundle arises from the hippocampal formation?

359. A young man received a head injury in a football game, which later resulted in the development of seizure activity and the loss of his short-term memory. Which is the likely structure affected by this injury?

360. As a result of a vascular occlusion, a 64-year-old woman developed a homonymous hemianopsia. Which structure was affected by this occlusion?

361. From which region do neurons play an important role in transmitting information from the reticular formation to widespread areas of the cerebral cortex and, additionally, project their axons to the neostriatum?

Questions 362–368

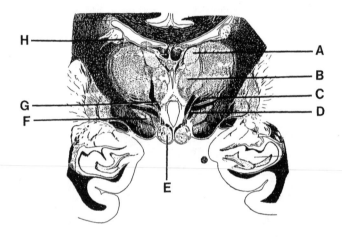

362. An elderly man suffered a stroke that was limited mainly to the globus pallidus, resulting in a hyperkinetic disorder. This was due mainly to the degeneration of fiber bundles that arise from the globus pallidus, which supply the ventrolateral (VL) and ventral anterior (VA) nuclei of the thalamus. Which fiber bundle would be affected by the stroke?

363. A 72-year-old male sustained a vascular occlusion involving a region of his forebrain. Afterward, he displayed symptoms of dyskinesia, which was later diagnosed as hemiballism. Which structure would be damaged by the vascular occlusion?

364. A person had a stroke involving the ventral aspect of the diencephalon, resulting in significant damage to the mammillary bodies. As a result, there was considerable loss of input that normally supplies a major target region of the mammillary bodies. Which structure is now deprived of such input?

365. In the case described in question 364, there was considerable degeneration in the major efferent pathway of the mammillary bodies. Which pathway was degenerated?

366. As a result of an injury involving the temporal lobe, a person suffered changes in personality and autonomic functions. These changes were due in part to the loss of input to the medial hypothalamus. Which fiber bundle normally transmits information from parts of the temporal lobe to the medial hypothalamus?

367. An experiment was performed to determine the effects of converging inputs from the cerebellum and basal ganglia on neurons in the ventrolateral thalamic nucleus. In order to conduct this experiment, the investigator had to stimulate the pathway that transmits information from the cerebellum and basal ganglia. Which pathway was stimulated?

368. A vascular lesion affecting a middle-aged woman resulted in the development of changes in affective responses and related aspects of emotionality, characterized by a flattened affect. The neurologist attributed the flattened affect to the loss of communication between the affected structure and the prefrontal cortex. Which of the structures was affected by the lesion?

Questions 369–375

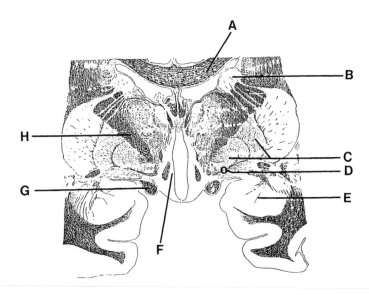

369. A 68-year-old male was taken to the emergency room after having a stroke while working in his office. Several days later, he presented with a UMN paralysis of the right hand and right leg as well as a motor aphasia. An MRI indicated that the stroke involved structures situated within the forebrain. Which structure was affected by the stroke?

370. A patient suffered from epilepsy for approximately 10 years and had been successfully treated with drugs. In recent months, the intensity of the seizures became significantly worse, spreading to both hemispheres of the brain, as drug treatment proved ineffective. In order to block the spread of the seizures, surgery was indicated. Which structure was now the subject of the surgical procedure?

371. A patient presented with a hypokinetic movement disorder. Both the neurosurgeon and the neurologist recommended a surgical lesion of the major output pathway of the basal ganglia in order to alleviate his condition. In which pathway was the surgical lesion placed?

372. A new procedure was developed for the treatment of Parkinson's disease. It involved the direct administration of dopamine, a dopamine agonist, or a dopamine precursor to the brain structure whose dopamine concentrations have been depleted as a result of the disease. Which structure received delivery of these compounds?

373. A patient was sent to be examined by an endocrinologist after complaining of excessive thirst and increased excretion of urine. The patient was then referred to a neurologist and neuroradiologist, who detected the presence of a secondary brain lesion after viewing an MRI of the patient's brain. Where would the possible locus of the lesion that could account for these deficits be?

374. After receiving a neurological examination, a patient was told that he was suffering from psychomotor seizures induced by the presence of a brain tumor. The patient also presented with an altered personality state characterized by marked irritability with heightened anger in response to circumstances normally considered to be innocuous. Where would the most likely locus of the tumor be?

375. A patient was referred to a neurologist after complaining that he could not see out of the right half of each eye. The examination, coupled with an MRI, revealed the likely presence of a brain lesion causing the right homonymous hemianopsia. Which structure was affected by the lesion?

Questions 376–379

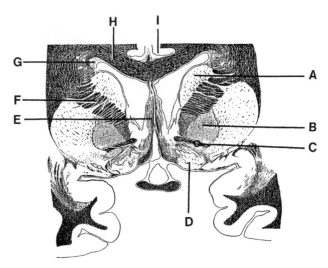

376. A patient who had been suffering from Huntington's disease died and an autopsy was performed. The neuropathologist noted marked degeneration in the forebrain. Which forebrain structure showed marked neuronal loss?

377. After displaying progressive memory loss over a period of several months, an elderly patient was referred to a neurologist, who concluded that the patient was suffering from Alzheimer's disease. Several years later, the patient died and an autopsy was performed, indicating a significant loss of cholinergic neurons in specific regions of the forebrain. Which structure most likely exhibited the greatest loss of cholinergic neurons?

378. Which structure receives major GABAergic input from neurons originating in the neostriatum?

379. Which structure (considerably larger in nonhumans, such as the rat, cat, and monkey) constitutes a component of the limbic system and receives a major afferent projection from the hippocampal formation?

DIRECTIONS: Each item below contains a question or incomplete statement followed by suggested responses. Select the **one best** response to each question.

Item 380–384

Susan is a 32-year-old woman, who recently stopped taking her birth control pills in order to become pregnant. However, after several months, her menstrual period failed to resume. Prior to beginning the birth control pills several years before, she had been having normal cycles. She also noticed headaches, which had been increasing in severity over the past several months. Recently, she became aware of difficulty with her peripheral vision. Thinking that she might be pregnant, she sought the attention of her gynecologist. Her doctor ran a pregnancy test, which was negative. The doctor told her that there might be another cause for the absence of her menstrual cycle, and she tested Susan's blood for levels of various hormones. When Susan returned to find out the results of the tests, her gynecologist told her that the level of the hormone prolactin was high. Susan remembered her headaches and visual symptoms, and informed her doctor, who promptly referred her to a neurologist. The neurologist listened to Susan's story and examined her. She found only that Susan was unable to see fingers in the temporal fields (lateral half of each visual field) of both of her eyes. The remainder of her neurologic exam was normal. The neurologist told Susan that she would like to order an MRI test of her head, in order to find out why she had the headaches, visual problem, and high prolactin levels.

380. A tumor in which area could cause a high prolactin level?
a. Adenohypophysis
b. Neurohypophysis
c. Amygdala
d. Hippocampus
e. Adrenal gland

381. What type of neurologic visual loss can cause a loss of peripheral vision?
a. Central scotoma
b. Superior quadrantanopsia
c. Bitemporal hemianopsia
d. Homonymous hemianopsia
e. Papilledema

382. A lesion adjacent to which structure caused Susan's visual problem?
a. Optic nerve
b. Optic radiations
c. Retina
d. Optic chiasm
e. Lateral geniculate nucleus

383. Which hypothalamic nucleus regulates prolactin secretion?

a. Suprachiasmatic nucleus
b. Preoptic nucleus
c. Paraventricular nucleus
d. Supraoptic nucleus
e. Arcuate nucleus

384. Which neurotransmitter system regulates prolactin secretion?

a. Tuberoinfundibular dopaminergic system
b. Nigrostriatal dopaminergic system
c. Mesolimbic dopaminergic system
d. Mesocortical dopaminergic system
e. Mesostriatal dopaminergic system

Item 385–389

Norma is a 75-year-old woman who had a stroke several months ago, manifested by numbness on her right side, including her arm, face, trunk, and leg. The numbness improved somewhat over time, but did not completely disappear. One day, she noticed that brushing her right arm against a door was very painful. Thinking that perhaps this was "in her mind," she tried touching the right arm with her left hand, and this, too, was painful. Fearful that she might be having another stroke, she went immediately to see her neurologist at the local hospital. Norma's neurologist examined her and found that sensation for a pin, temperature, and vibration were diminished on the entire right side of her body. The degree of sensory loss was unchanged from an examination several months before. However, she had a large amount of discomfort with any type of stimulus, accompanied by some emotional disturbance. The discomfort was far out of proportion to the degree of the stimulus (e.g., a light touch to her right arm would engender a scream similar to that elicited by a knife). The remainder of her examination was normal. The neurologist told Norma that he didn't think she had had another stroke, but would order a head CT to be sure there was no tumor or bleeding. In addition, he told her that if the head CT showed nothing new, she could begin a new medication that would help with the pain.

385. What was the most likely location of the old stroke?

a. Right precentral gyrus
b. Left precentral gyrus
c. Right ventral thalamus
d. Left ventral thalamus
e. Left cerebral peduncle

386. Which two nuclei mediating sensation of the arms, face, legs, and trunk may have sustained damage from the original stroke?

a. Lateral and medial geniculate nuclei of the thalamus
b. Ventral posterior lateral and ventral posterior medial nuclei of the thalamus
c. Putamen and globus pallidus
d. Caudate and putamen
e. Anterior and lateral dorsal nuclei of the thalamus

387. Which pathway mediating pain is the afferent input into the infarcted area?

a. Fasciculus gracilis
b. Fasciculus cuneatus
c. Spinocerebellar tract
d. Spinothalamic tract
e. Corticospinal tract

388. Surgical stimulation of various regions of the CNS has been shown to alleviate pain. Which of the following is the locus of an area producing analgesia?

a. Anterior nucleus of the thalamus
b. Caudate nucleus
c. Anterior horn of the spinal cord
d. Globus pallidus
e. Periaqueductal gray

389. Of the neurotransmitters implicated in pain modulation, which one of the following may be targets of pain-alleviating drugs?

a. Aspartate
b. Glutamate
c. Epinephrine
d. Dopamine and norepinephrine
e. Opiates and serotonin

Anatomy of the Forebrain

Answers

357–361. The answers are 357-A, 358-E, 359-C, 360-D, 361-B. (*Nolte, pp 375–387, 417–421, 538–561.*) This section is taken at the level of the posterior thalamus and, because of the oblique cut, also includes parts of the midbrain and pons. The pulvinar (A), a very large nucleus situated at this level of the thalamus, projects extensively to wide regions of the inferior parietal lobule. The fornix (E), situated just below the corpus callosum, arises from the hippocampal formation and supplies the septal area, anterior thalamic nucleus, and mammillary bodies. The hippocampal formation (C) is associated with a number of different processes, including short-term memory and as a seizure focus during temporal lobe epilepsy. Thus, a lesion of this structure will likely produce deficits in short-term memory, and trauma to this region will result in temporal lobe epilepsy. The lateral geniculate nucleus (D), situated in the far VL aspect of the posterior thalamus, is a relay nucleus for the transmission of visual information to the cortex. Damage to this structure would result in a homonymous hemianopsia. The centromedian (CM) nucleus (B), identified by its encapsulated appearance, can be found in posterior levels of the thalamus, where it receives inputs from the brainstem reticular formation and projects to the neostriatum as well as to wide regions of the cerebral cortex.

362–368. The answers are 362-D, 363-F, 364-A, 365-G, 366-H, 367-C, 368-B. (*Nolte, pp 375–394, 451–467, 538–545, 548–555.*) This section is taken at the level of the mammillary bodies (at ventral levels) and includes parts of the anterior thalamus (at dorsal levels). The lenticular fasciculus (D), situated just below the thalamic fasciculus and immediately above the subthalamic nucleus at the level of this brain section, arises from the dorsomedial aspect of the medial pallidal segment and projects to the VL, VA, and CM nuclei of the thalamus. Damage to the neurons of the medial pallidal segment would cause degeneration of the efferent projections from this region, one pathway of which is the lenticular fasciculus. The subthalamic nucleus (F), which lies on the dorsal surface of the internal capsule, maintains reciprocal connections with the globus pallidus through a pathway called the *subthalamic fasciculus.* Damage to the subthalamic nucleus has been associated with the onset of hemiballism. The anterior nucleus of the thalamus (A), which lies at the rostral end of the thalamus in a dorsomedial position, receives a major input from the mammillary bodies via the *mammillothalamic tract.* The mammillary bodies (E), situated at the base of the posterior aspect of the hypothalamus, are the origin of the mammillothalamic (G) tract, which innervates the anterior thalamic nucleus. The region immediately below the tail and body of the caudate nucleus is occupied by a major output pathway of the medial amygdala (within the temporal lobe), the *stria terminalis* (H). It supplies the medial preoptic region, bed nucleus of the stria terminalis, and medial hypothalamus. The *thalamic fasciculus* can be seen in sections taken through the caudal half of the thalamus and is clearly visualized in a position dorsal to the subthalamic nucleus and lenticular fasciculus. The *thalamic fasciculus* (C) also projects to the ventral lateral and ventral anterior thalamic nuclei. While many of the fibers contained in this bundle arise from the medial pallidal segment, others arise directly from the dentate nucleus of cerebellum. A large nuclear mass situated in the medial aspect of the posterior two-thirds of the thalamus is the mediodorsal thalamic nucleus (B). This nucleus projects extensively to wide regions of the frontal lobe, including the prefrontal cortex. In turn, the prefrontal region of the cortex and adjoining regions of the frontal lobe project their axons back to the mediodorsal nucleus. Thus, there are reciprocal connections linking the mediodorsal nucleus and rostral portions of the frontal lobe. Because of the major input to the prefrontal cortex from the mediodorsal nucleus and since the prefrontal cortex plays an important role in the regulation of affective processes, damage to the mediodorsal nucleus would clearly alter emotional responses associated with the prefrontal cortex.

369–375. The answers are 369-H, 370-A, 371-D, 372-B, 373-F, 374-E, 375-G. *(Nolte, pp 239–240, 261, 507–515, 517–523, 538–561. Waxman, p 249.)* This section is taken from rostral levels of the diencephalon. Corticobulbar and corticospinal fibers contained within the internal capsule (H) arise from the deeper layers of the cerebral cortex (i.e., layers V–VI). A lesion of the internal capsule would produce a UMN paralysis of the contralateral side of the body because of disruption of corticospinal fibers as well as damage to some corticobulbar fibers contained within the internal capsule. In this instance, there was damage associated with corticobulbar fibers descending from the motor speech area, resulting in a motor aphasia. Fibers associated with the corpus callosum (A) arise from more superficial layers of the cortex (i.e., layers II–III) and project to the homotypic region of the contralateral cortex. Because this commissure represents the principal means by which one side of the cortex communicates with the other, surgical disruption of these fibers is carried out when all means of drug therapy have been shown to be ineffective and when seizures are shown to have spread to the cortices on both sides of the brain. Fibers of the ansa lenticularis (D) arise from the ventral aspect of the medial pallidal segment and can be visualized at more anterior levels of the pallidum. It represents a major output pathway of the basal ganglia and its axons supply the VL, VA, and CM nuclei of the thalamus. The caudate nucleus (B) receives dopaminergic inputs from the substantia nigra. Loss of dopamine levels in the caudate is associated with Parkinson's disease, and experimental strategies have been applied to treat this disorder through replenishment of dopamine in the caudate nucleus.

Different cells of the paraventricular nucleus of the hypothalamus (F), situated in the dorsomedial region at anterior levels, synthesize oxytocin and vasopressin. These hormones are transported down their axons to the posterior pituitary. Loss of vasopressin would result in excessive thirst and increased urine secretion, since vasopressin acts as an antidiuretic hormone. Although the marked changes in emotionality could be accounted for by damage to either the medial hypothalamus or the amygdala (E), psychomotor seizures are typically associated with temporal lobe structures and not with the hypothalamus. Thus, the correct answer in this case is (E). Different fiber groups of the amygdala provide major inputs into the medial and lateral regions of the hypothalamus and thus constitute a significant modulator of hypothalamic functions, including rage and aggression. The optic tract (G) arises from the retina. Each optic tract represents fibers associated with the visual fields of the opposite side. Therefore, a lesion of the optic tract will result in a homonymous hemianopsia.

376–379. The answers are 376-A, 377-D, 378-B, 379-E. (*Nolte, pp 277–278, 380–388, 544–561. Waxman, p 199.*) This section is taken at the level of the septum pellucidum, the anterior commissure, and the substantia innominata. While a variety of structures may show degeneration in Huntington's disease, it is generally agreed that Huntington's disease is associated with loss of GABAergic neurons situated principally in the caudate nucleus (A). Fibers from the region of the basal nucleus of Meynert located in the substantia innominata (D) (at the base of the brain in the far rostral forebrain) send a cholinergic projection to wide areas of the neocortex. Loss of these cholinergic neurons has generally been associated with the presence of Alzheimer's disease. The globus pallidus (B) receives GABAergic inputs from the neostriatum (i.e., caudate nucleus and putamen), and these inputs represent the principal afferent supply of the neostriatum to the pallidum. The septal area (E), seen at this level of the forebrain as a thin structure separated by the lateral ventricles on both sides, receives major inputs from the hippocampal formation and is a principal component of the limbic system.

380–384. The answers are 380-a, 381-c, 382-d, 383-e, 384-a.
(Adams, pp 676–678. Afifi, pp 404–409. Kandel, pp 544, 978–980.) The MRI of Susan's head revealed a pituitary microadenoma, a benign tumor arising from the anterior pituitary or adenohypophysis. This particular tumor consisted of cells that secrete the hormone prolactin, which is not only the stimulating factor for lactation, but inhibits menstruation when levels are high. It is common for this tumor's symptoms to be manifested during the childbearing years. The visual problem is called *bitemporal hemianopsia.* Since the pituitary gland is in very close proximity to the optic chiasm, pituitary tumors often invade this structure. Since only the medial fibers (which perceive the temporal field of each eye) in each optic nerve cross, these are the fibers damaged by these tumors, and the patient will be unable to see either temporal visual field. Neither central scotoma (an island of visual loss surrounded by normal vision in one eye), which is usually seen with lesions of the retina or optic nerve nor papilledema (blurring of the optic disc margin when viewed by fundoscopic examination due to increased intracranial pressure) would be caused by damage to the optic chiasm. The optic chiasm can be compressed by pituitary tumors, causing bitemporal hemianopsia (see the answer for the previous question). The prolactin-releasing factor is found in the arcuate nucleus of the hypothalamus and activates the lactotropic cells of the anterior pituitary gland. Several different peptides, including dopamine, have the capacity to raise the level of prolactin in the blood. Specifically, the tuberoinfundibular dopaminergic system regulates prolactin secretion through direct projection to the pituitary. For this reason, a newer treatment for prolactin-

secreting microadenomas is the drug bromocriptine, a dopamine agonist commonly used in the treatment of Parkinson's disease. By giving a dopamine agonist, serum prolactin increases, inhibiting production by the tumor cells, and eventually the tumor size shrinks. This has become either an alternative or a first-line treatment prior to trying radiation or surgery.

385–389. The answers are 385-d, 386-b, 387-d, 388-e, 389-e. *(Kandel, pp 446–450, 454–460, 473–475, 480–487, 874–875.)* Norma's head CT showed an old stroke in her left ventral thalamus and no new lesions. A stroke involving the ventral posterolateral nucleus of the thalamus, especially several months after the stroke, can produce an entity called the *Déjérine-Roussy syndrome,* or *thalamic pain syndrome.* Although there is sensory loss on the contralateral side, there is pain or discomfort out of proportion to the stimulus on the affected side of the body. Emotional disturbance aggravates the response. Some patients describe the sensation as knifelike or hot. As the deficit (numbness) resolves, the pain may lessen. This syndrome may also occur in lesions of the parietal white matter and is thought to occur as a result of an imbalance of afferent sensory impulses. Sensation of the limbs and trunk are projected through the ventral posterior lateral nucleus of the thalamus to the somatosensory cortex. Sensory information from the face is carried through the trigeminal system to the ventral posteromedial nucleus, from which it is projected to the somatosensory cortex. The spinothalamic tract is the only sensory pathway listed that mediates pain. The periaqueductal gray is one area of many that produces analgesia when stimulated in both animals and humans. It is an area with a high density of opiate receptors and opioidergic neurons and is thought to represent a key area in gating pain. Many neurotransmitters have been implicated as pain modulators, including the opiates and enkephalins, norepinephrine, serotonin, substance P, GABA, and acetylcholine. Most analgesic medications are designed to target a particular aspect of the pain pathway. In more recent years, the advent of a class of drugs called *tricyclic antidepressants* has added another dimension to medical pain treatment. The methylated forms of these medications are useful blockers of serotonin reuptake. Since serotonin is known to be a pain modulator, it is thought that blocking the reuptake of serotonin enhances its action and facilitates the action of intrinsic opiates to relieve pain. This is a common class of drugs used to treat chronic pain, since these medications are not addictive.

Motor Systems

Questions

DIRECTIONS: Each item below contains a question or incomplete statement followed by suggested responses. Select the **one best** response to each question.

390. A patient delays initiation of movement, displays an uneven trajectory in moving her hand from above her head to touch her nose, and is uneven in her attempts to demonstrate rapid alternation of pronating and supernating movements of the hand and forearm. Which of the following regions would most likely contain the lesion?

a. Hemispheres of the posterior cerebellar lobe
b. Flocculonodular lobe of the cerebellum
c. Vermal region of the anterior cerebellar lobe
d. Fastigial nucleus
e. Ventral spinocerebellar tract

391. Spasticity may result from a lesion of which of the following structures?

a. Ventral horn cells
b. Corpus callosum
c. Postcentral gyrus
d. Internal capsule
e. Substantia nigra

392. In studying the functional relationships between the motor cortex and the spinal cord, which of the following effects of motor-cortical stimulation on synaptic potentials would an investigator be likely to observe?

a. The largest potentials would be seen in spinal motor neurons that innervate proximal muscles
b. The largest potentials would be seen in spinal motor neurons that innervate distal muscles
c. The potentials seen in spinal motor neurons that innervate proximal and distal muscles would be approximately equivalent
d. The largest potentials would be seen in spinal sensory neurons that carry information from spindle afferents to the cerebellum
e. The largest potentials would be seen in spinal sensory neurons that carry information from proprioceptors to the thalamus

393. Which of the following statements correctly characterizes the properties of neurons in the motor cortex?

a. In the resting state, the membranes of motor cortex neurons are more permeable to sodium than to potassium ions
b. Motor cortex neurons receive information from the muscle to which they project or from a region of skin that is related to the function of that muscle
c. Motor cortex neurons have reciprocal connections with the red nucleus
d. Motor cortex neurons that excite alpha motor neurons generally have little effect upon gamma motor neurons that project to the same muscle group
e. Motor neurons of the cerebral cortex have reciprocal, monosynaptic connections with neurons in the cerebellar cortex

394. Paralysis of the right side of the lower face, right spastic paralysis of the limbs, deviation of the tongue to the right with no atrophy, and no loss of taste from any region of the tongue will likely result from a lesion of which of the following structures?

a. Internal capsule of the right side
b. Internal capsule of the left side
c. Right pontine tegmentum
d. Base of the medulla on the right side
e. Base of the medulla on the left side

395. A 74-year-old female was brought to the hospital after she suffered a stroke. Several days later, a neurological examination revealed that she was unable to perform certain types of learned, complex movements (referred to as *apraxia*). Which region of the cerebral cortex was affected by the stroke?

a. Precentral gyrus
b. Postcentral gyrus
c. Premotor cortex
d. Prefrontal cortex
e. Cingulate gyrus

396. In which of the following structures do the overwhelming majority of fibers that supply the basal ganglia terminate?

a. Paleostriatum
b. Neostriatum
c. Subthalamic nucleus
d. Substantia nigra
e. Claustrum

397. Which of the following best characterizes neurons in the neostriatum?

a. Inhibited by γ-aminobutyric acid (GABA) released at corticostriate terminals
b. Inhibited by GABA released at nigrostriatal terminals
c. Inhibited by substance P released at corticostriate terminals
d. Excited by acetylcholine (ACh) released from hypothalamic-caudate terminals
e. Excited by glutamate released at corticostriate terminals

398. Which of the following is the primary transmitter released from terminals of both neostriatal and paleostriatal neurons?

a. Glycine
b. Enkephalin
c. Dopamine
d. GABA
e. Glutamate

399. Since motor dysfunctions associated with disturbances of basal ganglia are expressed on the contralateral side of the body, which of the following is the most appropriate conclusion regarding the projections of the basal ganglia?

a. Fibers to the spinal cord that are crossed
b. Fibers to motor nuclei of the brainstem whose axons then project to the contralateral spinal cord
c. Fibers to structures that ultimately influence motor regions of the ipsilateral cerebral cortex
d. Axons to the cerebellum, whose outputs are known to modulate the contralateral side of the body
e. Fibers directly to the contralateral motor cortex

400. Which of the following structures provides the major input to the flocculonodular lobe?

a. Clarke's nucleus dorsalis of the spinal cord
b. Red nucleus
c. Vestibular nuclei
d. Cerebral cortex
e. Midbrain reticular formation

401. Which of the following is lost or reduced in Huntington's disease?

a. Dopamine in the neostriatum
b. Substance P in the substantia nigra
c. ACh and GABA in intrastriatal and cortical neurons
d. Serotonin in the neostriatum
e. Most of the pallidal neurons

402. A patient was admitted to the local hospital for treatment of a vascular occlusion within the forebrain. An MRI indicated that the damage was limited to the subthalamic nucleus. As a result of this lesion, which of the following disorders is likely to be present in the patient?

a. Torsion dystonia
b. Tremor at rest
c. Hemiballism
d. Spastic paralysis
e. Tardive dyskinesia

403. A patient is given medication for the treatment of choreiform movements. Which of the following strategies is the neurologist likely to apply?

a. ACh blockers because there is an excess of this transmitter in the caudate nucleus
b. Dopamine blockers because there is too low a ratio of ACh to dopamine in the neostriatum
c. Serotonin blockers because there is too low a ratio of serotonin to ACh and dopamine in the neostriatum
d. Substance P antagonists because the ratio of substance P to ACh is too high in the neostriatum
e. Norepinephrine antagonists because the ratio of norepinephrine to ACh is too high in the subthalamic nucleus

404. A 65-year-old male has been under long-term treatment for an anxiety disorder. Recently, the psychiatrist observed that he began to develop symptoms of tardive dyskinesia. This disorder is most likely the result of which of the following alterations?

a. A reduction in serotonin receptors in the neostriatum
b. A change in ACh receptors that causes a hypersensitivity to ACh
c. A change in enkephalin receptors that causes a hypersensitivity to enkephalin
d. A change in GABA levels in the basal ganglia
e. A change in dopamine levels in the limbic system

405. The neurotoxin 1-methyl-4-phenyl-1,2,3,6-tetrahydropyridine (MPTP) has recently been applied experimentally with considerable success as a model for the study of which of the following diseases?

a. Huntington's disease
b. Hemiballism
c. Parkinson's disease
d. Tardive dyskinesia
e. Dystonia

406. The dorsal spinocerebellar tract, the ventral spinocerebellar tract, and the cuneocerebellar tract, in a general sense, show convergence in their projections to the cerebellum. Which of the following is the principal region within the cerebellum where these fibers converge?

a. Anterior lobe
b. Posterior lobe
c. Flocculonodular lobe
d. Fastigial nucleus
e. Dentate nucleus

407. Information arising from the cerebral cortex is known to reach the cerebellum. Which of the following best describes the distribution of these fibers?

a. Somatotopically distributed only to the anterior lobe
b. Somatotopically distributed only to the vermal region of the anterior and posterior lobes
c. Somatotopically distributed to the cerebellar hemispheres
d. Not somatotopically organized but do project to the hemispheres of the anterior and posterior lobes
e. Distributed mainly to the interposed and dentate nuclei

408. Which of the following best characterizes a cerebellar glomerulus?

a. Mossy fiber terminals, Golgi axons, and axon terminals of granule cells
b. Climbing fiber terminals, Golgi axons, and granule cell dendrites
c. Mossy fiber terminals, Purkinje cell axons, and granule cell dendrites
d. Mossy fiber terminals, Golgi and granule cell dendrites, and Golgi cell axon terminals
e. Climbing fiber terminals, Golgi cell dendrites, Purkinje cell dendrites, and axon terminals of parallel fibers

Item 409–411

The cerebellum contains a number of important feedback relationships with different regions of the CNS. In each of the following circuits, one or more of the structures has been omitted. Indicate the structure(s) that must be added to complete that circuit.

409. Frontal lobe → deep pontine nuclei → cerebellar cortex → _____ ?
_____ → _____ ? _____ → motor cortex (frontal lobe)

a. Fastigial nucleus → red nucleus
b. Interposed nuclei → red nucleus
c. Dentate nucleus → ventrolateral (VL) nucleus of the thalamus
d. Dentate nucleus → ventral anterior (VA) nucleus of the thalamus
e. Purkinje cell axons → reticular formation of pons

410. Red nucleus → inferior olivary nucleus → cerebellar cortex of the anterior and posterior lobes → _____ → red nucleus

a. Fastigial nucleus
b. Interposed nuclei
c. Dentate nucleus
d. Purkinje cells of the cerebellar hemispheres
e. Vestibular nuclei

411. Spinal cord (via dorsal and ventral spinocerebellar tracts) → anterior lobe of the cerebellum → _____ → reticular formation and vestibular nuclei → spinal cord

a. Fastigial nucleus
b. Globose nucleus
c. Emboliform nucleus
d. Dentate nucleus
e. Red nucleus

412. Based upon your knowledge of the anatomic and neurophysiologic relationships of the anterior lobe of the cerebellum, which of the following best describes what would occur following electrical stimulation of the medial vermal aspect of the cerebellar cortex of the anterior lobe?

a. Produce movement of the arms
b. Produce spasticity
c. Cause tonic seizures to occur
d. Modulate extensor muscle tone
e. Have little effect upon muscle tone

413. A man presents with a wide-based, ataxic gait during his attempts at walking. He also is unsteady, sways when standing, and displays a tendency to fall backward or to either side in a drunken manner. In which of the following structures is a lesion most likely located?

a. Hemispheres of the posterior cerebellar lobe
b. Anterior limb of the internal capsule
c. Dentate nucleus
d. Anterior lobe of the cerebellum
e. Flocculonodular lobe of the cerebellum

Item 414–418

Sam is a 62-year-old man, previously healthy, who was brought to a neurologist by his daughter because of increasing difficulty walking. His daughter noticed that for the past year, he had difficulty getting out of a chair and took a lot of time to begin to walk. When he did walk, he walked with a slow, shuffling gait. In addition, she had noticed some changes in his face, and that he had been drooling excessively. His signature on checks became progressively smaller from the beginning of his name to the end, and he had developed a new tremor. She brought him in to make sure this wasn't just "aging." The neurologist examined Sam and noticed immediately that Sam's facial expression was masklike, with few eyeblinks. When asked to write a sentence, the letters became progressively smaller toward the end of the sentence. His speech was soft and monotonous, and he had a slow, resting pill-rolling tremor in both of his hands. He had very little spontaneous movement, and his arms, legs, and trunk were stiff. When the neurologist tried to flex his arm, he felt many catches, similar to a cogwheel. There was no weakness, sensory problems, or abnormalities in his reflexes. When asked to walk, Sam took many tries to rise from his chair. When he finally stood up, his posture was stooped and flexed. His gait was slow, his feet shuffled when he walked, and his arms didn't swing with his steps. The neurologist told Sam's daughter that she was correct that this wasn't aging and explained to her all of the details about a new medication that Sam needed to take.

414. Damage to which structure in particular causes Sam's problem with movement?

a. Substantia gelatinosa
b. Substantia nigra, pars reticularis
c. Substantia nigra, pars compacta
d. Caudate nucleus
e. Thalamus

415. What is the blood supply of the main structure damaged?

a. Lenticulostriate branches of the middle cerebral and anterior cerebral arteries
b. Perforating branches of the basilar and vertebral arteries
c. Anterior choroidal artery and anterior cerebral artery
d. Posteromedial branches of the posterior cerebral and posterior communicating arteries
e. Anterior cerebral and anterior communicating arteries

416. What neurotransmitter is deficient?

a. Norepinephrine
b. Glutamate
c. Dopamine
d. ACh
e. GABA

417. Which of the following is a precursor to the deficient neurotransmitter and can be given as a medication to improve Sam's movement?

a. Tyrosine
b. Choline
c. Acetyl-CoA
d. Tryptamine
e. L-dopa

418. The antagonism of which enzyme by drugs will increase the amount of the deficient neurotransmitter?

a. Choline acetyltranferase
b. Monoamine oxidase
c. GABA transaminase
d. Acetylcholinesterase
e. Tyrosine hydroxylase

Item 419–424

John is a 57-year-old man who has always been a very heavy drinker, often consuming 2 pints of whiskey per day, for many years. Upon the urging of his wife, he decided to seek medical attention for help with problems with his gait, which has steadily worsened over the past several months. He noticed that he now needs to stand with his feet far apart in order to maintain his balance and that he waddles when he walks. The doctor who evaluated him tested his memory and speech carefully, as well as his cranial nerves, and was unable to find any deficits. There was no weakness, sensory loss, or abnormalities in his reflexes. When asked to touch the doctor's finger and then his nose, John missed his nose slightly, but rapidly corrected the movement on both sides. When asked to slide his right heel down his left shin, his heel slid sideways and clumsily across the bone until it reached his ankle. The response with the left heel was similar. When asked to walk, John walked with his feet very far apart. If he attempted to walk in a tandem fashion, with one heel in front of the other toe, he began to fall, and the doctor needed to catch him. The doctor ordered an MRI of John's head.

419. What term could one use for John's gait?

a. Stiff
b. Festinating
c. Ataxic
d. Spastic
e. Shuffling

420. A gait problem of this type could be caused by lesions in which system(s)?

a. Cerebellar tracts only
b. Posterior columns only
c. Corticospinal tracts
d. Both the cerebellar and the posterior column systems
e. Spinothalamic system

421. Where in the brain would a neurologist expect to visualize the lesion on an MRI scan?

a. Red nucleus
b. Cerebellar vermis
c. Substantia nigra
d. Internal capsule
e. Basilar pons

422. The region of the affected area is associated with which functional division of the cerebellum?

a. Cerebrocerebellum
b. Spinocerebellum
c. Dentate nucleus
d. Superior cerebellar peduncle
e. Brachium pontis

423. To which deep cerebellar nucleus does the damaged region project?

a. Globose
b. Dentate
c. Fastigial
d. Vestibular
e. Emboliform

424. Which cell type most likely sustained the most damage from John's alcohol consumption?

a. Schwann cell
b. Pyramidal cell
c. Stellate cell
d. Anterior horn cell
e. Purkinje cell

Item 425–429

Louise is an 86-year-old woman who has had difficulty with high blood pressure, high cholesterol, diabetes, strokes, and blood clots in her legs for many years. One day, her grandson arrived at her apartment in a senior citizen center for his weekly visit and found her lying unconscious on the floor. He immediately called an ambulance to take her to the nearest emergency room. The paramedics in the ambulance gave Louise some medications, including glucose, but she did not awaken. She was taken to the nearest emergency room, where a physician was called to evaluate her. She was breathing on her own and had a pulse, but could not be aroused to any stimulus. Her arms and legs were stiff and would not move in response to a painful stimulus. Her eyes moved in response to moving her head. Finally, in response to a very loud shout and pinch on the arm, she briefly opened her eyes; however, she immediately shut them again. Further attempts to arouse Louise were unsuccessful. She was taken for a CT scan of her head, and then taken to an intensive care unit.

425. An acute stroke in which portion of the CNS could cause this scenario?

a. Right frontal lobe
b. Left frontal lobe
c. Right temporal lobe
d. Pons and midbrain
e. Right occipital lobe

426. What was the cause of the stiffness in Louise's arms and legs?

a. Infarction of the corticospinal tracts bilaterally in the pons
b. Damage to the basal ganglia
c. Infarction of the precentral gyrus
d. Infarction of the internal capsules bilaterally
e. Thalamic infarction

427. Infarction of which artery may cause this picture?

a. Anterior cerebral artery
b. Middle cerebral artery
c. Anterior choroidal artery
d. Basilar artery
e. Lenticulostriate branches of the middle cerebral artery

428. If the stroke occurred in the brainstem, which region is most likely affected?

a. Facial nerve nucleus
b. Trochlear nerve nucleus
c. Reticular formation
d. Trigeminal system
e. Medial longitudinal fasciculus

429. What are the main monoaminergic systems of the region infarcted?

a. Dopamine
b. Norepinephrine
c. Serotonin
d. GABA
e. Norepinephrine and serotonin

Motor Systems

Answers

390. The answer is a. *(Nolte, pp 485–492.)* The classic appearance of a patient with a lesion of the cerebellar hemispheres is one in which voluntary and skilled movements are affected. They are uncoordinated, and there are errors in the range, force, and direction of movement. The relationships between the cerebellum and the motor regions of the cerebral cortex have been disrupted. Lesions of other regions, such as the flocculonodular lobe, vermal region of the anterior cerebellar cortex, or fastigial nucleus, produce different symptoms (disturbances of balance, muscle tone, or nystagmus). Although pure lesions limited to the ventral spinocerebellar tract have not been reported, it is likely that such a lesion could not account for the symptoms indicated in this question. Information carried by this tract concerns activity of Golgi tendon organs of muscles of the lower limbs.

391. The answer is d. *(Nolte, pp 269–271, 439–448.)* A UMN paralysis occurs following a lesion of the internal capsule. Such a lesion disrupts not only fibers destined for the spinal cord, but others that project to parts of the reticular formation and activate inhibitory reticulospinal mechanisms. Loss of such inhibitory input to spinal cord motor neurons then leads to increased levels of excitation of these neurons. The behavioral manifestation of this process is spasticity. Lesions of ventral horn cells produce a flaccid paralysis. Lesions of the postcentral gyrus primarily produce sensory loss, not spasticity. Since the corpus callosum is concerned with interhemispheric transfer of information, a lesion of this bundle will not produce spasticity. A lesion of the substantia nigra will result in Parkinson's disease, which is associated with tremors at rest and rigidity, but not spasticity.

392. The answer is b. *(Kandel, pp 764–777.)* The largest synaptic potentials produced by cortical stimulation would most likely be seen in spinal motor neurons that innervate distal muscles. One of the primary functions of the corticospinal tract is to control the distal muscles of the hands and fingers. Penfield and others constructed a homuncular map from stimulation studies of the cortex. Such studies reveal that the region of the cortex that is associated with the hands and fingers is considerably larger than those regions that are associated with the proximal musculature. Accordingly, stimulation of the hand region of the cortex would activate more fibers than other cortical regions. It is likely that more ventral horn neurons (located in a lateral position) innervate distal musculature than neurons (located in a medial position) innervate proximal musculature. Since the size of the synaptic potential is a function of both the number of fibers that provide a converging input into a given region and the number of cells that discharge in response to that converging input, it is reasonable to conclude that the largest potentials would be observed following stimulation of the cortical regions associated with the distal musculature. Since neurons situated in the motor cortex project their axons to motor horn cells and interneurons but not to sensory neurons of the dorsal horn (although the component of the corticospinal tract that arises from the parietal lobe does project to the dorsal horn), stimulation of the motor cortex could produce only weak potentials at best among sensory neurons in the dorsal horn.

393. The answer is b. (*Kandel, pp 150–164, 764–777.*) Motor cortex neurons receive information from the muscle to which they project or from a region of skin related to the function of that muscle. The anatomic pathway includes dorsal column–medial lemniscal fibers that terminate in the ventral posterolateral (VPL) nucleus of the thalamus. Fibers from the VPL nucleus then project to the postcentral gyrus. Fibers from a given region of the primary sensory cortex project to the region of the primary motor cortex whose projection target in the spinal cord involves the same muscle group (or body part) from which the sensory stimulus originated. All other choices are incorrect. The properties of membrane potentials of neurons in the motor cortex follow the same principles as those found elsewhere in the nervous system; namely, in the resting state, the cell membrane is more permeable to potassium than to sodium. The red nucleus does not have an ascending projection (and, therefore, cannot be reciprocally connected with the motor cortex). Its fibers project, instead, to the spinal cord and lower brainstem. In general, corticospinal fibers that activate alpha motor neurons that innervate a given muscle group will also synapse with gamma motor neurons associated with that same muscle group. Coactivation of both alpha and gamma motor neurons is an important principle because it enables muscle spindles to react to changes in the length of the muscle even during the process of movement of the limb associated with that muscle. The projection to the cerebellum from the motor cortex is disynaptic. Projections from the cerebellum to the motor cortex synapse in the dentate nucleus and the ventrolateral nucleus of the thalamus.

394. The answer is b. *(Kandel, pp 1306–1309.)* This constellation of deficits, including paralysis of the lower right face, paralysis of the lower right limbs, and right deviation of the tongue, requires a lesion located in the left internal capsule. Since the motor fibers from the cortex that supply all three of these regions (i.e., limbs, lower face, and tongue) are all crossed, a lesion of the internal capsule will produce each of these deficits. Also, recall that the tongue will deviate to the side of the lesion when the lesion affects the LMN (i.e., cranial nerve XII) directly. When it affects the UMN (i.e., fibers in the internal capsule), inputs into the contralateral nucleus of cranial nerve XII are affected. Thus, the tongue in this instance will deviate to the side opposite the lesion. A lesion of the pontine tegmentum will not affect descending corticospinal or corticomedullary fibers, since these fibers are contained in the basilar part of the pons. A lesion of the medulla would be too caudal to affect cortical fibers that terminate on cells of the facial nucleus whose axons innervate muscles of the lower face.

395. The answer is c. *(Kandel, pp 654–672, 770–777.)* The premotor areas play an important role in the programming or sequencing of responses that compose complex learned movements. They receive significant inputs for this process from the posterior parietal lobule and, in turn, signal appropriate neurons in the brainstem and spinal cord (both flexors and extensors). Lesions of the postcentral gyrus produce a somatosensory loss. Lesions of the precentral gyrus produce paralysis. Neither lesions of the prefrontal cortex nor those of the cingulate gyrus have been reported to produce apraxia.

396. The answer is b. *(Kandel, pp 853–864.)* The neostriatum (i.e., caudate nucleus and putamen) constitutes the principal, if not exclusive, receiving area for afferent fibers to the basal ganglia. The subthalamic nucleus and the substantia nigra share reciprocal connections with the paleostriatum (i.e., globus pallidus) and the neostriatum, respectively. However, these areas receive few, if any, fibers from the cerebral cortex or the centromedian nucleus of the thalamus, which are the major afferent sources to the basal ganglia. Functions of the claustrum are not well understood, but it is believed to be more closely associated with the neocortex than with the basal ganglia.

397. The answer is e. (*Kandel, pp 853–864.*) The cerebral cortex is a principal source of afferent fibers to the neostriatum and utilizes glutamate as its transmitter, which is excitatory to caudate neurons. Thus, neither GABA nor substance P is a transmitter from the cortex to the neostriatum; nor is GABA a transmitter released from the nigrostriatal terminals. Projections from the hypothalamus to the caudate nucleus have never been demonstrated and, presumably, do not exist.

398. The answer is d. (*Kandel, pp 853–864.*) The major transmitter released at terminals of neostriatal and paleostriatal fibers is GABA. Thus, the output of the basal ganglia is mainly inhibitory. This suggests that thalamic influences upon the cortex are generated through the process of disinhibition, whereby neurons of the basal ganglia are inhibited. The presence of glycine in striatal neurons has yet to be demonstrated. Enkephalins are released from terminals of neostriatal-pallidal fibers but not from other efferent neurons of the striatum. Dopamine is released from the brainstem and some adjoining hypothalamic neurons but certainly not from striatal neurons. The neostriatum receives cortical inputs that utilize glutamate, but the release of GABA from terminals of striatal efferent fibers has not been demonstrated.

399. The answer is c. (*Kandel, pp 853–864.*) The basic principle governing how the basal ganglia control motor activity is that they do so by modulating neurons of the motor cortex and premotor areas (of the ipsilateral side) via synaptic connections in the VL and VA nuclei of the thalamus. One can see from the circuits:

globus pallidus → ventrolateral nucleus → area 4 of cortex (medial segment) (VL)
globus pallidus → ventral anterior nucleus → area 6 of cortex (medial segment) (VA)

that damage to the basal ganglia on one side of the brain will affect cortical neurons on the same side. This will result in dyskinesia expressed on the contralateral side of the body because the corticospinal tract is crossed. The other possibilities listed in the question are not viable. Projections of the basal ganglia to the brainstem nuclei are minimal. The basal ganglia do not project fibers down to the spinal cord, nor do they project to the cerebellum.

400. The answer is c. (*Kandel, pp 833–846.*) The principal source of afferent fibers to the flocculonodular lobe is the vestibular complex, in particular, the inferior and medial vestibular nuclei. For this reason, this lobe of the cerebellum is sometimes referred to as the *vestibulocerebellum*. The red nucleus and cerebral cortex project topographically (via relays in the inferior olivary nucleus and deep pontine nuclei, respectively) to the anterior and posterior lobes. Pathways arising from the spinal cord, such as the spinocerebellar tract, project to the anterior lobe. Other fibers arising from the spinal cord enter the cerebellum through a relay in the inferior olivary nucleus. Such fibers terminate in both anterior and posterior lobes.

401. The answer is c. (*Kandel, pp 864–866.*) In Huntington's disease, the essential neurochemical change is in the basal ganglia, where there is a significant reduction in the two transmitters ACh and GABA. In particular, there are reduced levels of choline acetyltransferase, glutamic acid decarboxylase, and GABA.

402. The answer is c. (*Kandel, pp 864–866.*) A lesion of the subthalamic nucleus results in hemiballism, a form of dyskinesia in which the patient displays severe involuntary movements. It is believed to occur as a result of an imbalance in the output signals of the basal ganglia. There is a change in the relationship between efferent pathways associated with the two pallidal segments (i.e., a direct pathway from the medial pallidal segment to the VL and VA nuclei of the thalamus versus an indirect pathway, involving connections between the lateral pallidal segment, subthalamic nucleus, and substantia nigra). Thus, in hemiballism the indirect pathway is disrupted, resulting in a change in the output signals of the pallidum to the thalamus.

403. The answer is b. (*Kandel, pp 861–866.*) Choreiform movements have generally been associated with damage to the neostriatum (the cortex and the globus pallidus have occasionally been implicated). Normally, there is a balance in what seems to be opposing effects of ACh, dopamine, and GABA in the neostriatum. In this disorder, the levels of ACh and GABA are significantly reduced. This creates an imbalance in which dopamine levels now become (relatively) too high. Accordingly, effective pharmacologic treatment involves the use of dopamine receptor blockers.

404. The answer is d. (*Kandel, p 1201. Gilroy, pp 172–174. Greenberg, pp 253–255.*) Tardive dyskinesia, a disorder involving involuntary movements of the mouth, face, and tongue, is caused by long-term treatment with antipsychotic drugs. This treatment is likely to involve GABA neurons in the basal ganglia because both GABA and the enzyme that synthesizes it, glutamic acid decarboxylase, are depleted after long-term treatment with antipsychotic drugs. It was previously thought that dopamine receptor hypersensitivity could account for the appearance of this disorder because it could be brought on with haloperidol treatment. However, a dopamine receptor hypothesis is not probable because this form of dyskinesia does not always appear when supersensitivity is present following long-term drug treatment. Moreover, supersensitivity can be reversible following discontinuation of the drug, while tardive dyskinesia would still be present. Other transmitter systems have not been implicated in this disorder.

405. The answer is c. *(Kandel, pp 862–864.)* MPTP was discovered by accident when drug abusers who were using a synthetic heroin derivative developed signs of Parkinson's disease. It was discovered that their drug included the contaminant MPTP. As a consequence, MPTP has been applied systemically in a number of experimental animals, resulting in significant decreases in dopamine content of the brain due to the loss of dopaminergic neurons in the substantia nigra. These animals also developed symptoms similar to those seen in Parkinson's patients. For these reasons, this drug is currently being used for research purposes in order to develop a better understanding of this disease and to establish possible drug therapies for its treatment and eventual cure.

406. The answer is a. *(Nolte, pp 473–485.)* One of the most important features of the anterior lobe of the cerebellum is that it receives major inputs from structures that mediate information concerning muscle spindle and Golgi tendon organ activity (sometimes referred to as *unconscious proprioception*). The pathways that mediate unconscious proprioception include the dorsal and ventral spinocerebellar tracts and the cuneocerebellar tract. Accordingly, the cerebellar anterior lobe is sometimes referred to as the *spinocerebellum*. The fastigial and dentate nuclei receive their principal inputs from the cerebellar cortex, and their axons project out of the cerebellum. The posterior lobe receives few, if any, inputs from pathways that mediate unconscious proprioception information.

407. The answer is c. *(Kandel, pp 833–846. Nolte, pp 480–484.)* A unique feature of the connections between the cerebral cortex and the cerebellum is the somatotopically organized projection from the cerebral cortex largely to the cerebellar hemispheres (some fibers terminate in the vermis). The somatotopic maps are arranged in both anterior and posterior lobes in a manner that has the distal musculature functionally represented in the lateral aspect of the hemispheres, while the proximal musculature is represented toward or in the vermal region. Because of this somatotopic arrangement, the lateral hemispheres are concerned with functions associated with detailed movements of the limbs, while more medial regions are concerned with regulation of the proximal musculature (e.g., postural mechanisms).

408. The answer is d. *(Kandel, pp 835–837.)* The cerebellar glomerulus consists of mossy fiber terminals, Golgi dendrites, axon terminals of Golgi cells, and granule cell dendrites. The flow of information in the glomerulus is as follows: (1) Information reaches the cerebellar cortex through mossy fibers. (2) Axon terminals of mossy fibers terminate upon dendrites of either granule or Golgi cells. (3) Collaterals of parallel fibers (axons of granule cells) may contact dendrites of Golgi cells, whose axons then feed back onto the granule cells. (4) Mossy fiber terminals synapse with Golgi cell dendrites, whose axons then make synaptic contact with the granule cell (feed-forward mechanism). The axons of the granule cells run parallel to the cortex and perpendicular to the orientation of the Purkinje cell dendrites with which they synapse. The circuitry for feedback and feed-forward mechanisms is as follows:

Feedback mechanism:
mossy fiber axon terminal → granule cell dendrites → granule cell axon
    → Golgi cell dendrites → Golgi cell axon → (inhibits) granule cell

Feed-forward mechanism:
mossy fiber axon terminal → Golgi cell dendrites → Golgi cell axon
    → (inhibits) granule cell

409–411. The answers are 409-c, 410-b, 411-a. *(Kandel, pp 833–846.)* For each of these questions, the central point relates to the projection targets of the relevant deep cerebellar nuclei and their relationship to their afferent sources. In question 409, note that the inputs from the frontal lobe eventually reach the cerebellar cortex (which involves the cerebellar hemispheres of the anterior and posterior lobes to a large extent). Because many of these cerebellar afferents terminate in the lateral aspect of the hemisphere, the return (or feedback) pathway will initially involve Purkinje cell axons that synapse with cells in the dentate nucleus. Fibers of the dentate nucleus then supply the VL nucleus of the thalamus, which, in turn, supplies the primary motor cortex. Question 410 concerns the feedback pathways associated with the red nucleus. Inputs to the cerebellum from the red nucleus utilize the inferior olivary nucleus as a relay. These inputs supply the anterior and posterior cerebellar lobes in a topographic manner. Since many of these fibers are distributed to an intermediolateral position within the cerebellar cortex, Purkinje cells from this area supply the interposed (i.e., globose and emboliform) nuclei. The interposed nuclei, in turn, supply the red nucleus via the superior cerebellar peduncle. In question 411, the issue concerns the relationship of the cerebellum to those spinal cord mechanisms relating to descending fibers of the vestibulospinal and reticulospinal systems. Recall that many of the spinocerebellar fibers are distributed to the medial vermal region of the anterior lobe. Thus, the return flow of information to the spinal cord with respect to the regulation of muscle tension will involve the vestibulospinal and reticulospinal systems. To achieve this objective, the Purkinje cells of the medial (vermal and paravermal) regions of the cerebellar cortex project to the fastigial nucleus. The fastigial nucleus, in turn, projects to both the reticular formation and the vestibular nuclei, which then complete the feedback circuit by sending their axons down to the spinal cord.

412. The answer is d. *(Kandel, pp 833–846.)* This experiment was actually carried out many years ago by several investigators. They observed that stimulation of the medial vermal region of the cerebellar cortex could either inhibit or facilitate extensor muscle tone, depending on the precise site of stimulation. It is most likely that stimulation directly affected local populations of Purkinje cells, which then inhibited other local populations of neurons within the fastigial nucleus. Since the fastigial nucleus (as well as the other deep cerebellar nuclei) has excitatory effects upon its target neurons, inhibition or excitation of the fastigial nucleus following local stimulation of the cerebellar cortex would result in either decreased or increased activation of the vestibulospinal system. Thus, such a mechanism could account for the changes of muscle tone that are seen after stimulation of the anterior vermal region of the cortex.

413. The answer is e. *(Nolte, pp 488–492.)* Since the flocculonodular lobe receives and integrates inputs from the vestibular system, it is understandable why lesions that disrupt this integrating mechanism for vestibular inputs would result in difficulties in maintaining balance. Indeed, this is a classic feature of lesions of the flocculonodular lobe but is not associated with lesions in the hemispheres of the posterior lobe, the anterior limb of the internal capsule, or the dentate nucleus, which are functionally linked to the frontal lobe. Lesions of the anterior lobe also do not affect mechanisms of balance.

414–418. The answers are 414-c, 415-d, 416-c, 417-e, 418-b. *(Adams, p 1074. Kandel, pp 861–866, 1306–1309.)* Sam has Parkinson's disease, a degenerative condition caused by progressive loss of dopaminergic cells in the substantia nigra, pars compacta. This is an area that controls the speed and spontaneity of movement, so damage to this area can produce deficits that include a slow, shuffling gait with a tendency to move progressively faster (festinating gait); problems with maintaining size in handwriting, with a tendency to write with small letters (micrographia); masklike facial expression with a paucity of eyeblinks; and difficulty getting out of a chair. Other problems include a soft, monotonous voice; muscle rigidity (lead-pipe rigidity); a tremor at rest that is "pill-rolling"; and a combination of a tremor and rigidity, especially in the arms, which, when flexion is attempted, elicits a "cogwheeling" property. Failure to swallow with a normal frequency makes drooling a problem. Dementia (senility) is also a problem with Parkinson's patients, especially later in the course of the disease. The blood supply to the substantia nigra arises from the posterior circulation, specifically the posteromedial branches of the posterior cerebral artery and branches of the posterior communicating artery. The lenticulostriate branches of the middle cerebral artery supply other portions of the basal ganglia, such as the striatum and the globus pallidus. The anterior choroidal artery also supplies some of the telencephalic nuclei of the basal ganglia. The majority of cells that are lost in this disease are dopaminergic cells in the substantia nigra, pars compacta. Only the pars compacta region of the substantia nigra contains dopaminergic neurons. Medications are currently available to lessen the symptoms of Parkinson's disease. Some of these medications contain various concentrations of L-dopa, an immediate precursor to dopamine. Dopamine itself doesn't cross the blood-brain barrier, so it cannot be directly replaced. Medications that antagonize the breakdown of catecholamines by monoamine oxidase can increase the amount of dopamine available for the remaining cells in the substantia nigra.

419–424. The answers are 419-c, 420-d, 421-b, 422-b, 423-c, 424-e. *(Kandel, pp 833–849, 879–885. Adams, pp 89, 118, 1156–1158.)* An ataxic gait is an unsteady gait. Gaits due to motor weakness or spasticity tend to involve circling of the weak leg (circumduction); festinating or shuffling, which are often due to parkinsonism or disease of the basal ganglia and involve a stooped posture with shuffling of the feet and very small steps. An ataxic gait may result from motor incoordination due to cerebellar disease or from lack of proprioception in the lower extremities due to disease in the posterior column system (gait becomes unsteady when a patient is unable to detect the location of his or her feet). Degeneration of both systems may occur due to alcoholism, although in this case we are told that John does not have any sensory deficits when this modality is tested in isolation. This is an example of alcoholic cerebellar degeneration. It is caused by degeneration (probably through nutritional deficiency) of neurons in the cerebellar cortex, particularly of the Purkinje cells, and is usually restricted to anterior and superior parts of the vermis, as well as anterior portions of the anterior lobes. For this reason, most of the deficits in this syndrome involve midline structures such as the trunk, which are represented most in the vermis (whose major projection is to the fastigial nucleus). Trunk instability usually causes problems with gait. In addition, because the cerebellar homunculus represents the legs in the anterior portion of the anterior lobe, the legs are affected more than the arms. Loss of volume within the vermis of the cerebellum is readily visualized, especially on an MRI of the brain, because this technique allows good visualization of the posterior fossa. If these changes are visualized, then the condition is most likely chronic (as also indicated by the history) and most likely irreversible. However, it is important to make sure that the patient is well nourished, takes vitamins, and stops drinking in order to prevent other neurologic problems from occurring. Damage to other brain regions listed do not cause such effects. The spinocerebellum receives sensory inputs from the spinal cord and is instrumental in controlling posture and movement. It includes the vermis and the intermediate hemisphere. The cerebrocerebellum consists of the lateral hemispheres and is instrumental in the planning of movement. The dentate nucleus comprises the cell bodies that form the superior cerebellar peduncle. The brachium pontis corresponds to the middle cerebellar peduncle. The spinocerebellar cortical (Purkinje) cells project mainly to the fastigial nucleus. Purkinje cells are found in the cerebellar cortex. None of the other choices are cells that are found in the cerebellum.

425–429. The answers are 425-d, 426-a, 427-d, 428-c, 429-e. (*Adams, pp 347, 350. Kandel, pp 887–888, 898–902, 1307–1311.*) The CT scan of Louise's brain revealed a large, acute stroke of her upper pons and midbrain. Strokes of these areas often result from occlusion of the basilar artery and can produce coma or a variant of hypersomnia called *akinetic mutism* or *coma vigil*. An EEG of a patient like this shows a pattern associated with slow-wave sleep, but eye movements are preserved. It is likely that the corticospinal tracts within the pons were damaged during this very large stroke, causing the increased tone from lack of inhibition, as well as the lack of movement in Louise's arms and legs. Infarctions of perforators of the basilar artery, supplying the reticular formation of the pons, may cause coma. These perforators also supply the corticospinal tracts, causing the increased tone and weakness of Louise's legs, so a large stroke may involve both functions. Coma occurs because there is damage to the brainstem tegmentum, which is a major component of the ascending reticular activating system. Although it is not known exactly which area is precisely responsible for consciousness, lesions of this region, as well as projections from the medial regions of the midbrain reticular formation can produce coma. The two main monoaminergic systems of the reticular formation are the noradrenergic and the serotonergic systems, originating in the locus ceruleus and raphe nuclei, respectively. The mesolimbic, mesostriatal, and mesocortical dopaminergic systems are located within the ventrorostral aspect of the brainstem, but not within the reticular formation.

Higher Functions

Questions

DIRECTIONS: Each item below contains a question or incomplete statement followed by suggested responses. Select the **one best** response to each question.

Item 430–431

A 67-year-old man suffers an infarct of the geniculothalamic branch of the posterior cerebral artery. In particular, there is involvement of nuclei of the posterior thalamus.

430. Which of the following would be the most likely effect of such an infarct?

a. Emotional volatility in response to an innocuous statement
b. Short-term memory loss that occurs about one week following the infarct
c. Long-term memory loss that occurs about one month following the infarct
d. Severe pain triggered by cutaneous stimuli applied to the patient
e. Spastic paralysis of the contralateral limbs

431. To which region would the neurons affected by this infarction normally project?

a. Hypothalamus and midbrain
b. Parietal and occipital cortices
c. Precentral and postcentral gyri
d. Basal ganglia and premotor cortex
e. Prefrontal cortex and medial aspect of the frontal lobe

Item 432–434

A 52-year-old woman has an infarct involving a branch of the posterior communicating artery, causing damage to the ventral anterior (VA), ventrolateral (VL), dorsomedial, and anterior thalamic nuclei.

432. Which of the following is the most likely clinical manifestation of this infarct?

a. Hemiparesis and neuropsychological impairment
b. Loss of sleep and apnea
c. Loss of appetite and thermoregulation
d. Total blindness of the contralateral eye
e. Marked endocrine dysfunction

433. What functions are associated with the inputs to the VA nucleus?

a. Somatosensory functions
b. Motor functions
c. Autonomic functions
d. Auditory and taste functions
e. The regulation of sleep

434. Which of the following would be considered a primary output of the VA nucleus?

a. Prefrontal and premotor cortices
b. Precentral and postcentral gyri
c. Posterior parietal lobe
d. Middle temporal gyrus
e. Wernicke's area

Item 435–437

A patient has an infarct involving the medial branches of the basilar root of the posterior cerebral artery. The primary region affected includes nuclei of the medial thalamus.

435. Which of the following effects would likely result from the infarct?

a. Grand mal epilepsy
b. Severe acute depression and hyperphagia
c. Drowsiness and abnormalities in memory and attention
d. Marked somatosensory loss, including pain and temperature
e. UMN paralysis

436. The probable basis for the effects of the infarct is the loss of processing of information from which of the following structures?

a. Hypothalamus
b. Parietal cortex
c. Reticular formation
d. Basal ganglion
e. Hippocampal formation

437. Which of the following structures constitutes the major output of the mediodorsal thalamic nucleus?

a. Precentral gyrus
b. Postcentral gyrus
c. Prefrontal cortex
d. Posterior parietal lobe
e. Temporal lobe

438. Which of the following structures provides the primary input to the superior temporal gyrus?

a. Centromedian thalamic nucleus
b. Medial geniculate thalamic nucleus
c. Lateral geniculate thalamic nucleus
d. Dorsomedial thalamic nucleus
e. Anterior thalamic nucleus
f. VA thalamic nucleus

439. Of the following thalamic nuclei, which nucleus contains neurons that have properties of both specific and nonspecific thalamus?

a. Centromedian thalamic nucleus
b. Medial geniculate thalamic nucleus
c. Lateral geniculate thalamic nucleus
d. Dorsomedial thalamic nucleus
e. Anterior thalamic nucleus
f. VA thalamic nucleus

440. Which one of the following thalamic nuclei makes local connections with other thalamic nuclei and, additionally, projects to the basal ganglia?

a. Centromedian thalamic nucleus
b. Medial geniculate thalamic nucleus
c. Lateral geniculate thalamic nucleus
d. Dorsomedial thalamic nucleus
e. Anterior thalamic nucleus
f. Pulvinar

441. A middle-aged male was having difficulty sleeping and was referred to a sleep clinic. The diagnostician specifically sought to determine whether the patient showed rapid eye movement (REM) sleep on the recorded EEG activity. What kind of activity would the diagnostician look for in order to determine the presence of REM sleep?

a. Slow-wave EEGs
b. Sleep spindles
c. Low-voltage EEGs
d. High-voltage biphasic waves
e. An increase in most skeletal muscle tone

442. An investigator sought to study the neurophysiological properties of neurons that have been shown to regulate REM sleep. Where would he be likely to place his recording electrodes?

a. Spinal cord–medulla border
b. Rostral aspect of the medulla
c. Rostral aspect of the pons
d. Tectal aspect of the rostral midbrain
e. Hypothalamic-thalamic border

443. A study was conducted using a first-year medical student as a subject in order to identify the EEG pattern present during relaxed periods of wakefulness. Assuming that the student was "normal," which of the following EEG rhythms would be likely to be present during this period?

a. α rhythms (8–13 Hz)
b. β rhythms (13–30 Hz)
c. θ rhythms (4–7 Hz)
d. δ rhythms (0.5–4 Hz)
e. Spike and wave activity

444. A patient is confused and displays localized jerks in his right hand, which progress to jerks of the entire arm with a brief loss of consciousness. Which of the following best characterizes this disorder?

a. Generalized seizure
b. Absence seizure
c. Simple partial seizure
d. Complex partial seizure
e. Petit mal epilepsy

445. The display shown by the patient described in question 444 is then followed by his falling to the ground with a further loss of consciousness in which all of his extremities are extended and rigid, and jerks of these limbs are displayed as well. Which of the following best characterizes this disorder?

a. Generalized seizure
b. Absence seizure
c. Simple partial seizure
d. Complex partial seizure
e. Petit mal epilepsy

446. Vasopressin is released from the posterior pituitary. However, it is synthesized elsewhere. In which of the following structures is it synthesized?

a. Mammillary bodies
b. Lateral hypothalamus
c. Supraoptic hypothalamic nucleus
d. Ventromedial hypothalamic nucleus
e. Posterior hypothalamus

447. Which of the following statements concerning temperature regulation is correct?

a. Stimulation of the posterior hypothalamus results in panting, dilation of blood vessels, and suppression of shivering
b. Neurons in the anterior hypothalamus respond to local warming of hypothalamic tissue but not to warming of the skin
c. Stimulation of the anterior hypothalamus may produce constriction of blood vessels and shivering
d. Neurons in the preoptic region and septal area act in concert to intensify increases in body temperature generated by pyrogens
e. Temperature regulation requires the integration of skeletomuscular, endocrine, and autonomic responses

448. The supraoptic nucleus is most closely associated with which of the following structures?

a. Feeding behavior
b. Temperature regulation
c. Sexual behavior
d. Short-term memory functions
e. Water balance

449. Following a routine examination, a tumor was detected mainly in the lateral hypothalamus in a 26-year-old male. Sometime afterward, he began to display a significant change in behavior. Which of the following disorders best characterizes this behavior?

a. Hyperphagia
b. Alcoholism
c. Hypersexuality
d. Aphagia
e. Hypertension

450. A number of investigations have provided strong evidence that the suprachiasmatic nucleus plays an important role in specific functions. Which of the following functions is most closely associated with the suprachiasmatic nucleus?

a. Water intake
b. Food intake
c. Hypertension
d. Circadian rhythms
e. Short-term memory

451. A 49-year-old male showed changes in emotional behavior over the past few months. Several characteristics of his behavior included heightened sexuality, a very placid appearance, and making physical contact with almost anything that he could touch. The neurologist's diagnosis was that the patient was exhibiting a Klüver-Bucy syndrome. An MRI was given to the patient and a small vascular lesion was detected. Which of the following structures is most likely to contain the lesion?

a. Septal area
b. Amygdala
c. Cingulate gyrus
d. Medial hypothalamus
e. Lateral hypothalamus

452. Which of the following best reflects an anatomical or functional property of the central nucleus of amygdala?

a. Projects its axons to the medial hypothalamus via the stria terminalis
b. Is a major receiving area for information concerning tertiary auditory and visual signals
c. Has high concentrations of enkephalins, somatostatin, and dopamine
d. Is a primary location of norepinephrine-containing cell bodies in the forebrain
e. Projects axons that directly inhibit spinal motor neurons

453. Which of the following best characterizes a major hypothesis underlying neurochemical and related theories of schizophrenia?

a. Basically caused by environmental factors rather than genetic ones
b. Linked to increases in brain dopamine levels
c. Linked to increases in brain serotonin levels
d. Linked to decreases in brain endorphin levels
e. Linked to decreases in brain neuropeptide levels

454. While the hippocampal formation has few if any direct (monosynaptic) connections with the lateral hypothalamus, it is known to modulate functions associated with the hypothalamus. Which of the following structures forms the underlying anatomical synaptic relay subserving regulation of the hypothalamus by the hippocampal formation?

a. Cingulate gyrus
b. Habenular nucleus
c. Mediodorsal thalamic nucleus
d. Septal area
e. Bed nucleus of the stria terminalis

455. Which of the following constitutes the Papez circuit?

a. Hippocampal formation → mammillary bodies → anterior thalamic nucleus → prefrontal cortex → hippocampal formation
b. Hippocampal formation → septal area → hypothalamus → hippocampal formation
c. Hippocampal formation → mammillary bodies → anterior thalamic nucleus → cingulate gyrus → hippocampal formation
d. Amygdala → hippocampal formation → mammillary bodies → amygdala
e. Prefrontal cortex → hippocampal formation → septal area → medial hypothalamus → prefrontal cortex

Questions 456–457

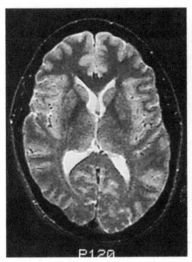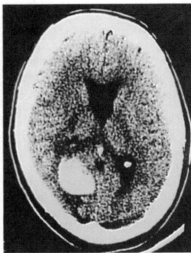

456. The T2-weighted MRI scan on the left side of the figure is of a normal patient. In the CT scan on the right side, the patient sustained a right cerebral hemorrhage, indicated by the large white area. Which of the following deficits most likely resulted from the cerebrovascular accident?

a. Right homonymous hemianopsia
b. Left homonymous hemianopsia
c. Loss of intellectual and emotional processes
d. Aphasia
e. Hemiparesis of the right side of the body

457. Based on the figure, which of the following blood vessels was affected by the cerebrovascular accident?

a. Anterior cerebral artery
b. Middle cerebral artery
c. Posterior cerebral artery
d. Superior cerebellar artery
e. Striate arteries

Questions 458–459

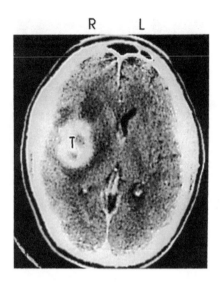

R   L

458. The CT scan shown here reveals that the patient has a glioma (T) on the right side of the brain. Which of the following has the patient likely sustained?

a. A UMN paralysis of the left side
b. Dyskinesia
c. Intention tremor
d. Upper left quadrantanopia
e. Upper right quadrantanopia

459. Which of the following structures was most likely damaged by the tumor?

a. Lentiform nucleus only
b. Internal capsule only
c. Thalamus only
d. Lentiform nucleus and internal capsule
e. Lentiform nucleus, internal capsule, and thalamus

Questions 460–461

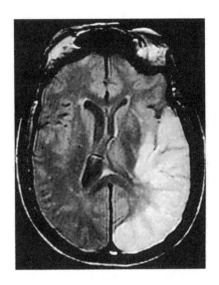

460. The patient whose CT scan is shown in the figure sustained an occlusion of a major artery on the left side of the brain. Which of the following deficits was most likely to be present in this patient?

a. A right homonymous hemianopsia only
b. Aphasia only
c. A right homonymous hemianopsia coupled with aphasia
d. Marked intellectual deficits
e. Marked intellectual deficits coupled with hemiballism

461. Which of the following blood vessels in this figure was occluded?

a. Anterior cerebral artery
b. Middle cerebral artery
c. Posterior cerebral artery
d. Posterior choroidal artery
e. Superior cerebellar artery

Questions 462–463

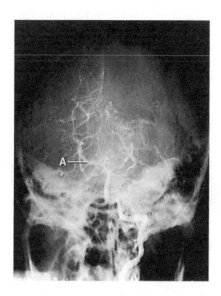

462. The vertebral angiogram in the figure reveals the effects of a severe motorcycle accident upon a 21-year-old woman. As a result of the accident, from which of the following does she most likely suffer?

a. A UMN paralysis of the right side of the body
b. A right homonymous hemianopsia
c. A left upper quadrantanopia
d. Aphasia
e. Dyskinesia

463. Which of the following arteries was occluded on the left side and labeled in the figure on the normal side as **A?**

a. Vertebral
b. Basilar
c. Middle cerebral
d. Anterior cerebral
e. Posterior cerebral

464. The MRI scan in the following figure reveals a large chromophobe adenoma (T) of the pituitary that impinges on the adjoining brain tissue. Which of the following dysfunctions resulted from this tumor?

a. Binasal hemianopsia
b. Bitemporal hemianopsia
c. Loss of the accommodation reflex
d. Loss of the pupillary light reflex
e. Loss of conjugate gaze

Item 465–470

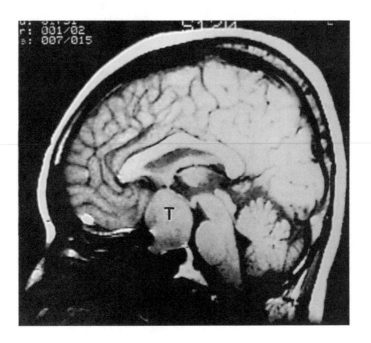

June is a 65-year-old woman who was previously healthy. One day, while taking a walk in the park, she noticed her right fingers twitching, then her right hand, then her arm and shoulder, followed by a march of twitches down her leg. She did not remember any more than this, because she lost consciousness. An onlooker saw her drop to the ground and deviate her neck backward, while making a high-pitched noise. Then both of her arms and legs began to jerk for approximately 1 to 2 minutes, stopping abruptly. She had lost control of her bladder during this event. When the onlooker attempted to speak to June to ask her if she was okay, she was unresponsive. The onlooker called an ambulance, which brought June to the nearest hospital. A doctor met June at the emergency room entrance and asked her what had happened. By this time, June was slightly drowsy, but able to answer questions appropriately. Her speech was fluent and grammatically correct. She knew the month, but not the day of the week or where she was. She moved the left side of her body better than her right, but had too much difficulty following commands for an effective motor examination. The remainder of her examination was normal. The doctor ordered a CT of June's head and drew some blood.

465. From which area of the brain did June's seizure begin?

a. Left precentral gyrus
b. Right precentral gyrus
c. Right temporal lobe
d. Left temporal lobe
e. Thalamus

466. What could account for June's loss of consciousness following the seizure?

a. Involvement of the reticular activating system
b. Head trauma
c. Bilateral postictal suppression
d. Thalamic involvement
e. Brain hemorrhage from the seizure

467. Which of the following could explain the march of twitching that June experienced?

a. Proximity of the body part to the spinal cord
b. Proximity of the body part to the cerebral cortex
c. Somatotopic representation within the brainstem
d. Somatotopic representation within the basal ganglia
e. Somatotopic representation within the precentral gyrus

468. Which cell type is the predominant cause of the seizure?

a. Basket cell
b. Purkinje cell
c. Stellate cell
d. Schwann cell
e. Pyramidal cell

469. A burst of what type of potentials may initiate an epileptic seizure?

a. Inhibitory postsynaptic potentials (IPSPs)
b. Membrane potentials
c. Resting potentials
d. Excitatory postsynaptic potentials (EPSPs)
e. Nernst potential

470. Which of the following chemical mechanisms could underlie seizure generation?

a. Na^+ channel blockade
b. γ-aminobutyric acid (GABA) inhibition
c. Glutamate inhibition
d. Aspartate inhibition
e. Substance P inhibition

Item 471–475

Helen is a 76-year-old woman who has had high blood pressure and diabetes for more than 10 years. One day, as she was reaching for a jar of flour to make an apple pie, her right side suddenly gave out, and she collapsed. While trying to get up from the floor, she noticed that she was unable to move her right arm or leg. Helen attempted to cry for help because she was unable to reach the telephone; however, her speech was slurred and rather unintelligible. She lay on the floor and waited for help to arrive. Helen's son began to worry about his usually prompt mother when she didn't arrive with her apple pie. After several attempts to telephone her apartment without getting an answer, he drove there and found her lying on the floor. She attempted to tell him what had happened, but her speech was too slurred to comprehend. Assuming that his mother had had a stroke, the son called an ambulance to take her to the nearest emergency room. A neurology resident was called to see Helen in the emergency room because the physicians there likewise thought that she had had a stroke.

The resident noted that Helen followed commands very well, and, although her speech was very slurred, it was fluent and grammatically correct. The lower two-thirds of her face drooped on the right, but when she was asked to raise her eyebrows, her forehead appeared symmetric. Her tongue pointed to the right side when she was asked to protrude it. Her right arm and leg were severely, but equally, weak; her left side had normal strength. She felt a pin and a vibrating tuning fork equally on both sides.

471. Where in the CNS did Helen's stroke occur?

a. Left precentral gyrus
b. Right precentral gyrus
c. Left basilar pons or left internal capsule
d. Right putamen or globus pallidus
e. Left thalamus

472. A CT scan revealed a new infarct in the left internal capsule. Which artery was occluded, causing the stroke?

a. Lenticulostriate branches of the middle cerebral artery
b. Posterior cerebral artery
c. Anterior cerebral artery
d. Vertebral artery
e. Posterior choroidal artery

473. Damage to which two tracts caused Helen to be weak on her right side?

a. Spinothalamic and corticospinal tracts
b. Spinothalamic and corticobulbar tracts
c. Corticospinal and corticobulbar tracts
d. Corticospinal and spinocerebellar tracts
e. Corticospinal and rubrospinal tracts

474. Which of the following could explain why Helen's forehead was spared from weakness?

a. The forehead is innervated by different fibers originating in the postcentral gyrus
b. There are two cranial nerves innervating the forehead
c. The forehead is represented bilaterally at the cortical level
d. The forehead is stronger than the rest of the face
e. Thalamic regions receiving inputs from the forehead contain few inhibitory neurons

475. How can Helen's speech deficit be classified?

a. Wernicke's aphasia
b. Broca's aphasia
c. Anomia
d. Dysarthria
e. Conduction aphasia

Item 476–480

Lindsey is a 12-year-old girl who has never had medical problems. One day, while in the kitchen with her mother, she told her mother that she felt very frightened all of a sudden and had a funny feeling in her stomach. Immediately after this, she turned her head to the right, stared persistently, and began to chew. Her mother called her name several times, but Lindsey, who was usually a very obedient child, did not answer. After approximately 1 minute of staring, Lindsey slowly turned her head back to her mother. Apparently confused, she asked her mother where she was. Over the next 10 to 15 minutes, she became less and less confused, and by the time she was in the car being driven to the pediatrician by her mother, she felt like she was back to normal. The pediatrician listened to Lindsey's mother's story when they arrived. He examined Lindsey and could find no abnormalities on general physical examination or on neurologic examination. The pediatrician told her mother that he would refer Lindsey to a pediatric neurologist for further evaluation, as well as further evaluation of the need for medication.

476. What type of problem did Lindsey most likely have?

a. Attention deficit disorder (ADD)
b. Temporary psychosis
c. Conversion disorder
d. Epilepsy
e. Schizophrenia

477. From which area of the brain is this problem most likely emanating?

a. Medulla
b. Occipital lobe
c. Temporal lobe
d. Thalamus
e. Midbrain

478. If the amygdala is involved with this problem, which two major efferent pathways from this structure may be affected?
a. Corticospinal tract and stria terminalis
b. Mammillothalamic tract and stria terminalis
c. Medial forebrain bundle and stria terminalis
d. Ventral amygdalofugal pathway and stria terminalis
e. Corticospinal tract and mammillothalamic tract

479. If the hippocampal formation is involved in this problem, which structures may be damaged?
a. Hippocampus, dentate gyrus, and subiculum
b. Hippocampus, amygdala, and subiculum
c. Hippocampus, fornix, and amygdala
d. Hippocampus, fornix, and habenulae
e. Hippocampus, dentate gyrus, and fornix

480. If Lindsey's problem continues with a high frequency, what ongoing problem may she eventually develop?
a. Hemiparesis
b. Diminished memory function
c. Diminished sensation
d. Improved attention
e. Dyslexia

Item 481–485

Jane is a 75-year-old woman who has taken medication for high blood pressure and high cholesterol for the past 10 years. One morning, upon awakening, she attempted to get up from her bed, only to find that she had difficulty walking, but didn't know why. When she tried to walk, her left leg collapsed beneath her. Jane couldn't understand why she was having so much difficulty walking, because she felt fine. Thinking that perhaps something was wrong, she edged her way across the floor to her telephone and called for an ambulance. Jane hadn't noticed until now that her speech was slightly slurred. She was taken to the nearest emergency room for an evaluation. Upon arriving in the emergency room, the staff, noting that her face drooped on the left and that she persistently looked to her right side, called a neurologist to see Jane. The neurologist tested Jane's language functions by asking her to name objects, repeat sentences, and write sentences, and thought that all of these tests were normal. Her speech was mildly slurred, and she had a right gaze preference. She would not cross the midline with her eyes when asked to look to the left, but instead, immediately returned her eyes to their right-sided gaze. When asked to raise her left hand, she raised her right hand. The neurologist asked Jane if her left hand belonged to her and she replied, "No, it's yours." When asked to fill in the numbers of a clock, Jane put numbers 1 through 12 on the right side of the clock. When asked to bisect a line, she placed the perpendicular line on the right side. She did not blink to hand waving in the temporal visual field of her left eye and the nasal visual field of her right eye. Other cranial nerves were normal, except for a left facial droop that spared the forehead. Her left arm and leg were markedly weak, and the muscle tone was flaccid (floppy). All reflexes were depressed on the left side and normal on the right. The neurologist thought that all sensory modalities were depressed on the left side. The neurologist ordered a CT scan of Jane's head and admitted her to the hospital for further workup and treatment.

481. What kind of neurologic deficits does Jane have?

a. Left hemiparesis, hemineglect, left homonymous hemianopsia, left hemisensory loss
b. Left hemiparesis, right superior quadrantanopsia
c. Left hemiparesis, left hemisensory loss, hemineglect, left superior quadrantanopsia
d. Left hemisensory loss, hemineglect, bitemporal hemianopsia
e. Left hemisensory loss, hemineglect, left superior quadrantanopsia

482. Where in the nervous system has the damage occurred?

a. Left temporal and parietal lobes
b. Right frontal and temporal lobe
c. Right frontal and parietal lobes
d. Left frontal and parietal lobes
e. Left occipital lobe

483. If this damage was caused by a stroke, which artery became occluded?

a. Right anterior cerebral artery
b. Left anterior cerebral artery
c. Right posterior cerebral artery
d. Right middle cerebral artery
e. Left middle cerebral artery

484. Damage to which fibers caused Jane's inability to blink in response to the hand waving in her left temporal visual field?

a. Left facial nerve
b. Right oculomotor nerve
c. Left optic nerve
d. Optic chiasm
e. Right optic radiations

485. Damage to which specific area caused Jane's inability to notice the left side of her body?

a. Left anterior frontal cortex
b. Right anterior frontal cortex
c. Right posterior frontal cortex
d. Right posterior parietal cortex
e. Right anterior parietal cortex

Item 486–490

Morris is a 79-year-old man who was brought to the emergency room because his family was worried that he suddenly was not using his right arm and leg and seemed to have a simultaneous behavior change. He was unable to write a reminder note to himself, even with his left hand, and he put his shoes on the wrong feet. A neurologist was called to the ER to examine the patient. A loud bruit was heard with a stethoscope over the left carotid artery in his neck. When asked to show the neurologist his left hand, he pointed to his right hand, since it could not move. The neurologist asked him to add numbers, and he was unable to do this, despite having spent his life as a bookkeeper. Morris was unable to name the fingers on either hand, and he could not form any semblance of a letter using his left hand. Morris's eyes did not blink when the neurologist waved his hands close to them in the left temporal and right nasal visual fields. The right lower two-thirds of his face drooped. There was some asymmetry of his reflexes between the right and left sides, and there was a positive Babinski response of his right toe.

486. Where in the CNS is the damage?

a. Right frontal and parietal lobes
b. Left frontal and parietal lobes
c. Right frontal lobe
d. Left frontal lobe
e. Right temporal lobe

487. Assuming that Morris had a stroke, which artery has become occluded?

a. Left anterior cerebral
b. Right anterior cerebral
c. Right middle cerebral
d. Left middle cerebral
e. Left posterior cerebral

488. Damage to which area of the brain caused Morris's inability to move his right side?

a. Right precentral gyrus
b. Left precentral gyrus
c. Right angular gyrus
d. Left angular gyrus
e. Left supramarginal gyrus

489. Damage to which region caused Morris's inability to tell right from left and his inability to write, even with his nondominant hand?

a. Left parietal
b. Left frontal
c. Right frontal
d. Left temporal
e. Right temporal

490. Damage to which structure caused the visual defect?

a. Right optic nerve
b. Left optic nerve
c. Optic chiasm
d. Right optic radiations
e. Left optic radiations

Item 491–494

Bob is a 75-year-old male college graduate who was brought to a neurologist by his family because he was having problems with his gait, suffered from urinary incontinence for the past six months, and recently began to have problems with his short-term memory and paying his bills. The gait problem manifested itself mainly as difficulty climbing stairs and frequent falls. Bob had no past medical history other than a subarachnoid hemorrhage resulting from a ruptured cerebral aneurysm many years earlier. When the neurologist examined Bob, she found that he could not remember three objects five minutes after they were shown to him, even when he was prompted. He was unable to figure out how many quarters were in $1.75, and he spelled the word *world* incorrectly. A grasp reflex (squeezing the examiner's hand as a reflex reaction to stroking of the palm) was present. Although his motor strength was full in all of his extremities, when asked to walk, he took many steps in the same place without moving forward, then started to fall. His cranial nerve, sensory, and cerebellar examinations were normal.

491. Bob has a grasp reflex and dementia. A lesion in which of the following regions can cause this deficit?

a. Occipital lobe
b. Frontal lobe
c. Medulla
d. Thalamus
e. Pons

492. You are asked to evaluate Bob with the neurologist. The nurse in the office asks if you would like to order a CT scan, and you request one. The CT scan shows that all the ventricles are dilated, especially the frontal horns of the lateral ventricles, without any evidence of obstruction by a tumor. What would be a possible mechanism underlying the enlargement of the ventricles?

a. Decreased CSF absorption
b. Low blood pressure
c. Decreased CNS blood flow
d. Decreased intracranial pressure
e. High blood pressure

493. If there is diminished CSF absorption, where does the blockage occur?

a. Pyramidal cells
b. Renshaw cells
c. Arachnoid villi
d. Purkinje cells
e. Sagittal sinus

494. Where would the greatest damage be done by the expanding ventricles?

a. Thalamus
b. Brainstem
c. Pituitary gland
d. Parietal cortex
e. Deep frontal white matter (corona radiata)

Item 495–499

Joe is a 75-year-old man who is right-handed and was told in the past by his internist that he had an irregular heartbeat. Unfortunately, Joe decided that he didn't wish to learn anything further about this condition, so he didn't return to this physician, and it remained untreated. One morning, he awoke to find that his face drooped on the right side and that he couldn't move his right arm or right leg. When he tried to call an ambulance for help, he had a great deal of difficulty communicating with the operator because his speech was slurred, nonfluent, and missing some pronouns. The call was traced by the police; an ambulance arrived at his house and took him to an emergency room. A neurologist was called to see Joe in the emergency room. When he listened to Joe's heart, he detected an irregular heartbeat. It was very difficult to understand Joe's speech because it was halting, with a tendency to repeat the same phrases over and over. He had a great deal of difficulty repeating specific sentences given to him by the neurologist, but he was able to follow simple commands such as "Touch your right ear with your left hand." His mouth drooped on the right when he attempted to smile, but his forehead remained symmetric when he wrinkled it. He couldn't move his right arm at all, but he was able to wiggle his right leg a little bit.

495. What kind of language problem does Joe have?

a. Dysarthria
b. Wernicke's aphasia
c. Broca's aphasia
d. Alexia
e. Pure word deafness

496. Which area of the brain was damaged?

a. Internal capsule and thalamus
b. Right occipital lobe
c. Pontine reticular formation
d. Corpus callosum
e. Left precentral gyrus and Broca's area

497. Which artery was blocked when the event occurred?

a. Anterior cerebral artery
b. Posterior cerebral artery
c. Anterior inferior cerebellar artery
d. Middle cerebral artery
e. Basilar artery

498. Which structure best relates to Joe's facial weakness?

a. Peripheral nerve VII
b. Central nerve VII
c. Nerve XII
d. Nerve V
e. Oculomotor nerve weakness

499. With which hand does Joe most likely write?

a. Right
b. Left
c. Ambidextrous (both)
d. Cannot be determined

500. A 68-year-old man went to a sleep clinic after he had repeated episodes of loud snoring during sleep, coupled with sudden periods of restlessness and cessation of breathing. After extensive analysis, the physicians concluded that the patient's problem was not a result of obstructive sleep. Instead, it was judged that this condition reflected central sleep apnea due to loss of chemoreceptor sensitivity of the neuronal control mechanisms governing respiration. Which of the following sites within the CNS is most closely associated with these effects?

a. Dorsal horn of the thoracic spinal cord
b. Reticular formation of the medulla
c. Midbrain periaqueductal gray
d. Hippocampal formation
e. Border of occipital and parietal lobes

Higher Functions

Answers

430–431. The answers are 430-d, 431-b. *(Afifi, pp 235–252, 266–271. Simon et al., p 203.)* The infarct caused damage to posterior thalamic nuclei. When these structures are damaged, a disorder referred to as *thalamic pain* can ensue. In this condition, light cutaneous stimulation is sufficient to produce severe pain. The projections from nuclei situated in this region project principally to the parietal and occipital lobes and play a role in the regulation of pain (although the precise mechanisms remain unknown). The other processes offered as alternate choices have not been shown to be related to functions of the posterior thalamus.

432–434. The answers are 432-a, 433-b, 434-a. *(Afifi, pp 235–252, 266–271.)* Damage to the VA, VL, dorsomedial, and anterior thalamic nuclei would most likely result in motor impairment such as a hemiparesis (because of the connections of these nuclei with the motor and premotor cortices). Damage to the dorsomedial nucleus could also be linked with neuropsychological impairment because of its connections with the prefrontal cortex and adjoining regions of the frontal lobe. The other processes mentioned in question 432 have not been shown to be related to these groups of nuclei. As noted earlier, the VA nucleus is associated with motor functions, not only in its projections to motor regions of the cerebral cortex—the premotor and prefrontal cortices—but also in the inputs that it receives from structures associated with motor functions such as the globus pallidus and substantia nigra.

435–437. The answers are 435-c, 436-c, 437-c. *(Afifi, pp 235–252, 266–271.)* An infarct that affects the medial thalamus, which includes the dorsomedial nucleus and midline thalamic and intralaminar nuclei, can result in abnormalities in memory, attention, and drowsiness. The other choices offered for question 435 have not been shown to be related to functions associated with medial thalamic structures. A key input into the medial thalamus is the reticular formation. In this manner, the medial and intralaminar thalamus represent a relay from reticular formation to the cerebral cortex. Since a major function of the reticular function is to regulate states of sleep and wakefulness, these thalamic nuclei thus contribute to these states. When these nuclei are damaged, this mechanism is affected, resulting in drowsiness. Because of the connections of the medial thalamus with much of the frontal lobe, including the prefrontal cortex, damage to the medial thalamus would also affect the functions of these cortical regions, which involve memory and other cognitive processes.

438. The answer is b. *(Afifi, p 250.)* The superior temporal gyrus is the primary auditory receiving area in the cerebral cortex. Accordingly, the primary afferent source to this region arises from the medial geniculate nucleus, which constitutes a specific thalamic relay for processing of auditory information.

439. The answer is f. *(Afifi, pp 242–245, 249–251. Kandel, pp 341–345.)* The term "*specific*" *thalamic nuclei* refers to those nuclei of the thalamus that project to specific regions of the cerebral cortex. The term "*nonspecific*" *thalamic nuclei* refers to those thalamic nuclei that have widespread projections to large areas of the cerebral cortex. The VA nucleus has properties of both the specific and the nonspecific thalamus. This means that, on the one hand, the VA nucleus receives motor inputs from the basal ganglia, including the substantia nigra, and projects its axons to an important motor region of the brain—the premotor cortex. In this context, the VA nucleus functions as a relay nucleus for the transmission of information associated with motor functions. On the other hand, the VA nucleus also receives various inputs from other thalamic nuclei (such as the centromedian nucleus) and projects its axons in a widespread manner to other parts of the frontal lobe, including the prefrontal cortex. In this context, the VA nucleus can modulate a wide variety of neurons in the cerebral cortex, both directly and indirectly, which is characteristic of nonspecific thalamic nuclei.

440. The answer is a. *(Afifi, pp 242–245, 249–251. Kandel, pp 341–345.)* The centromedian nucleus is a classical nonspecific thalamic nucleus. It can modulate cortical activity by making local connections with specific thalamic nuclei and therefore modify the specific thalamic inputs to different regions of the cerebral cortex. In addition, the centromedian nucleus also projects to the putamen. This projection is sometimes referred to as the *thalamostriatal projection*. Since the centromedian nucleus receives considerable inputs from the cerebral cortex, this connection to the putamen provides a basis by which the cerebral cortex can influence the basal ganglia in addition to its direct projections to the neostriatum.

441. The answer is c. *(Kandel, pp 937–940.)* REM sleep is characterized by a low-voltage EEG pattern typical of an alert person. For this reason, REM sleep is sometimes referred to as *paradoxical sleep*. Other EEG patterns, such as slow waves, high-voltage EEGs, and sleep spindles, occur at other stages of sleep. In addition, REM sleep is characterized by a general loss of skeletal muscle tone, with the exception of the eye muscles, which govern the REMs.

442. The answer is c. *(Kandel, pp 940–943.)* Animal research studies have indicated that the region of the rostral pons bordering on the caudal midbrain contains special sets of cholinergic neurons that are maximally active during REM sleep (and during wakefulness, as well). These neurons are located in the reticular formation. One group of neurons has been identified as the nucleus reticularis pontis oralis. Other neurons include the region of the pedunculopontine nucleus. It appears that these cholinergic neurons depolarize GABAergic neurons, which prevent rhythmic firing of reticular formation neurons. This latter effect allows for the asynchronous firing of thalamocortical neurons that take place during periods of wakefulness and REM sleep.

443. The answer is a. *(Kandel, pp 916–917.)* During states of quiet wakefulness or drowsiness, the EEG pattern becomes slower (8 to 13 Hz; average amplitude of 50 V) than what is seen during an alert state. This pattern is called an α wave.

444. The answer is d. *(Kandel, pp 910–918. Simon, pp 47, 258.)* This person displays a complex partial seizure, which is characterized by a confusional state with brief losses of consciousness. It is called a partial seizure because the seizure involves a localized region, reflected by jerks of the muscles of a specific part of the body. The focus of this seizure is typically in the temporal lobe, such as the amygdala, hippocampal formation, or adjoining cortical regions. A simple partial seizure does not involve loss of consciousness. Absence seizures are nonconvulsive seizures and are also called *petit mal epilepsy*. Generalized seizures typically involve all of the limbs. The patient falls to the ground and loses consciousness.

445. The answer is a. *(Kandel, pp 910–918. Simon, pp 47, 258.)* The seizure described in this patient has progressed from a complex partial seizure to a generalized seizure. As indicated previously, this type of seizure involves all of the limbs. The patient falls to the ground and typically loses consciousness. As stated in the answer to question 444, the other choices involve seizures that are characterized differently than what was described in the progression of this case.

446. The answer is c. *(Kandel, p 979.)* Certain magnocellular neurons of the hypothalamus synthesize the hormones vasopressin and oxytocin. These include the paraventricular and supraoptic nuclei. The cell bodies of the magnocellular neurons that produce vasopressin are found mostly within the supraoptic nucleus. Vasopressin is important because it makes the membranes of the convoluted tubules and collecting ducts of the kidneys more permeable to water. This results in water conservation.

447. The answer is e. *(Kandel, pp 1000–1002.)* The process of temperature regulation requires the integration of autonomic, skeletomuscular, and endocrine responses. For example, dilation of blood vessels of the skin (an autonomic response) facilitates heat loss, while constriction of these vessels helps to conserve heat. Panting and shivering (skeletomuscular responses) aid in the processes of heat loss and conservation (heat generation), respectively. Finally, when an organism is exposed to cold for long periods of time, there is an increase in thyroxine release from the anterior pituitary gland, which helps to increase body temperature by increasing metabolism. The classic interpretation of the role of the hypothalamus in temperature regulation has been that the anterior hypothalamus constitutes a heat loss center, while the posterior hypothalamus is a heat conservation center. Although such a generalization is somewhat oversimplified, the general phenomenon has been demonstrated. For example, stimulation of the anterior hypothalamus has been shown to dilate blood vessels and inhibit shivering, and lesions of this region produce hypothermia. Stimulation of the posterior hypothalamus produces heat conservation by constricting blood vessels and causing shivering. Neurons in this region respond to both local warming of hypothalamic tissue as well as warming of the skin. Neurons in both the septal and the preoptic regions constitute antipyretic areas, in that they respond to increases in fever by limiting the magnitude of the fever. Activation of these antipyretic regions is thought to occur through a mechanism utilizing the peptide vasopressin. The precise mechanism by which these regions become activated remains unknown.

448. The answer is e. *(Kandel, p 979.)* The supraoptic nucleus, like the paraventricular nucleus, contains magnocellular neurons that synthesize vasopressin and oxytocin and transport these hormones down their axons to the posterior pituitary. For this reason, the supraoptic nucleus plays a significant role in the regulation of water balance. There is no evidence to support the notion that the supraoptic nucleus has a role in feeding behavior, temperature regulation, sexual behavior, or short-term memory functions.

449. The answer is d. *(Kandel, pp 1002–1003.)* Lesions of the lateral hypothalamus are likely to produce aphagia. Feeding behavior is elicited by stimulation of the lateral hypothalamus. Neurons in this region respond to the sight or taste of food. Since drinking is also associated with lateral hypothalamic functions, a lesion of this structure would also disrupt this behavior. Lesions of the lateral hypothalamus do not produce either hypertension or sexual behaviors. The neurons regulating these functions are elsewhere within the hypothalamus.

450. The answer is d. *(Kandel, pp 45, 322, 937, 946.)* Recent studies have demonstrated that the suprachiasmatic nucleus controls the biologic clock of internal circadian rhythms. During the light phase of the light-dark cycle, metabolic activity (measured by ^{14}C-2-deoxyglucose autoradiography) within the suprachiasmatic nucleus is significantly increased. In contrast, during the dark phase, there is very little metabolic activity.

451. The answer is b. *(Kandel, p 988.)* In this syndrome, produced experimentally in monkeys and also seen in cats, there is an extreme change in the personality of the animal. Its responses to emotion-laden stimuli are much reduced. It appears very tame. Aggressive tendencies are not evident. It also manifests oral tendencies and displays hypersexuality. This syndrome is the result of lesions of the temporal lobe in which parts of the amygdala are involved. Lesions of other regions such as the hypothalamus, cingulate cortex, or septal area do not produce the Klüver-Bucy syndrome.

452. The answer is c. *(Cooper, pp 275–276, 295; Nolte, pp 556–561.)* One of the most interesting discoveries concerning the amygdala made in recent years is that the central nucleus contains high concentrations of a number of peptides. These include enkephalins and somatostatin, in particular. This region also receives large numbers of dopaminergic axon terminals. The central nucleus does not project its axons to the medial hypothalamus. It does not receive auditory or visual signals, nor does it project to the spinal cord, where it could inhibit spinal motor neurons. It receives norepinephrine-containing fibers from the brainstem rather than being a source of this neurotransmitter.

453. The answer is b. (*Kandel, pp 1200–1204.*) There have been a variety of neurochemical and related theories of schizophrenia that have evolved over the past three decades. Unfortunately, each of these theories has had its limitations. Nevertheless, one of the more popular theories has been that schizophrenia is linked to increased levels of brain dopamine. The hypothesis suggests that schizophrenia results from overstimulation of the brain by the dopaminergic system. Support for this view comes from the observation that antipsychotic agents are known to block dopamine receptors. Co-twin behavioral and developmental studies have shown that, while environmental factors are certainly important in the ontogeny of schizophrenia, genetic factors are also quite significant in the development of this disease. Other researchers have suggested that schizophrenia may bear some relationship to decreased levels of serotonin in the brain, as evidenced by the hallucinogenic effects of LSD, which binds to serotonin receptors. Other investigations have shown that opioid peptide blockade by naloxone is effective in reducing hallucinations, which suggests that increased levels of endorphins may be linked to this disorder. Investigations involving neuropeptides have indicated that neuropeptides such as cholecystokinin (CCK) is colocalized with dopamine in brain neurons. In this fashion, CCK may function as a neuromodulator for dopamine, in which case increased levels of CCK may be linked with schizophrenia in the same fashion as are increased levels of dopamine.

454. The answer is d. (*Nolte, pp 548–560.*) A major target of efferent fibers from the hippocampal formation is the septal area. Fibers located in the precommissural fornix supply the septal area in an extensive and topographical manner. In turn, the septal area projects significant numbers of fibers to the lateral (and medial) regions of the hypothalamus. In this manner, the septal area serves as a relay for the transmission of signals from the hippocampal formation to the hypothalamus. The hippocampal formation does not project to the habenular nuclei, mediodorsal nucleus, or the bed nucleus of the stria terminalis. Moreover, the cingulate gyrus does not project directly to the hypothalamus.

455. The answer is c. (*Kandel, pp 987–988. Nolte, p 554.*) For many years, it was believed that a neural circuit composed of the hippocampal formation → mammillary bodies → anterior thalamic nucleus → cingulate gyrus → hippocampal formation played a major role in the regulation of emotional behavior. More recent studies by a number of investigators have revealed that neither the mammillary bodies nor the anterior thalamic nucleus appears to contribute to the regulation of emotional behavior. Instead, it is believed that this circuit may subserve functions more closely related to short-term memory.

456. The answer is b. *(Kandel, pp 544, 1306–1309. Nolte, pp 418–424.)* The cerebrovascular accident produced damage of the right primary visual cortex. Therefore, this would result in a homonymous hemianopsia of the left visual fields. Since the damage was confined to the occipital lobe, there would be little effect upon other processes such as speech, motor functions, or intellectual activities.

457. The answer is c. *(Kandel, pp 544, 1306–1309. Nolte, pp 120–133.)* The occipital lobe is supplied by the posterior cerebral artery. The calcarine cortex (primary visual cortex) is supplied by a branch of this artery, the calcarine artery. The anterior cerebral artery supplies the medial aspect of the frontal lobe and the anterior-medial aspect of the parietal lobe. The middle cerebral artery supplies the lateral aspect of the frontal and parietal lobes. The superior cerebellar artery supplies the dorsolateral aspect of a portion of the pons and the cerebellum. The striate arteries arise from the anterior and middle cerebral arteries and supply portions of the internal capsule and neostriatum.

458. The answer is a. *(Kandel, pp 854–857. Nolte, pp 390–393, 451–467.)* The tumor is situated in the lentiform nucleus and internal capsule. Therefore, corticospinal fibers will be affected, causing a UMN paralysis of the left side. Dyskinesia would not be seen because any effects normally seen in association with damage to the basal ganglia would be masked by the effects of the damage to the internal capsule. Since the cerebellum was not involved, there would be no intention tremor. Neither would there be any visual deficits from this glioma since optic nerve fibers are not involved.

459. The answer is d. *(Kandel, pp 854–857. Nolte, pp 390–393, 451–467.)* As noted in the preceding answer, the tumor involves the lentiform nucleus of the basal ganglia and the internal capsule as well. At the stage when the CT scan was taken, the tumor had not involved the thalamus.

460. The answer is c. (*Nolte, pp 418–423, 515–529.*) The arterial occlusion involves both the temporal and the occipital regions of the cortex. Therefore, it would affect Wernicke's area as well as primary visual areas of the occipital lobe. The patient would most likely present with receptive aphasia as well as a right homonymous hemianopsia. The lesion would not likely produce marked intellectual deficits, since the prefrontal cortex was spared; nor would it produce hemiballism, since there was no damage to the subthalamic nucleus.

461. The answer is b. (*Kandel, pp 1305–1309. Nolte, pp 120–128.*) Although the tissue affected involves parietal, temporal, and occipital lobes, the primary artery affected is the middle cerebral artery. The unusual feature of this occlusion is that it appears that the middle cerebral artery extends more caudally than usual. Nevertheless, the middle cerebral artery is the only one of the choices presented that could account for the damage to the temporal and parietal cortices. The anterior cerebral artery supplies the medial aspects of the frontal and parietal lobes; the posterior cerebral artery supplies the occipital cortex (visual areas); the posterior choroidal artery mainly supplies part of the tectum, the medial and superior aspects of the thalamus, and the choroid plexus of the third ventricle. The superior cerebellar artery supplies the dorsolateral aspect of a portion of the pons and the cerebellum.

462. The answer is b. (*Kandel, pp 1305–1309. Nolte, pp 120–128, 421–425.*) An arterial occlusion compromised the blood supply to the occipital lobe on the left side of the brain. Therefore, it would result in a right homonymous hemianopsia with no motor deficits (since no motor regions of the brain are affected).

463. The answer is e. (*Kandel, pp 1303–1311. Nolte, pp 117–128, 131–135.*) This vertebral angiogram is an anterior view of the back of the brain. It reveals an occlusion of the left posterior cerebral artery (A). It should be noted that the posterior cerebral arteries are formed from the bifurcation of the basilar artery. As the basilar artery runs in a caudal direction, It passes laterally to form the vertebral artery on each side.

464. The answer is b. (*Kandel, p 544. Nolte, pp 422–424.*) This large pituitary tumor is seen to compress the optic chiasm. Damage to the chiasm affects the crossing fibers of the nasal retina, which convey information from the temporal visual fields. This results in a bitemporal hemianopsia. Since some parts of the optic nerves are spared, pupillary reflexes are preserved. The neuroanatomic substrates for conjugate gaze (i.e., frontal eye fields, pontine gaze center, medial longitudinal fasciculus, and nuclei of cranial nerves III, IV, and VI) are unaffected by the tumor; the mechanism of conjugate gaze remains intact.

465. The answer is a. *(Kandel, pp 388, 759, 920.)* June had a seizure, which began focally on the left motor strip (the left precentral gyrus), moved up the motor strip, then secondarily generalized, or spread throughout the cortex. The phenomenon whereby there is twitching of an extremity that spreads to other areas on that extremity or other areas of the body is called a *Jacksonian march.* This phenomenon is named for Hughlings Jackson, a neurosurgeon who was instrumental in mapping out the cerebral cortex and describing the somatotopic organization of the cortex of the prefrontal gyrus called a *homunculus* (meaning "little man"). Observing patients with a Jacksonian march helped him to identify areas represented at each location of the motor strip.

466. The answer is c. *(Kandel, pp 919–927.)* Very often, there is inhibition following a seizure, which accounts for drowsiness or a postictal state after the seizure has finished. Sometimes, epileptic discharges spread to other areas of the cortex, recruiting contiguous areas of the cortex through callosal, commissural, and sometimes thalamic circuits to eventually involve a large area of the cortex, causing the movements of the entire body. This occurs with a generalized seizure. If the cortices of both hemispheres become involved, there may be impairment or loss of consciousness. The cells (often pyramidal cells) in the cortex can generate a seizure through high-frequency, synchronous discharges in large groups. If the seizure begins focally, as this one did, there may be a *Todd's paralysis,* as June had, where there is transient paralysis of the involved motor area during the postictal period.

467. The answer is e. *(Kandel, pp 759, 919–927.)* There is somatotopic organization of the motor strip, and cortical neurons are included among the most likely to generate seizures, making this area the most likely to cause such a pattern.

468. The answer is e. *(Kandel, pp 919–927.)* The pyramidal cell is a cell in the cortex that uses glutamate, an excitatory neurotransmitter, whereas most other types of cortical neurons use GABA, an inhibitory neurotransmitter. The spike, one identifying feature of an epileptic seizure seen on an

EEG recorded on the scalp, is initiated by a depolarization shift, which is thought to be generated by EPSPs.

469. The answer is d. *(Kandel, pp 925–927.)* Excitatory postsynaptic potentials are considered to be an initiating cellular event for a seizure. To become a seizure, however, the cellular discharges require enhancement and synchronization.

470. The answer is b. *(Kandel, pp 922–925.)* Since seizure generation requires excitation, or a loss of inhibition, the only correct choice is the inhibition of GABA, an inhibitory neurotransmitter. All the other choices cause inhibition only. Many new anticonvulsant medications are currently being designed to either enhance GABA activity or inhibit the excitatory neurotransmitter glutamate.

471. The answer is c. *(Kandel, pp 758–765.)* A CT scan of Helen's head was done in the emergency room, which showed a new infarct or stroke in the genu and anterior portion of the posterior limb of the left internal capsule. This is the region of the internal capsule through which most of the fibers of the corticospinal and corticobulbar tracts pass in a somatotopically organized fashion before entering the brainstem. Because most of these fibers pass through a very small region, a small infarct can cause deficits in a wide distribution of areas. In this case, Helen had weakness in her face and tongue, causing her slurred speech, in addition to weakness of her arm and leg. In addition, since somatosensory fibers destined for the postcentral gyrus occupy a position in the internal capsule caudal to the corticospinal tract fibers, these fibers were spared and Helen had no sensory deficits. The only other area in the CNS that can cause a pure motor hemiparesis is the basilar pons, an area through which corticospinal and corticobulbar fibers also run. The vascular supply of this region consists of perforators from the basilar artery, which are small and subject to atherosclerotic disease.

472. The answer is a. *(Kandel, pp 1303–1307.)* The internal capsule is supplied primarily by the lenticulostriate branches of the middle cerebral artery. In addition, portions of the posterior limb of the internal capsule are supplied by the anterior choroidal artery, a branch of the internal carotid artery. Both the lateral striate branches and the anterior choroidal artery are small branches of larger arteries and are more susceptible to damage (atherosclerosis) from high blood pressure and diabetes than the larger vessels.

473. The answer is c. (*Kandel, pp 757–763.*) The corticospinal and corticobulbar tracts contain motor fibers originating in the precentral gyrus, mediating voluntary motor function of the face, arms, legs, and trunk. They pass through the internal capsule to the crus cerebri in the midbrain. The spinothalamic tract is a sensory tract and could not cause the observed deficits. The rubrospinal tract affects only the spinal cord.

474. The answer is c. (*Afifi, p 349.*) Helen's forehead was unaffected by the lesion because the forehead is bilaterally represented on the cortex, so the right side retains innervation despite a lesion in the left internal capsule. Motor fibers from each side pass into the internal capsule ipsilaterally, so a lesion in the internal capsule will not affect the forehead. This type of finding is called a *central seventh nerve lesion*, because it represents a lesion in the CNS superior to the level of the seventh nerve nucleus, where the fibers from both sides of the forehead coalesce.

475. The answer is d. (*Adams, p 1383.*) Dysarthria is slurred speech, occurring from lesions affecting innervation of the tongue, lips, and palate. We are given evidence that her tongue was weak in that it pointed to the right. The interruption of fibers traveling to the hypoglossal nerve from the left side eventually innervates the right genioglossus muscle, which pulls the tongue to the left. Dysarthria is a motor phenomenon, unlike aphasia, which is a disruption of language. Language is primarily generated in the cerebral cortex; therefore, because the lesion spares the cortex, there were no signs of aphasia.

476. The answer is d. (*Adams, pp 321–322.*) This is an example of a complex partial seizure, most likely originating in the temporal lobe. A seizure is a paroxysmal derangement of the CNS due to rhythmic, synchronous discharges from cerebral neurons, causing changes in consciousness, sensation, and/or behavior. Complex partial seizures often start with a warning, or "aura." Since limbic structures are often involved, the seizure can include emotions, feelings of deja vu or jamais vu, or gastrointestinal sensations. Because olfactory pathways end in the temporal lobe, patients may experience smells as well. The seizure itself involves impairment of consciousness of some form, often manifested as staring, in addition to various stereotyped, automatic behaviors called *automatisms*. The latter may be manifested as chewing, repetitive swallowing, hand gestures, or vocalizations. These usually occur during the seizure, but may occur after it. After the seizure ends (the seizures usually last one to two minutes), the patient is often in a confused or postictal state for several minutes, or even up to several hours. Occasionally, a patient may manifest aggressive behavior while in the postictal state. Unless a structural lesion, such as a tumor, is present, the physical examination is usually normal. Verification of the diagnosis of epilepsy is done with the help of an EEG, which records potential differences of summed cortical action potentials over the scalp of a patient. Often, an epileptic spike, or sharp wave, is seen over the area from which the seizures arise. Epilepsy patients usually also have a CT scan or MRI to make certain that there is no structural lesion causing the seizures.

477. The answer is c. (Adams, pp 321–322.) Seizures similar to this one often begin with abnormal neuronal discharges in temporal lobe structures, which include the amygdala or hippocampus. These structures tend to have a lower threshold for this type of activity than other structures in the brain.

478. The answer is d. (Afifi, pp 435–438.) The major descending pathways from the amygdala are the stria terminalis and the ventral amygdalofugal pathway. The medial forebrain bundle is a major pathway of the lateral hypothalamus. The mammillothalamic and corticospinal tracts do not involve the amygdala.

479. The answer is a. (Afifi, pp 425–443.) The hippocampal formation includes the hippocampus, the dentate gyrus, and the subiculum. All of the other structures listed are within the limbic system but do not lie within the hippocampal formation.

480. The answer is b. (Kandel, pp 988–992, 1228–1237.) Since memory is a function that is mediated by the limbic system, a structure most likely involved in the generation of these seizures, it is possible that Lindsey will have memory problems in the future if she has frequent seizures. Early studies of patients who have undergone resection of portions of one or both temporal lobes have demonstrated the presence of memory deficits.

481. The answer is a. (Kandel, pp 1306–1309. Adams, pp 456–457.) Jane was not only unable to move her left side (hemiparesis), but ignored its existence (anosagnosia or the syndrome of hemineglect, see answer to question 485). Even though she neglected her left side, the blink reflex should still be intact if she only neglected the side. Therefore, a visual field deficit, called a *homonymous hemianopsia*, was present on the left side, in which the left temporal and right nasal fields were damaged. There may also have been some degree of primary sensory loss, which can be difficult to evaluate when a patient neglects the same side.

482. The answer is c. *(Adams, pp 443–446, 456–457.)* Jane's deficits resulted from lesions of the posterior frontal cortex, as well as from some contribution of corticospinal tract fibers to the parietal lobe and deeper motor cortical structures. In addition, the neglect and hemisensory loss resulted from damage to the parietal cortex. The homonymous hemianopsia resulted from damage to the deep portion of the parietal lobe where the optic radiations pass to the superior and inferior banks of the visual cortex, causing the visual field defect.

483. The answer is d. *(Kandel, pp 1303–1307.)* The posterior frontal lobe, as well as the parietal lobe, are supplied by the middle cerebral artery. Areas supplied by this artery, such as primary and supplementary motor areas, and the primary and secondary somatosensory cortices may be affected. As a result, the patient may have left-sided weakness, UMN facial weakness that spares the forehead, and hemisensory loss.

484. The answer is e. *(Kandel, pp 544–545, 1303–1307.)* If the lesion is deep enough, the patient may have a visual field cut, called a *homonymous hemianopsia*, where fibers traveling from the optic chiasm to the occipital cortex within the optic radiations are interrupted, and the patient doesn't see the left temporal and the right nasal visual field. It is common for patients with neglect not to notice the areas of blindness because they ignore the left side. Patients with this problem are usually advised not to drive a car.

485. The answer is d. *(Kandel, pp 1303–1307. Adams, pp 456–457.)* Jane's problem is an example of the syndrome of hemineglect, which arises from a lesion of the posterior parietal lobe. This area is essential for spatial organization. If this area, usually on the nondominant (right) side, is no longer functioning, the patient will live in a world that consists solely of a right side. Patients with the syndrome of hemineglect will look only to the right side (if the lesion is on the right), and when asked to look to the left, often will not cross the midline with their eyes. Especially when the lesion is acute, these patients will not acknowledge any person or objects on their left side, and it is not unusual for a patient to, for example, complain of losing her glasses when they are on a table on the left side. Since these patients see only the right side of everything, they will put all of the numbers of a clock on the right side of the clock and will bisect a line on its right side. In addition, they will comb only the right side of their hair, dress the right side of their bodies, and shave the right side of their faces. When confronted with a left-sided entity, such as a left arm, they will often ignore the question or may even go as far as claiming it belongs to someone else. In resolving lesions where the patient now has sensation and acknowledgment on the left side, she may still display extinction to double simultaneous stimuli where, if both sides are touched simultaneously, the patient feels the touch only on the right side and "extinguishes" the stimulus on the left. However, it is important to remember that neglect can resemble weakness because the patient won't move the left side.

486. The answer is b. (*Adams, pp 443–445, 453–459.*) This case is an example of a lesion of the left (usually dominant) parietal lobe, most often in the angular gyrus, with some involvement of the precentral gyrus in the posterior frontal lobe. There is contralateral UMN weakness (with a positive Babinski sign), as well as several cortical sensory defects—specifically, right-left confusion, agraphia (inability to write, independent of motor weakness), acalculia (the inability to calculate), and finger agnosia (the inability to designate the fingers). The latter four elements are sometimes referred to as the *Gerstmann syndrome* by neurologists, and all represent spatial discriminatory functions of the parietal lobe (often the dominant parietal lobe, which is usually the left). The parietal lobe also subserves other visual-spatial functions such as construction of complex drawings. There are other locations within the CNS where UMN weakness can occur; however, the combination with parietal lobe signs can occur only in this location. If the damage was slightly more extensive, it may have involved Broca's area, causing aphasia.

487. The answer is d. (*Kandel, pp 1303–1309.*) The artery serving this region (both posterior frontal and parietal lobes) is the left middle cerebral artery, which originates at Willis's circle. Because it continues in a nearly straight line from the internal carotid artery, it is a common route for small emboli formed from blood clots in the internal carotid artery. The bruit noted over the right common carotid artery in this patient is most likely a result of a thrombus (clot) that occludes part of the lumen of the artery. These emboli can occlude the middle cerebral artery because it is considerably smaller than the internal carotid artery. Since the middle cerebral artery has many branches through which an embolus may travel, but the territory of this stroke is large, it is likely that the embolus lodged in a more proximal location in this case.

488. The answer is b. *(Kandel, pp 1303–1309.)* Morris's leg weakness included a positive Babinski sign, which is a UMN sign. Although this type of weakness may occur in several locations in the CNS, the combination with the cortical parietal signs can occur only in the left precentral gyrus if there is to be one lesion.

489. The answer is a. *(Adams, pp 443–445, 453–459.)* These deficits are visual-spatial in nature and are characteristic of damage to the dominant parietal lobe.

490. The answer is e. *(Kandel, pp 1303–1309.)* The visual defect that Morris experienced is a homonymous hemianopsia, resulting from damage to the optic radiations traveling from the lateral geniculate nucleus to the visual cortex in the occipital lobe. These split so that inferior images are carried through the parietal lobe and superior images through the temporal lobes, but in large infarcts the defect is more likely to involve more fibers of this tract. Since the optic radiations carry representations of the ipsilateral temporal field and the contralateral nasal field (only the nasal field fibers cross), this defect is noted clinically as the inability to detect objects in the regions described. Often, the patient will only notice bumping into objects on the side ipsilateral to the stroke, since turning of the eyes can compensate for the nasal field defect.

491. The answer is b. *(Rowland, pp 277–293.)* This case is an example of a condition called *normal-pressure hydrocephalus.* This may be caused by various nonprogressive meningeal and ependymal diseases, such as chronic meningitis and subarachnoid hemorrhages, which can initially block CSF absorption. Initially, the CSF pressure is high, which results in the enlargement of the ventricles. The CSF pressure becomes normal because the CSF absorption begins again. However, the enlarged ventricles, despite normal CSF pressure, cause hydrostatic impairment to the central white matter surrounding the ventricles. Maximal ventricular expansion is usually located in the frontal lobes with preservation of the cortical gray matter and other subcortical structures. As a result, patients with this condition have diminished frontal lobe functions, namely, gait problems without any weakness, as well as urinary incontinence and dementia. Frontal lobe dysfunction can also cause the reappearance of primitive reflexes, which disappear shortly after birth, such as the grasp reflex. Late in the course of normal-pressure hydrocephalus, the patient may develop *frontal lobe incontinence,* where he or she becomes indifferent to the incontinence, much like a very small child. Headaches are rare in this particular type of hydrocephalus. Normal-pressure hydrocephalus is usually diagnosed with a thorough neurological examination, in addition to a head CT, which shows enlarged ventricles and, occasionally, interstitial fluid within the white matter adjacent to the lateral ventricles. (Measurement of CSF pressures with a lumbar puncture and radionuclide cisternography—a procedure where a radionuclide is injected intrathecally, and its distribution is observed over a period of 24 hours—is also helpful.) Occasionally, shunting procedures, which allow the CSF to drain into the peritoneal cavity or the blood, are helpful if performed early in the course of this condition.

492. The answer is a. (*Rowland, pp 277–293.*) The major mechanism underlying hydrocephalus is decreased absorption of CSF. In the case of normal-pressure hydrocephalus, the problem is described in the answer for question 491. Another cause of decreased absorption is obstruction of CSF flow by a tumor. Low blood pressure does not cause enlarged ventricles. High blood pressure causes hydrocephalus only as a result of hypertensive crisis, but not chronically. Decreased blood flow in the brain can actually be used as a temporizing measure to acutely decrease intracranial pressure in emergencies, in order to make room for expanding tissue through the mechanism of decreasing P_{CO_2} in the brain with a ventilator.

493. The answer is c. (*Rowland, pp 277–293.*) The major location for reabsorption of CSF is the arachnoid villi within the ventricular system. In the case of this particular patient, there was a history of a subarachnoid hemorrhage, which may have caused obstruction within this area.

494. The answer is e. (*Rowland, pp 277–293.*) The frontal horns of the lateral ventricles are the area of greatest expansion; thus, the expansion would affect the adjoining white matter of the frontal lobe. The other areas listed are subcortical and gray matter areas, which are located further from the expanding frontal horns and are less affected. The pituitary gland is quite distant from the frontal horns as well.

495. The answer is c. (*Gilroy, pp 6–9. Rowland, pp 7–10.*) The language problem is an example of Broca's aphasia, a deficit seen with lesions of Broca's area and manifested by defects in the motor aspect of speech, leaving the patient's speech halting and nonfluent. People with Broca's aphasia tend to repeat certain phrases, as well as leave out pronouns. Since the language centers are usually located on the dominant side of the brain (the left side for a right-handed person), this lesion must be on the left side of Joe's brain. Wernicke's aphasia is a problem with the sensory aspect of speech, where the patient can speak fluently, but the speech sounds like gibberish. The area of disruption in this type of aphasia is usually in Wernicke's area, a region of the posterior superior temporal lobe. Dysarthria is slurred speech, but makes grammatical sense. Alexia is the inability to read. Pure-word deafness is a type of sensory aphasia whereby language, reading, and writing are only mildly disturbed, but auditory comprehension of words is very abnormal. This arises from lesions of the posterior temporal lobe.

496. The answer is e. (*Gilroy, pp 225–230. Rowland, pp 7–10.*) Joe's condition is an example of a left inferior frontal lobe cortical stroke, including the region of Broca's area and the left precentral gyrus. The weakness on his right side confirms this, since the left side of the brain controls the right side of the body. The right leg is most likely less involved than the arm because the leg area of the precentral gyrus extends onto the medial aspect of the frontal lobe, an area served by a different artery than that serving the arm and face areas. The internal capsule contains motor fibers traveling to the cortex, but usually does not involve language. The thalamus contains many sensory, motor, and association areas, but only rarely causes language problems. Functions of the pontine reticular formation do not include language. The corpus callosum is a white matter structure that connects the hemispheres. Lesions of the posterior aspect may cause language problems, such as alexia without agraphia (the ability to write, but not to read), but would not cause both an aphasia and weakness.

497. The answer is d. (*Gilroy, pp 225–230, 235–239. Rowland, pp 7–10, 61–62.*) The middle cerebral artery subserves the precentral gyrus, the area that has been damaged. The damage can be more widespread, depending upon which portion of the vessel becomes occluded. The anterior cerebral artery supplies the orbitofrontal cortex, deep limbic structures, as well as the cingulate gyrus. The posterior cerebral artery supplies the thalamus, portions of the temporal lobes, and portions of the midbrain. The anterior inferior cerebellar artery supplies the lateral inferior pons and portions of the cerebellum. Perforating branches of the basilar artery supply medial portions of the brainstem. The irregular heartbeat observed in this case is an example of aerial fibrillation, a heart rhythm that is often recognized by being "irregularly irregular." This rhythm can cause strokes by throwing small blood clots or emboli from the heart to the cerebral blood vessels and occluding them.

498. The answer is b. (*Rowland, pp 7–11, 440–442.*) Joe's forehead didn't droop like the rest of his face because this region receives innervation from both sides of the cerebral cortex, giving this area a backup in case of damage. This can occur only when the lesion is above the level of nerve VII, where both sides no longer contribute to the innervation of the face. This type of weakness is called a *central nerve VII lesion,* because it occurs within the CNS. A *peripheral nerve VII lesion* is a lesion within the nerve VII nucleus, or distal. This type of lesion always involves the forehead in addition to the rest of the face. Nerve XII innervates the tongue and nerve V innervates sensation of the face, in addition to the muscles of mastication, but not the muscles of facial expression. The oculomotor nerve innervates four of the muscles that move the eyes.

499. The answer is a. (*Gilroy, pp 6–9. Rowland, pp 7–10.*) Joe is probably right-handed, which implies left-sided cerebral dominance. Since language is usually on the dominant side, and Joe's has an aphasia, his dominant cerebral hemisphere has been damaged. People who are left-handed may also have dominance of either side or may have mixed dominance. True ambidexterity is rare.

500. The answer is b. (*Gilroy, p 337. Kandel, pp 951–953.*) Sleep apnea can occur for several reasons. One common basis is an obstruction of the airways (called *obstructive sleep apnea*). In this case, as indicated in the statement of the question, the physicians ruled out this possibility. Another possible cause involves central sleep apnea. This is due to disruption of the mechanism involving chemoreceptors in the carotid body that monitors carbon dioxide and oxygen levels in the blood. Axons in the carotid body project via the glossopharyngeal nerve (IX) to the reticular formation of the medulla. Therefore, disturbances involving the carotid body could result in central sleep apnea. Here, inappropriate signals are sent to the medullary reticular formation, which, in part, projects caudally to ventral horn sites in the spinal cord, governing such muscles as those that regulate the diaphragm and, therefore, disrupt the normal breathing process.

Bibliography

Adams RD, Victor M, Ropper AH: *Principles of Neurology,* 6/e. New York, McGraw-Hill, 1997.

Afifi AK, Bergman RA: *Functional Neuroanatomy.* New York, McGraw-Hill, 1998.

Cooper JR, Bloom FE, Roth RH: *The Biochemical Basis of Neuropharmacology,* 7/e. New York, Oxford University Press, 1996.

DeArmond SJ, Fusco MM, Dewey MM: *Structure of the Human Brain: A Photographic Atlas,* 3/e. New York, Oxford University Press, 1989.

Gilroy, J: *Basic Neurology,* 3/e. New York, McGraw-Hill, 2000.

Greenberg DA, Aminoff MJ, Simon RP: *Clinical Neurology,* 5/e, New York, McGraw-Hill, 2002.

Kandel ER, Schwartz JH, Jessel TM: *Principles of Neural Science,* 4/e. New York, McGraw-Hill, 2000.

Kingsley RE: *Concise Text of Neuroscience,* 2/e. Philadelphia, Lippincott, Williams & Wilkins, 2000.

Martin JH: *Neuroanatomy,* 2/e, Stamford, CT, Appleton & Lange, 1996.

Nolte J: *The Human Brain: An Introduction to Its Functional Anatomy,* 4/e. St. Louis, MO, Mosby, 1999.

Purves D, Augustine GJ, Fitzpatrick D, Katz LC, LaMantia A-S, McNamara JO, Williams SM: *Neuroscience,* 2/e. Sunderland, Sinauer Associates, Inc., 2001.

Rowland, LP (ed): *Merritt's Textbook of Neurology,* 10/e. Philadelphia, Lippincott, Williams & Wilkins, 2000.

Siegel GJ, Agranoff BW, Albers RW, Fisher SK, Uhler MD: *Basic Neurochemistry,* 6/e. Philadelphia, Lippincott, Williams & Wilkins, 1999.

Simon RP, Aminoff MJ, Greenberg DA: *Clinical Neurology,* 4/e. New York, McGraw-Hill, 1999.

Villiger E, Ludwig E, Rasmussen AT: *Atlas of Cross Section Anatomy of the Brain.* New York, McGraw-Hill, 1951.

Index

A

Abducens nerve, 52, 59
Acetylcholine (ACh)
  in Alzheimer's disease, 100, 112
  function of, 17–18, 149
  in Horner's syndrome, 182, 206
  in Huntington's disease, 248, 261
  release of, 96, 109–110, 145, 148
Acetylcholinesterase, 110, 111
Action potential, 13–14, 70, 74, 79, 83, 210,
  220–221
Adenohypophysis, 237, 243–244
Adenosine triphosphate (ATP), 24
Aδ fibers, 130, 142
Adrenal medulla, 34
Agnosia, 306
Agraphia, 288, 306, 307
Akinesia, 42
Akinetic mutism, 267
Alar plate, 63, 66
Alcoholism, 253, 254, 266–267
All-or-none response, 74, 83
Alpha (α)–adrenergic receptors, 27, 103, 114
Alpha (α)–toxins, 97, 110–111
Alpha (α) wave, 272, 295
Alternating hypoglossal hemiplegia, 38
Alzheimer's disease, 19, 100, 112, 236, 243
Ambidexterity, 310
Amygdala
  central nucleus of, 275, 297–298
  function of, 5
  lesion in, 274, 297
  in seizure, 284–285, 304
  stroke effect on, 234–235, 242
  supplied by olfactory bulb, 218, 228–229
Amyotrophic lateral sclerosis (ALS), 18, 31,
  121–122, 134–135
Analgesia, 28, 214, 215, 224–225, 239, 244
  (See also Pain)
Anosagnosia, 285–286, 304–305
Ansa lenticularis, 234, 242
Anterior cerebellar lobe, 5, 42
Anterior cingulate gyrus, 4
Anterior commisure, 5, 47, 56
Anterior corticospinal tract, 128, 140
Anterior neuropore, 61, 65
Anterior spinocerebellar tract, 31
Anterior spinothalamic tract, 30
Anterior thalamic nuclei, 232, 241, 269–270,
  293
Antipsychotic drugs, 248, 261–262
Anxiety disorders, 102, 103, 113, 117
Aortic arch, 154, 187
Aphagia, 274, 297

Aphasia
  Broca's, 44, 290–291, 309
  motor, 234, 242
  Wernicke's, 44, 49, 57, 278, 300, 309
Apoptosis, 64, 66
Apraxia, 44, 246, 259
Arachnoid villi, 290, 308
Arcuate nucleus, 238, 243
Area postrema, 169, 196–197
Argyll Robertson pupil, 38, 172, 200
Astereognosia, 44
Astigmatism, 211, 221
Ataxia of movement, 125, 137, 253, 266
Atherosclerosis, 176, 203
Athetosis, 42
ATP (see Adenosine triphosphate)
Auditory function
  impaired, 49, 57, 167, 194, 198, 200
  thalamic relay for, 271, 294
Automatisms, 303
Autonomic nervous system
  disorders of, 37–38, 145–150
  divisions of, 32–33, 39–40
  functions of, 36–37
  neurotransmitters in, 36
  organs involved in, 33–36
  receptors in, 36
  in temperature regulation, 273, 296
Axon
  in cell body, 6
  damage to, 68, 76
  function of, 8–9
Axonal transport
  function of, 69, 77
  nerve pathways and, 67, 75
Axon hillock, 8, 72, 81
Axosomatic synapses, 85

B

Babinski's sign, 132, 144, 288, 306, 307
Bacterial meningitis, 53, 59–60
Baroreceptors, 37, 187
Basal ganglia
  disorders of, 42, 55, 247, 248, 260, 261
  fibers supplying, 246, 259
  function of, 5
  output of, 234, 242, 247, 260
Basal nucleus of Meynert, 100, 112
Basal plate, 62, 65
Basilar artery, 173, 176, 180, 201, 205,
  254–255, 267
Basilar pons, 6, 48, 56, 176, 202–203,
  282–283, 302
Bell's palsy, 178, 204–205

Beta (β)–adrenergic receptors, 27, 87, 91–92, 146, 148–149
Bilateral postictal suppression, 280–281, 301
Bipolar cell, 209, 216, 220, 226
Bipolar disorders, 108, 117
Bitemporal hemianopsia
  from optic chiasm damage, 52, 59, 212, 222
  pituitary tumors and, 237, 243, 280, 300–301
Bladder function, 35, 146, 149
  (*See also* Urinary incontinence)
Blink reflex, 287, 305
Blood-brain barrier, 54, 60
Blood pressure, 154, 162, 187, 191, 192
  (*See also* Hypertension)
Blood vessels, 34
Brachial plexus, 119, 133
Brain
  anatomy of, 1–6
  development of, 6
  tumors of, 47, 52, 53, 59–60, 218, 229
Brainstem
  anatomy of, 5–6
  auditory pathway of, 175, 202
  compression of, 168, 195
  infarction of, 168, 195–196
  lesions of, 38, 52, 58–59, 161, 167, 169, 171–177, 191, 197, 198–208
Broca's aphasia, 44, 290–291, 309
Broca's area, 3, 57, 290–291, 309
Bromocriptine, 244
Brown-Séquard's syndrome, 31, 125, 131, 137, 142–143

C
Calcarine fissure, 48, 56
Calcium channels, 79, 88, 92
cAMP, 87, 91–92
Carotid artery, internal, 212, 221–222
Carotid sinus, 154, 187
Carotid sinus reflex, 146, 148, 155–156, 187–188
Carrier proteins, 11
Catecholamines, 20–22, 107, 108, 117, 118
Catechol-O-methyltransferase, 107, 117
Caudate nucleus, 5, 46, 55, 234–235, 236, 242–243
Cδ fibers, 130, 142
Cell body, 6, 68, 76
Central canal, 128, 140
Central nerve VII lesion, 290–291, 303, 310
Central nervous system (CNS), 6, 10, 200
Central sleep apnea, 310
Centromedian (CM) thalamic nucleus, 231, 240, 271, 294
Cerebellar column system, 253, 266
Cerebellar glomerulus, 249, 263
Cerebellar vermis, 5, 253–254, 266

Cerebellum
  anatomy of, 5
  anterior lobe of, 249, 250, 262, 264
  damage to, 65
  disorders of, 42–43
  feedback relationships, 250, 263–264
  formation of, 63, 66
Cerebral cortex
  in Alzheimer's disease, 100, 112
  bladder control and, 146, 149
  connection to cerebellum, 249, 262–263
  damage to, 46, 49–50, 55, 57–58
  disorders associated with, 43–44
  epileptic discharges in, 301
  motor/sensory structures of, 1, 3–4, 303
  neurons in, 213, 224
  sense of smell and, 217, 219, 226–227, 229
  transmitters from, 247, 260
Cerebral hemorrhage, 276, 299
Cerebral peduncle, 52–53, 58, 183–184, 207
Cerebrospinal fluid (CSF)
  in bacterial meningitis, 53, 59–60
  formation of, 4
  in normal-pressure hydrocephalus, 289–290, 307–309
  reduced production of, 63, 66
  with subarachnoid hemorrhage, 53, 60
Cervical disk prolapse, 120, 134
Channel proteins, 11
Chlordiazepoxide, 102, 113
Chloride channels, 6, 26, 27, 74, 83
Cholecystokinin (CCK), 298
Chorea, 42
Choreiform movements, 248, 261
Chromatin, 8
Cingulate gyrus, 5, 47, 56
Circadian rhythms, 274, 297
Clarke's nucleus dorsalis, 127, 139, 193
Clonidine, 103, 113–114
Cognitive functions, 270, 293–294
Coma vigil, 267
Combined systems disease, 32
Complex partial seizure, 272, 284, 295, 303–304
Cones, 209, 216, 220, 226
Conjugate lateral gaze, 171, 198
Conscious proprioception
  dorsal funiculus and, 140
  loss of, 161, 175, 190–191, 201–202
  pathway for, 219, 229
Corneal reflex, 151, 186
Corona radiata, 290, 308
Corpus callosum, 4, 48, 56–57
Corticobulbar fibers, 164–165, 194
Corticobulbar tract, 180–181, 205, 282–283, 303
Corticospinal fibers, 128, 140, 164–165, 181–182, 194, 205–206

Corticospinal tract
  dysfunction of, 135, 144
  function of, 245, 257
  infarction of, 254–255, 267
  lesion of, 174, 180–181, 201, 205
  stroke damage to, 124, 136, 282–283, 303
Cranial nerve I, 171, 199–200
Cranial nerve III (oculomotor nerve), 52–53,
    59, 168–169, 172, 175, 183–184, 188,
    196, 199–200, 202, 206–207
Cranial nerve IV (trochlear nerve), 52, 59,
    156–157, 184–185, 188, 207–208
Cranial nerve V, 151, 164–166, 169, 170,
    186, 193, 194, 196, 198
Cranial nerve VI, 171, 198, 199
Cranial nerve VII (facial nerve), 51, 58, 151,
    152, 159, 171, 178, 182, 186, 189, 190,
    199–200, 204–206
Cranial nerve VIII, 52, 59, 170, 198
Cranial nerve IX (glossopharyngeal nerve),
    152–153, 158–159, 169, 171, 186,
    189–190, 197, 199–200
Cranial nerve X, 155–156, 187–188, 189
Cranial nerves, 6, 38, 51–52, 58–59
Crus cerebri, 166–167, 175, 195, 202
Cuneocerebellar tract, 31, 249, 262
Cytoskeleton, 8
Cytosolic proteins, 69, 76–77

D
Dandy-Walker syndrome, 61, 65
Deep cerebellar nuclei, 163–164, 191
Déjérine-Roussy syndrome, 238–239, 244
Dementia, 19, 289, 308
Demyelination, 74, 83, 121, 134, 135,
    141–142
Dendrites, 6, 8, 70, 79
Dentate gyrus, 285, 304
Dentate nucleus, 163–164, 192
Depolarization, 70, 72, 79–81, 302
Depression, neurotransmitter role in, 21, 23,
    98, 111
Descending inhibition, 213, 223
Diabetes, 178, 204
Diaphragm, loss of function from, 131, 142
Diencephalon, 4, 48, 56
Distal muscles, 245, 257–258
Dopamine
  biosynthesis of, 95, 99, 109, 112
  in central nucleus of amygdala, 275, 297
  function of, 20–21
  loss of, 46, 55
  in Parkinson's disease, 42, 252, 265–266
  prolactin and, 243–244
  replenishment of, 234–235, 242
  schizophrenia and, 275, 298
Dopamine blockers, 248, 261
Dorsal column nuclei, 213, 223

Dorsal columns, 30
Dorsal horn, 214–216, 224–226
Dorsal spinocerebellar tract, 249, 262
Dorsolateral medulla, 170, 197
Dorsomedial nucleus, 269–270, 293
Drowsiness, 270, 293–294
Dysarthria, 176–177, 282–284, 293–204, 303
Dyskinesias, 42
Dysphagia, 155–156, 187–188
Dysphonia, 170, 197

E
Edinger-Westphal nucleus, 183–184, 207
EEG activity
  in epileptic seizure, 301–302, 304
  in REM sleep, 272, 295
  in wakefulness, 272, 295
Emboliform nucleus, 163–164, 192
Emesis, 169, 196–197
Emotional behavioral
  brain disorder effect on, 47, 50, 56, 57,
    233, 235, 241, 242
  head injury effect on, 46, 55
  mediation of, 43, 298–299
Endocrine functions, 43, 273, 296
Endomorphin, 28
End plate potential (EPP), 16, 96, 109–110
Enkephalin, 24, 195, 275, 297
Enteric nervous system, 32–33
Enzymatic degradation, 98, 111
Epilepsy
  GABAergic circuits in, 19
  mechanisms of, 280–282, 301–302
  petit mal, 295
  seizure spread with, 48, 56–57
  surgery for, 234, 242
  temporal lobe, 43, 105, 114–115, 231,
    240, 284, 303–304
  treatment for, 107, 116–117, 118
Epinephrine, 22, 99, 111–112
Excitatory postsynaptic potential (EPSP), 16,
    74, 83, 282, 302
Excitotoxicity, 18
Extensor muscle tone, 250, 264
Eye movement
  control of, 33, 167, 168–169, 171,
    195–196, 199
  cranial nerve III and, 183–184, 199–200,
    206–207
  loss of, 156, 188

F
Facial nerve (cranial nerve VII), 51, 58, 152,
    159, 171, 178, 182, 186, 190, 199–200,
    204–206
Farsightedness, 210–211, 221
Fasciculus cuneatus, 123, 135
Fasciculus gracilis, 132, 143

Fastigial cerebellar nucleus, 163–164, 192, 253–254, 266–267
Feedback inhibition, 213, 223, 263
Feed-forward inhibition, 213, 223, 263
Flocculonodular lobe, 5, 43, 247, 251, 261, 265
Fluoro-Gold, 9, 67, 75
Fluoxetine (Prozac), 23, 111
Forebrain
    anatomy of, 4–5
    lesions of, 172, 199, 233, 241, 248, 261
Fornix, 4, 46, 48, 55, 56, 231, 240
Frey's syndrome, 38
Frontal lobe, 3, 4, 287–288, 289–290, 306, 307–308

G

GABA (γ-aminobutyric acid)
    function of, 19, 247, 260
    vs. glycine, 87, 90–91
    in Huntington's disease, 248, 261
    inhibition of, 282, 302
    loss of, 55
    in tardive dyskinesia, 248, 261–262
Gag reflex, 162, 191
Gait
    impaired, 43, 176–177, 203, 251, 253, 265, 266–267, 289, 308
    in Parkinson's disease, 252, 265
Gamma motor neurons, 125, 137–138
Ganglion cells, 209, 210, 215, 220–221, 225
Gap junctions, 15, 74, 83, 85, 89, 90
Gaseous neurotransmitters, 25
Gastrointestinal (GI) system, 32–33, 34–35, 51, 58
Generalized seizure, 273, 295–296, 301
Geniculate ganglion, 159–160, 190
Gerstmann syndrome, 306
Glaucoma, 211, 221
Glial cells, 10, 71, 80
Globose nucleus, 163–164, 192
Globus pallidus, 5, 236, 243
Glossopharyngeal nerve (cranial nerve IX), 152–153, 158–159, 169, 171, 186, 189–190, 197, 199–200
Glutamate
    categories of, 91
    in epilepsy, 107, 116, 302
    as excitatory transmitter, 214, 224, 247, 260
    function of, 18, 101, 112–113
    in neurodegeneration, 102, 113
    pyramidal cell use of, 301–302
    in stroke, 114
Glycine, 19–20, 87, 90–91
Goldman equation, 13, 73, 80, 82
Golgi apparatus, 8
Granulous cortex, 57
Grasp reflex, 289, 308

Guillain-Barré syndrome, 121, 130, 134, 141–142

H

Hallucinations
    olfactory, 218, 229
    reducing, 298
Headache
    glaucoma-related, 211, 221
    tumor-related, 47, 52
Head trauma, 184–185, 207–208, 217, 226–227, 279, 300
Hearing loss, 49, 57, 167, 194, 198, 200
Heart, 34
Hemiballism, 42, 232, 241, 248, 261
Hemineglect, 285–286, 304–306
Hemiparesis, 269–270, 285–286, 293, 304–305
Hemisensory loss, 285–286, 304–305
Hippocampal formation
    in Alzheimer's disease, 100, 112
    function of, 5, 43, 231, 240
    in hypothalamus regulation, 275, 298
    in seizure, 284–285, 304
Hirschsprung's disease (megacolon), 38
Histamine, 23, 106, 115–116
Homonymous hemianopsia
    from cerebral hemorrhage, 276, 299
    characteristics of, 285–286, 305
    from damaged lateral geniculate nucleus, 232, 240
    from head trauma, 279, 300
    from left brain artery occlusion, 278, 300
    from optic tract lesion, 235, 242, 307
Horizontal cells, 217, 227
Horner's syndrome, 33, 37, 38, 181, 201, 205–206
Horseradish peroxidase (HRP), 9, 67, 75
Huntington's disease
    caudate nucleus role in, 236, 242–243
    characteristics of, 42
    GABA levels in, 19, 46, 55
    glutamate levels in, 18
    neurotransmitter reduction in, 248, 261
    substance P levels in, 25
Hydrocephalus
    characteristics of, 63, 66
    noncommunicating, 53, 60
    normal-pressure, 289, 307–308
Hyperacusis, 178–179, 204
Hyperglycinemia, 20
Hypertension, 103, 106, 113–114, 115, 146, 149
Hypoglossal nerve, 52, 59
Hypoglossal nucleus
    lesion in, 176–177, 203–204
    tongue extrusion and, 161–162, 164, 191–192, 193

Hypothalamus
 function of, 4, 43, 147, 149–150
 paraventricular nucleus of, 234–235, 242
 regulation by hippocampal formation, 275, 298
 in temperature regulation, 273, 296
 tumor in, 274, 297
 vasopressin and, 273, 296

I
Imidazoleamines, 23
Immunocytochemical labeling, 68, 75
Indoleamines, 22–23
Infarct
 basilar artery, 254–255, 267
 brainstem, 168, 195–196
 corticospinal tract, 254–255, 267
 medial thalamus, 270, 293–294
 posterior cerebral artery, 269–271, 293–294
Inferior cerebellar peduncle, 5, 161–162, 164–165, 192–193
Inferior colliculus, 5, 166–167, 194
Inferior olivary nucleus, 157, 161–162, 189, 191
Inferior parietal lobule, 231, 240
Inferior vestibular nucleus, 161–162, 164, 191, 192–193
Inhibitory neurons, 213, 223
Inhibitory postsynaptic potential (IPSP), 17, 74, 83
Initial segment, 72, 81
Internal capsule
 anatomy of, 45–46, 55
 lesion of, 234, 241–242, 246, 259, 277, 299
 stroke in, 282–283, 302
Internal carotid artery, 212, 221–222
Interposed nuclei, 163–164, 192
Ion channels
 in all-or-none response, 83
 characteristics of, 15–17, 69, 77–78
 function of, 12
 modulation of, 26, 86, 90
 in second messenger systems, 88, 92–93
 (See also specific channels)
Ionotropic receptors, 25–26, 30, 88, 91, 93
Irregular heartbeat, 290, 310

J
Jacksonian march, 301
Jaw-closing reflex, 198
Joint capsules, 213, 223

K
Kainate, 26, 88, 93
Kidneys, 34
Klüver-Bucy syndrome, 43, 274, 297

L
Labyrinth organs, 51, 52, 59
Lambert-Eaton syndrome, 17
L-arginine, 105, 115
Lateral corticospinal tract, 31
Lateral gaze paralysis, 52, 59
Lateral geniculate nucleus, 212, 215, 222, 225, 231, 240
Lateral lemniscus, 175, 202
Lateral medullary syndrome, 38
Lateral spinothalamic tract, 30
Lateral vestibulospinal tract, 124, 136, 154, 187
L-dopa, 99, 112, 252, 265
Lectins, 9
Left-handedness, 310
Left ventral thalamus, 238–239, 244
Length constant, 70, 78–79
Lenticular fasciculus, 232, 240–241
Lentiform nucleus, 277, 299
Lesions
 of amygdala, 274, 297
 of brain base, 212, 222
 of brainstem, 38, 52, 58–59, 161, 167, 169, 171–177, 191, 198–208
 central seventh nerve, 290–291, 303, 310
 of corticobulbar tract, 180–181, 205
 of corticospinal tract, 180–181, 205
 of flocculonodular lobe, 251, 265
 of forebrain, 172, 199, 233, 241, 248, 261
 of hypoglossal nucleus, 176–177, 203–204
 of internal capsule, 234, 241–242, 246, 259, 277, 299
 of medial lemniscus, 161, 164–166, 175, 191, 193, 194, 201–202
 of medulla, 176, 202–203
 of midbrain, 156–157, 172, 183–184, 188, 199–200
 in oculomotor nerve (cranial nerve III), 183, 206–207
 of optic tract, 235, 242, 307
 peripheral seventh nerve, 310
 of pons, 156, 178, 188, 204–205
 in posterior cerebellar lobe, 245, 257
 of posterior frontal cortex, 285–286, 305
 of skull base, 159, 190
 of visual pathway, 40–41
Ligand gating, 70, 79
Limbic cortex, 4
Limbic system, 5, 43
Lissauer's marginal zone, 126, 138
Lithium, 108, 117
Locked-in syndrome, 180, 205
Lower motor neurons (LMNs)
 function of, 130, 142
 paralysis of, 125, 127, 136, 137, 139
 weakness of, 178, 204–205

Lungs, 34
Lysosomes, 8

M
Magnetic resonance imaging (MRI), 68, 75
Mammillary bodies, 58, 232–233, 241
Mammillothalamic tract, 241
Mastication, 51, 58, 165–166, 194, 200–201
Medial geniculate thalamic nucleus, 168, 195,
    271, 294
Medial lemniscus
    left, 176–177, 203
    lesion of, 161, 164–166, 175, 191, 193,
        194, 201–202
Medial longitudinal fasciculus (MLF)
    damage to, 164, 176–177, 193, 203
    function of, 127, 139–140, 161, 191
Medial medullary syndrome, 38, 176, 203
Medial thalamus, 270–271, 293–294
Medial vermal region, 250, 264
Medial vestibulospinal nucleus, 161–162, 191
Medial vestibulospinal tract, 139, 155, 187
Mediodorsal thalamic nucleus, 46, 55–56,
    232–233, 241
Medulla, 6, 176, 202–203
Melatonin, 112
Membrane potential, 12–17, 73, 74, 82–83
    (See also Resting membrane potential)
Memory
    epilepsy and, 285, 304
    medial thalamus infarct effect on, 270,
        293–294
    Papez circuit and, 51, 58
    short-term, 46, 55, 231, 240, 299
Meningitis, 53, 59–60, 307
Mental retardation, 61, 65
Messenger RNA (mRNA), 76, 77
Metabotropic receptors, 26–28, 30, 88, 91,
    93
Meyer-Archambault loop, 222
Micrographia, 265
Midbrain
    damaged nerve in, 183–185, 207–208
    lesion of, 156–157, 172, 183–184, 188,
        199–200, 206–207
    stroke of, 254–255, 267
Midbrain periaqueductal gray
    analgesia and, 5, 214, 215, 224–225
    opioid receptors in, 104, 114
    tumor of, 166–167, 195
Middle cerebellar peduncle, 5, 165, 194
Middle cerebral artery, 278, 282–283,
    285–288, 290–291, 300, 302, 305–307,
    309–310
Miosis, 181, 205–206
Mitochondria, 8
Mitral cells, in olfactory function, 216, 218,
    226, 228

Monoamine oxidase, 252, 266
Monoamines, 107, 117, 256, 267
Morphine, 28, 104, 106, 114, 115–116
Motor aphasia, 234, 242
Motor cortex, 246, 258–259
Motor root, 51, 58
Motor systems
    basal plate cells and, 62, 65
    damage to, 110
    disorders of, 46, 55
    dysfunction of, 76
    function of, 42–43, 46, 55
    stroke effect on, 48, 56
    VA nucleus and, 269–270, 293
MPTP (1–methyl-4–phenyl-1,2,3,6–tetra-
    hydropyridine), 249, 262
Multiple sclerosis (MS), 38, 74, 83, 122, 135,
    183, 207
Muscle spindles, 128, 141
Myasthenia gravis, 15, 17, 97, 110
Myelin, 68, 76
Myelination, 6, 10, 64, 66
Myopia (nearsightedness), 210, 221

N
Na^+,K^+-ATPase, 12
Naloxone, 28
Neostriatal fibers, 247, 260
Neostriatum
    damage to, 248, 261
    function of, 246, 259
    GABAergic inputs from, 236, 243
    neurons in, 247, 260
Nernst equation, 12, 73, 80, 82
Nerve cell body (see Soma)
Neural crest cells, 62, 65
Neural tube, 7
Neuroglia, 10
Neuronal membrane
    depolarization of, 15, 70, 79–80, 92
    function of, 11–12
    hyperpolarization of, 79, 80, 87, 92
    repolarization of, 70, 79
    resting potential of, 13, 69, 73, 78, 82
    structure of, 11
    time constant of, 72, 81
Neurons
    components of, 8–9
    first-order sensory, 126, 138
    function of, 6
    impulse trigger zone for, 72, 81
    inhibitory, 213, 223
    injury to, 10, 18, 98, 111
    ion concentrations for, 14
    in REM sleep, 272, 295
    types of, 9–10
Neuropsychological impairment, 269–270,
    293

Neurotoxicity, 102, 113
Neurotransmitters
    in autonomic nervous system, 36
    blocking, 101, 112–113
    classes of, 17, 29
    detection of, 68, 75
    effects on calcium currents in heart, 146, 148–149
    excitatory, 214, 224
    function of, 14–15, 17
    individual types of, 17–25
    nitric oxide and, 106, 115
    in pain modulation, 244
    release of, 88, 92
Nicotinic ACh receptor, 25, 97, 110–111, 148
Nissl substance, 8
Nitric oxide, 29, 105, 106, 115
NMDA (N-methyl-D-aspartate) receptor
    activation of, 106, 116
    epilepsy and, 107, 116
    function of, 87, 88, 91, 93
    stroke and, 104, 114
Nociceptive transmission, blocking, 216, 225–226
Nodes of Ranvier, 8, 10, 14
Norepinephrine
    in blood pressure control, 146, 149
    conversion of, 99, 112
    degradation of, 107, 117
    depletion of, 108, 118
    effect on calcium current in heart, 146, 148–149
    in Horner's syndrome, 182, 206
    as neurotransmitter, 21
    removal from synaptic cleft, 108, 118
    in second messenger system, 87, 91–92
Normal-pressure hydrocephalus, 289, 307
Nucleus ambiguus, 155, 159, 161–162, 187–188, 189–190, 191
Nucleus cuneatus, 161, 191
Nucleus gracilis, 160, 190–191
Nucleus raphe magnus, 215, 225
Nystagmus, 41, 164, 193

O
Obstructive sleep apnea, 310
Occipital cortex, 3, 269, 278, 293, 300
Occipital lobe, 4
Oculomotor nerve (cranial nerve III), 51–52, 59, 168–169, 172, 175, 183–184, 196, 199–200, 202, 206–207
Oculomotor palsy, 202
Olfaction, 219, 229
Olfactory bulb/cortex, 4, 47, 56
Olfactory cilia, 217, 228
Olfactory glomerulus, 216, 218, 226, 228
Olfactory hallucinations, 218, 229

Olfactory nerve, peripheral neuropathy of, 47, 56
Oligodendrocyte, 6, 10
Olivocochlear bundle, 170, 198
Opiates, 239
Opioid peptides, 24, 104, 114, 298
Optic chiasm, 51–52, 59, 212, 222, 237, 243, 280, 300–301
Optic disk, neuritis of, 211, 221
Optic nerve, 212, 221–222
Optic radiations, 287–288, 307
Optic tract, 215, 225, 234–235, 242
Orbital frontal cortex, 49–50, 57
Otic ganglion, 158, 189–190
Oxytocin, 242, 297

P
Pacinian corpuscle, 130, 142
Pain
    modulation of, 104, 106, 114, 115–116, 161, 191, 195
    referred, 214, 224
    sensation of, 126, 132, 138, 143, 169, 196
    suppression of, 214–216, 224–226, 238–239, 244
Paleostriatal fibers, 247, 260
Pancoast tumor, 206
Panic disorder, 117
Papez circuit, 51, 58, 275, 298–299
Parabrachial nucleus, 172, 200
Paradoxical sleep, 295
Paralysis
    of contralateral limbs, 174, 201
    of extremities, 180, 205
    lateral gaze, 52, 59
    of lower motor neurons (LMNs), 125, 127, 136, 137, 139
    of upper motor neurons (UMNs), 44, 129, 137, 141, 167, 175, 194, 195, 202, 234, 241, 277, 299
Paramedian pontine reticular formation, 171, 199
Parasympathetic nervous system, 32, 39–40, 51, 58
Parietal cortex, 269, 285–286, 293, 305
Parietal lobe, 3, 4, 49–50, 58, 285–288, 305, 306, 307
Parkinson's disease
    characteristics of, 21, 42, 252, 265–266
    dopamine in, 168, 195, 234–235, 242
    GABAergic circuits in, 19
    study of, 249, 262
Pars compacta, 168, 175, 195, 202, 252, 265–266
Peptides, 107, 117, 145, 148, 275, 297
Peripheral nerve VII lesion, 310
Peripheral nervous system (PNS)
    characteristics of, 120, 133–134

Peripheral nervous system (PNS) (*Cont.*)
  components of, 10
  damage to, 10, 130, 141
  myelin formation in, 6, 10
Peripheral neuropathy, 47, 56, 68, 76
Petit mal epilepsy, 295
Phencyclidine (PCP), 107, 116
Phenylketonuria (PKU), 96, 109
Pituitary
  anterior, incomplete growth of, 63, 66
  chromophobe adenoma of, 280,
    300–301
  microadenoma of, 237, 243–244
Plasma membrane, 8
Polyproteins, 76
Pons
  anatomy of, 6
  dorsal, lesion in, 156, 188
  lesion of, 153–154, 156, 178, 187, 188,
    204–205
  lower, 159, 190
  rostral, 272, 295
  stroke of, 254–255, 267
Pontine reticular formation, 180–181, 205
Pontine tegmentum, 6, 180, 205
Posterior cerebellar lobe, 5, 42, 245, 257
Posterior cerebral artery
  cerebral hemorrhage and, 276, 299
  infarct of, 269–271, 293–294
  occlusion of, 279, 300
  substantia nigra supplied by, 252, 265
Posterior column system, 253, 266
Posterior communicating artery, 269–270, 293
Posterior frontal cortex, 285–286, 305
Posterior spinocerebellar tract, 30
Posttranslational importation, 69, 76
Potassium, equilibrium potential for, 73, 82
Potassium channels, 6, 26, 27, 70, 79, 80
Precentral gyrus
  function of, 3, 4
  seizure in, 280–281, 301
  in sensory neglect, 49–50, 58
  stroke of, 287–288, 290–291, 307, 309
Prefrontal cortex
  cognitive function and, 3, 4, 233, 241
  medial thalamus and, 270–271, 293–294
  olfactory sense and, 217, 226–227
  VA nucleus and, 270, 293
Preganglionic parasympathetic fibers,
    183–184, 207
Premotor cortex, 3, 246, 259, 270, 293
Pretectal area, 215, 225
Primary afferent fibers, 214, 224
Primary motor cortex, 49, 57
Primary somatosensory cortex, 49, 57
Prolactin, 237–238, 243–244
Proteins, 11, 69, 76–77
Pseudobulbar palsy, 55

Pseudocoma, 180, 205
Ptosis, 181–182, 205–206
Pulvinar nucleus, 231, 240
Pupillary light reflex, 172, 200
Purines, 24
Purkinje cell, 253–254, 267
Putamen, 5, 294
Pyramidal cell, 280–282, 301–302
Pyramidal tracts, myelination in, 42, 64, 66
Pyramids, 51, 58, 161–162, 191
Pyriform cortex, 218, 228–229

Q
Quandrantopia, 48, 56, 212, 213, 222
Quisqualate, 26, 88, 93

R
Raphe neurons, 98, 111
Rathke's pouch, 63, 66
Receptor cell, 209, 220
Receptors
  activation of, 106, 116
  in autonomic nervous system, 36
  characteristics of, 15, 86, 90
  detection of, 68, 75
  function of, 22–23
  opiate, 216, 225–226
  in second messenger system, 87, 88,
    91–93
  types of, 16, 25–28, 30, 91
Red nucleus, 168, 195, 201–202
Referred pain, 214, 224
REM sleep, 272, 295
Reproductive system
  female, 36
  male, 35
Reserpine, 108, 118, 146, 149
Respiratory system, 34, 37
Resting membrane potential, 13, 69, 73, 78,
    82, 83
Reticular formation, 254–256, 267, 270, 292,
    293–294, 310
Reticulospinal tract, 31
Retina, 209, 215, 217, 220, 225, 227
Retinitis pigmentosa, 209, 220
Rhodopsin, 220
Rhombic lips, 63, 66
Ribosomes, 8
Right-handedness, 291, 310
Rods, 209, 220
Roof plate, 63, 66
Rough endoplasmic reticulum (RER), 77
Rubrospinal tract, 31, 42, 124, 135–136

S
Saccule, 59
Salivation, 33–34, 158, 190
Saltatory conduction, 8, 10, 14

Schizophrenia, 19, 21, 118, 275, 298
Schwann cells, 6
Second messengers, 16, 27, 87, 88, 91–93, 115
Seizure
    complex partial, 272, 284, 295, 303–304
    generalized, 273, 295–296, 301
    initiating cellular event for, 282, 302
    of left precentral gyrus, 280–281, 301
    (*See also* Epilepsy)
Semicircular canals, 59
Senile dementia, 19
Sensory neglect, 44, 58
Sensory systems
    damage to, 110
    dysfunction of, 76
    function of, 40–41
Septal area, 236, 243
Septum pellucidum, 4
Serotonin
    biosynthesis of, 99, 112
    detection of, 68, 75
    as neurotransmitter, 22–23
    in pain treatment, 239
    receptors, 26
    role in depression, 23, 98, 111
    schizophrenia and, 298
Serotonin reuptake inhibitors (SSRIs), 23,
        111, 244
Short-term memory, 46, 55, 231, 240, 299
Skeletomuscular responses, in temperature
        regulation, 273, 296
Skull base, lesion of, 159, 190
Sleep
    apnea, 292, 310
    physiology of, 18
    REM, 272, 295
Sleep disorders, 99, 112
Smell
    brain tumor effect on, 218, 299
    physiology of, 4, 47, 56, 228
    prefrontal cortex and, 217, 226–227
Sodium channels, 6, 26, 72, 79, 81–82
Solitary complex, 161–162, 191
Solitary nucleus, 147, 149–150, 155, 187
    inputs received by, 147, 149–150
    loss of taste and, 158, 164, 172, 189, 193,
        200
    projections to/from, 155, 187
Soma (nerve cell body), 8
Somatosensory system, 4, 213, 224
Somatostatin, 275, 297
Spasticity, 245, 257
Speech function, 49, 57
    (*See also* Aphasia)
Spinal cord
    abdominal reflexes and, 119, 133
    anatomy of, 30–31
    cervical level of, 125, 137

Spinal cord (*Cont.*)
    compression of, 124, 136
    disorders of, 31–32
    hand injury and, 126, 138
    hemisection of right side of, 129, 141
    thoracic, 131, 142–143
Spinal motor neurons, 245, 257–258
Spinal nucleus of cranial nerve V, 164–165,
        193
Spinocerebellar tract, 124, 136
Spinocerebellum, 253–254, 262, 266–267
Spinothalamic tract, 123, 128, 132, 135, 140,
        143, 239, 244
Stapedius, 178–179, 204
Stria terminalis, 232–233, 241, 285
Stroke
    brainstem, 162, 166, 191–192, 194
    corticospinal tract, 124, 136, 282–283, 303
    dorsolateral medulla, 170, 197
    effects of, 47, 56, 104, 114, 124, 135, 136
    forebrain, 232–234, 238–239, 240–242,
        244
    hypoglossal nerve affected by, 52, 59
    left vertebral artery, 176, 202–204
    midbrain, 167, 195, 254–255, 267
    motor systems affected by, 48, 56
    pons role in, 153–154, 187, 282–283,
        302
    treatment for, 105, 114
Subarachnoid hemorrhage, 53, 60, 289,
        308
Subiculum, 285, 304
Substance P, 25, 126, 138, 214, 224
Substantia gelatinosa, 124, 136, 138
Substantia innominata, 236, 243
Substantia nigra, 5, 168, 175, 195, 202, 252,
        265–266
Subthalamic fasciculus, 241
Subthalamic nucleus, 232, 240–241
Superior cerebellar artery, 173, 200–201
Superior cerebellar peduncle, 5, 165–167,
        194–195
Superior colliculus, 5, 168, 174, 195, 201,
        215, 225
Superior oblique muscle, 184–185,
        207–208
Superior salivatory nucleus, 159, 190
Superior temporal gyrus, 4, 49, 57, 271, 294
Suprachiasmatic nucleus, 215, 225, 274, 297
Supraoptic hypothalamic nucleus, 273,
        296–297
Sympathetic fibers, interruption of, 181–182,
        205–206
Sympathetic nervous system, 32, 39–40
Synaptic boutons, 16
Synaptic transmission, 15–17, 85, 86, 89–90
Syphilis of central nervous system, 200
Syringomyelia, 32, 62, 65

T

Tabes dorsalis, 31
Tachykinins, 24–25
Tardive dyskinesia, 248, 261–262
Taste
    cranial nerves and, 152, 157–158, 161,
        186, 189, 191
    impaired, 158, 164, 172, 178–179, 189,
        193, 200, 204
Tegmentum, 5
Temperature regulation, 273, 296
Temporal lobe, 3, 4
Temporal lobe epilepsy, 43, 105, 114–115,
        231, 240, 284, 303–304
Tethered cord syndrome, 62, 65–66
Thalamic fasciculus, 232–233, 241
Thalamic nuclei, 269–271, 293–294
Thalamic pain, 238–239, 244, 269, 293
Thalamostriatal projection, 294
Thalamus, 4
Todd's paralysis, 301
Tongue deviation, 164, 193, 246, 249
Tremor
    of contralateral limb, 175, 201–202
    pill-rolling, 42, 265
Tricyclic antidepressants, 244
Trigeminal nerve, 52, 59, 161, 191
Trigeminal nucleus, 196
Trochlear nerve (cranial nerve IV), 156–157,
        184–185, 188, 207–208
Trochlear nucleus, 166–167, 195
Tryptophan hydroxylase, 99, 112
Tuberoinfundibular dopaminergic system,
        238, 243–244
Tufted cell, 228
Tumors
    of cerebral peduncle, 52, 58
    of hypothalamus, 274, 297
    of intraventricular foramen, 53, 60
    of lateral ventricle, 47, 56
    of midbrain periaqueductal gray, 166–167,
        195
    of optic chiasm, 52, 59
    Pancoast, 206
    of uncal region, 218, 229
2–deoxyglucose autoradiography, 68, 75
Tyrosine, 99, 111–112

U

Uncal region, 218, 229
Unconscious proprioception, 262

Unilateral sensory neglect, 44
Upper motor neurons (UMNs)
    in corticospinal tract, 132, 144
    deficit of, 125, 136–137
    paralysis of, 44, 129, 137, 141, 167, 175,
        194, 195, 202, 234, 241, 277, 299
    spasticity and, 257
Urinary incontinence, 289, 308
Utricle, 59
Uvula, deviation of, 158–159, 189–190

V

Vagus nerve, 51, 58
Vasopressin, 106, 115, 242, 273, 296, 297
Velocity detectors, 141
Ventral amygdalofugal pathway, 285
Ventral anterior (VA) nucleus, 269–271, 293,
        294
Ventral posterolateral thalamic nucleus, 219,
        229, 238–239, 244
Ventral posteromedial nucleus, 172, 200,
        238–239, 244
Ventral posteromedial thalamic nucleus, 158,
        189
Ventral spinocerebellar tract, 249, 262
Ventral tegmental area, 175, 202
Ventricular system (brain), 4, 5
Ventrocaudal pons, 171, 199
Ventrolateral (VL) nucleus, 269–270, 293
Vestibular nuclei, 247, 261
Vestibulocerebellum, 261
Vestibulospinal tracts, 31
Vigabatrin, 105, 114–115
Vision
    brain disruptions and, 48, 50, 56, 57–58,
        172, 199–200, 211–213, 221–222
    cranial nerve effect on, 52, 59, 156–157,
        171, 188, 198
    double, 52, 59, 183–185, 206–208
    lesions affecting, 40–41
    peripheral, 237, 243
Visual cortex, 40, 217, 222, 227–228, 276,
        299

W

Wallenberg's syndrome, 38
Wallerian degeneration, 10, 142
Weber's syndrome, 207
Wernicke's aphasia, 44, 49, 57, 278, 300,
        309
Wernicke's area, 49, 57